P9-DTI-568

Research Funding and Resource Manual

Mental Health and Addictive Disorders

Research Funding and Resource Manual

Mental Health and Addictive Disorders

Edited by

Harold Alan Pincus, M.D.

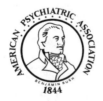

American Psychiatric Association
Washington, DC

Note: The findings, opinions, and conclusions of this report do not necessarily represent the views of the officers, trustees, or all members of the American Psychiatric Association. The views expressed are those of the authors of the individual chapters.

Copyright © 1995 American Psychiatric Association
ALL RIGHTS RESERVED
Manufactured in the United States of America on acid-free paper
First Edition
98 97 96 95   4 3 2 1

American Psychiatric Association
1400 K Street, N.W., Washington, DC   20005

Library of Congress Cataloging-in-Publication Data
Research funding and resource manual : mental health and addictive
    disorders / edited by Harold Alan Pincus.
        p.   cm.
    Includes bibliographical references and index.
    ISBN 0-89042-216-8
    1. Psychiatry—Research—United States.   2. Psychiatry—Research
grants—United States.   I. Pincus, Harold Alan, 1951–
    [DNLM: 1. Mental Disorders—economics.   2. Research Support—
economics.   3. Financing, Organized—economics.   WM 20 R43202
1995]
RC337.R473—1995
616.89'0072073—dc20
DNLM/DLC
for Library of Congress   95-23891
                                                                      CIP

British Library Cataloguing in Publication Data
A CIP record is available from the British Library.

To my family—Ellyn Roth and Zachary, Nathaniel, and Ezra Pincus-Roth—a very special resource.

Contents

Chapter 1

Chapter 2

Chapter 3

Chapter 4

Chapter 11

Chapter 12

Chapter 13

Appendixes

Contributors

Gene D. Cohen, M.D., Ph.D.
Director, Washington, DC, Center on Aging; Director, Center for Aging and Health, School of Medicine and Health Sciences, George Washington University, Washington, DC

Sharon Cohen, M.A.
Assistant Director, Division of Government Relations, American Psychiatric Association, Washington, DC

Jay Cutler, J.D.
Director, Division of Government Relations, American Psychiatric Association, Washington, DC

Christopher Dykton
Administrative Coordinator, Psychiatric Research Resource Center, American Psychiatric Association, Washington, DC

Theodora Fine, M.A.
Expert, PHS Office on Women's Health, Columbia, Maryland

Tricia Hill
Former Intern, Office of Research, Malad, Idaho

Vera Hollen
Senior Research Assistant, National Association of State Mental Health Program Directors Research Institute, Inc., Alexandria, Virginia

Peter S. Jensen, M.D.
Chief, Child and Adolescent Disorders Research Branch, Division of Clinical Treatment Research, National Institute of Mental Health, Rockville, Maryland

Cille Kennedy, Ph.D.
Assistant Director for Disability Research, Division of
Epidemiology and Services Research, National Institute of Mental
Health, Rockville, Maryland

Barry D. Lebowitz, Ph.D.
Chief, Mental Disorders of the Aging Branch, Division of Clinical
and Treatment Research, National Institute of Mental Health,
Rockville, Maryland

Theodore Lutterman
Director of Data Analysis, National Association of State Mental
Health Program Directors Research Institute, Inc., Alexandria, Virginia

Noel Mazade, Ph.D.
Executive Director, National Association of State Mental Health
Program Directors Research Institute, Inc., Alexandria, Virginia

Adrian R. Morrison, D.V.M., Ph.D.
Former Director, Program for Animal Research Issues, National
Institute of Mental Health, Rockville, Maryland; Professor of
Behavioral Neuroscience, Department of Animal Biology,
University of Pennsylvania, Philadelphia, Pennsylvania

Evelyn S. Myers, M.A.
Editorial Consultant, Silver Spring, Maryland

Sandra L. Patterson
Managing Editor, *American Journal of Psychiatry*, American
Psychiatric Association, Washington, DC

Harold Alan Pincus, M.D.
Deputy Medical Director and Director, Office of Research, American
Psychiatric Association, Washington, DC

Carol A. Steele
Program Manager, Research Training, American Psychiatric
Association, Washington, DC

Jane Steinberg, Ph.D.
Acting Director, Division of Clinical and Treatment Research,
National Institute of Mental Health, Rockville, Maryland

Joyce West, M.P.P.
Research Coordinator, Office of Research, American Psychiatric
Association, Washington, DC

***Robert M. Wettstein*, M.D.**
Co-Director, Law and Psychiatry Program, and Chair, Psychosocial IRB, Department of Psychiatry, University of Pittsburgh, School of Medicine, Pittsburgh, Pennsylvania

***Deborah A. Zarin*, M.D.**
Deputy Medical Director and Associate Director, Office of Research, American Psychiatric Association, Washington, DC

Introduction

The American Psychiatric Association's (APA) Office of Research was established in 1985 to provide a leadership role for the Association in advancing science policy issues in psychiatric research, in systematizing and overseeing the APA's scientific assessment programs (e.g., DSM-IV, practice guidelines), and in conducting coordinated research at the APA. From its inception, this office has served as a repository of information and a locus for communication regarding research funding opportunities, research training issues, and a broad array of other policies that affect the conduct of science in psychiatry. These policies range from academic-industry relations to human subjects and animal research, scientific misconduct, and other ethical issues.

Thanks to the very generous support of the van Ameringen Foundation, the Office of Research was able in 1989 to establish the Psychiatric Research Resource Center (PRRC) to study and accumulate research funding and policy information, systematizing this information, and providing it to junior investigators in the field. The PRRC maintains a number of databases cataloging this material; these are augmented by a library of additional reference information. The PRRC has established a two-way linkage with the research community, continually obtaining information to update our databases and resource materials and providing this information to individuals at all levels of research training and experience.

The work of the PRRC is augmented by other activities within the APA Office of Research and elsewhere within the APA that are described below. Perhaps most significant is the *Psychiatric Research Report (PRR)*, a quarterly newsletter that highlights science policy issues and provides information on the research activities of the APA and its components as well as providing timely information about funding and research training opportunities and important policy issues.

In the *Research Funding and Resource Manual: Mental Health and Addictive Disorders (RFRM)*, we have attempted to capture the broad array of information that is available through the databases of the PRRC and the *PRR* in a single volume. We hope this volume will serve as a reasonably encyclopedic reference and guide to the varied issues related to the needs of the mental illness and addictive disorders research community.

The *RFRM* consists of 13 chapters and six appendixes at the end of the book organized to reflect the overall "anatomy" of research funding sources and the "physiology" of the research funding process and relevant science policy issues. Most chapters are divided into two main parts: a narrative section devoted to specific research and policy, which generally discusses the background, policy information, and other substantive material; and a section that provides a list of organizational (e.g., federal agency or foundation) contacts, a bibliography, or other material that those interested may consult for more detailed information. The six appendixes list federal research contacts in a variety of areas. The *RFRM* is divided into the following chapters.

Chapter 1, "The 'Anatomy' of Research Funding of Mental Illness and Addictive Disorders," by Harold Alan Pincus, M.D., and Theodora Fine, M.A., is reprinted with permission from the *Archives of General Psychiatry*. It describes the level and sources of research funding for the fields of mental illness and substance abuse through a systematic survey of public and private funding entities, analyzes recent funding trends, and assesses policy issues affecting research support. The overall research funding "anatomy" also serves as a structure for much of the remainder of the *RFRM*.

Chapter 2, "Successful Research Grant Applications," by Jane Steinberg, Ph.D., and Cille Kennedy, Ph.D., focuses on the strategies for preparing research grant applications, especially those to be funded by the federal government. Part of this chapter is devoted to the federal research grant application and review process. The resource section includes a glossary of grant terms frequently used in the federal grant process and definitions of federal grant mechanisms used by the National Institutes of Health.

Chapter 3, "Federal Funding and Psychiatric Research," by Christopher Dykton, explores the history of federal research funding, notes overall trends, and briefly overviews the federal budgeting and allocation process. The resource section of this chapter comprehensively lists profiles of the federal agencies that provide research funding for areas of mental health and substance abuse research interest. This section outlines the points of contact, agency mission, and areas of interest to investigators and notes recent program announcements sponsored by each federal agency.

Chapter 4, "Foundations and Nonprofit Research Support," by Theodora Fine, M.A., is similar in structure to the chapter on federal funding. This chapter defines the different types of nonprofit funding organizations, their management structure, the grant decision-making process, and ways of identifying foundations for potential research support. The resource section of this chapter provides 1) profiles of foundations that support mental health and substance abuse research (cross-referenced with subject listing), 2) a list of foundations supporting broad biomedical or disease-specific research with mental health components, and 3) a list of local foundations that have supported psychiatric research.

Chapter 5, "Research Capacities and Activities of State Mental Health Agencies," by Theodore Lutterman, Vera Hollen, and Noel Mazade, Ph.D., provides an overview of mental health research efforts conducted or funded by state mental health agencies, elucidates different models of state funding for mental health research, and lists factors influencing state funding. Appended to this chapter are points of research contact at state mental health agencies.

Chapter 6, "Industry and Academia Collaboration in Psychiatric Research," by Joyce West, M.P.P., Deborah A. Zarin, M.D., Tricia Hill, and Harold Alan Pincus, M.D., discusses the growth in cooperation between private industry (especially pharmaceutical and biotechnology) and academic research. This chapter further describes goals, models, and problems (especially conflict of interest issues) of this collaboration. The resource section provides research contacts for pharmaceutical corporations involved with psychopharmacological development.

Chapter 7, "Research Opportunities in Child and Adolescent Mental Disorders," by Peter S. Jensen, M.D., focuses on federal support for research on child and adolescent mental disorders, describing broad and cross-cutting areas of particular interest. The resource section provides the research contacts in various federal agencies, with a brief description of the activities of these programs.

Chapter 8, "Aging and Psychiatric Research," by Gene D. Cohen, M.D., Ph.D., Barry D. Lebowitz, Ph.D., and Theodora Fine, M.A., addresses the federal interest in funding research on mental disorders associated with aging. The resource section of this chapter provides the research contacts in various federal agencies interested in aging, with a brief description of the activities of these federal programs and a list of organizations involved in aging and psychogeriatric issues.

Chapter 9, "How to Publish in the Scientific Literature," by Sandra L. Patterson, advises the psychiatric researcher on the ways to get research findings published by addressing manuscript preparation, the peer review process, how and which journal to approach, the revision process, and ethical considerations. Resources 9–1, compiled by Laura Little, lists over 100 journals where mental health and substance abuse investigators may publish their findings.

Chapter 10, "Issues in Psychiatric Research Training," by Harold Alan Pincus, M.D., and Carol A. Steele, aims to demystify the prospect of a psychiatric research career by noting opportunities in the field, describing elements that go into becoming a psychiatric researcher, and suggesting approaches to choosing and using a research training program. There is no resource section; the reader is referred to the *Directory of Psychiatric Research Fellowships*, published by the APA Office of Research.

Chapter 11, "Research Ethics and Human Subject Issues," by Robert M. Wettstein, M.D., addresses the ethical issues associated with conducting research involving human subjects, such as institutional review boards, informed consent, privacy and confidentiality, and risk assessment. The appended resource section includes relevant publications and policy documents as well as points of contact in federal organizations that focus on ethical issues.

Chapter 12, "Animal-Based Research and the Animal Rights Movement," by Adrian R. Morrison, D.V.M., Ph.D., examines the relationship among biomedical research, animal welfare, and animal rights. The resource section provides information on publications addressing animal-based research issues and contacts at national organizations assisting biomedical researchers.

Chapter 13, "Influencing the Political Agenda on Behalf of Psychiatric Research," by Jay Cutler, J.D., and Sharon Cohen, M.A., serves as a missive to readers, urging them to advocate on behalf of psychiatric research. It addresses ways in which researchers can be actively involved in the legislative and federal research funding process by describing how Congress works and passes legislation and providing direct advice on how to address research concerns. The resource section has a bibliography of related publications and a question and answer section on protocol when meeting with members of Congress.

At the end of the book, six appendixes provide lists of federal contacts on specific research issues of mental health and substance abuse interest. The appendixes include contacts for research on AIDS, health and behavior, health services research, sleep, women's health issues, and neuroscience.

As noted earlier, the APA Office of Research serves as the principal locus of communication for the research community in psychiatry. In addition, through its responsibilities in overseeing DSM-IV, developing practice guidelines, and initiating the Psychiatric Research Network (a network of 1,000 practicing psychiatrists systematically reporting clinical and policy-relevant data), it also seeks to ensure that the fruits of research are applied for the benefit of patients and their families. Interested readers may wish to obtain further information on the following activities of the office:

- *Psychiatric Research Report*, which contains information about research training and research funding opportunities for psychiatrists as well as about science policy issues, is published quarterly by the office. APA members and those interested in a career in psychiatric research may request this newsletter free of charge.
- The Program for Minority Research Training in Psychiatry (PMRTP), initiated in 1989 in conjunction with the APA's Office of Minority/National Affairs and funded by the National Institute of Mental Health, is designed to encourage underrepresented minority men and women to enter careers in psychiatric research. The PMRTP provides support for short- and long-term research training at the medical school, residency, and postresidency (PGY-V or later) levels. Staff also organize regional and national competitions to enable qualified participants ("mini-fellows") to attend research-oriented meetings of psychiatric organizations. For further information, contact PMRTP at 1 (800) 852-1390.
- The Psychiatric Research Resource Center (PRRC), funded through a 6-year grant from the van Ameringen Foundation, Inc., aids the psychiatric research community and enhances the development of an enlarged cadre of psychiatric researchers. The PRRC maintains a database of programs funding and supporting

psychiatric research that is regularly published in *Psychiatric Research Report*, maintains information and other resources on funding and policy issues for the research community, and sponsors regional meetings of researchers to encourage recruitment and retention.

Acknowledgments

M any people have given a great deal of time, patience, and thought to the development of this manual. We would like to express our deep gratitude to editorial consultant Evelyn S. Myers, M.A., former managing editor of the *American Journal of Psychiatry*, for her diligent technical editing of the manuscript. The Office of Research staff over the past years—Wendy Davis, Sandy Ferris, Teddi Fine, Julie Kuzneski, David Lowenschuss, Jeanne Nevin, Carol Steele, Nancy Sydnor-Greenberg, Nancy Vetterello, Joyce West, and Deborah A. Zarin, M.D.—have provided invaluable support during the creation of this manual. Special thanks go to Nancy C. Andreasen, M.D., Ph.D., John J. Bartko, Ph.D., and Raymond Purkis, and to Carol Nadelson, M.D., Ronald McMillen, Claire Reinburg, Pam Harley, and the rest of the staff of the American Psychiatric Press, Inc., and to Carolyn Robinowitz, M.D., and Melvin Sabshin, M.D., for their unfailing assistance. Finally, we would like to express our appreciation to our contributors, who gave so generously of their time and energy as the manual was being prepared.

Comments and Questions

Although the Office of Research has made a great effort to verify and update the information in the *RFRM* (current as of May 1995), certain information may have changed or been updated by the time of publication. Please direct all questions and comments concerning the manual to the PRRC, Office of Research, American Psychiatric Association, 1400 K Street, NW, Washington, DC 20005, (202) 682-6292.

CHAPTER

1

The "Anatomy" of Research Funding of Mental Illness and Addictive Disorders

Harold Alan Pincus, M.D., and
Theodora Fine, M.A.

Mental illnesses and substance abuse exact an undeniable and substantial toll on human life and productivity, affecting not only those millions of Americans suffering from these disorders, but also their families and associates and, indeed, the nation's health and economy as a whole. The direct and indirect costs associated with

This chapter is adapted with permission from *Archives of General Psychiatry*, July 1992, Vol. 49, pp. 573–579. Copyright 1992, American Medical Association. Although data are derived from 1988, nonetheless this survey represents the most recent comprehensive assessment of psychiatric research funding available. Despite the organizational changes affecting the federal institutes, it is unlikely that there have been significant changes in distribution of funding sources since that time.

This work was supported by research contracts from the National Institute of Mental Health and the (former) Alcohol, Drug Abuse, and Mental Health Administration, Rockville, MD.

these disorders amount to more than \$1,000 for every man, woman, and child in the United States (American Psychiatric Association 1988). The Institute of Medicine has estimated that the economic consequences of the disorders under the [former] Alcohol, Drug Abuse, and Mental Health Administration (ADAMHA) purview are comparable to those of heart disease and cancer (Board of Mental Health and Behavioral Medicine 1984). Yet, numerous reports have underscored the inadequate resources available to support research on mental and addictive disorders (Board of Mental Health and Behavioral Medicine 1984; Freedman 1985; Institute of Medicine 1983, 1989; President's Commission on Mental Health 1978).

This article provides an evaluation of the state of support for mental and addictive disorder research in 1988, presenting findings from a study of the sources of financial support for such research. It examines the federal commitment to the field from the National Institute of Mental Health (NIMH), the National Institute on Alcohol Abuse and Alcoholism (NIAAA), and the National Institute on Drug Abuse (NIDA), the larger Public Health Service (PHS), Department of Health and Human Services, to other disparate federal agencies and departments. This article also reviews nonfederal sources of research support, that is, foundations and other philanthropic organizations, state government, and industry. It identifies the absolute dollars available to support the research endeavor and addresses the distribution of the sources of those dollars. Last, it assesses how this support compares with that available for the conduct of overall biomedical research.

The National Institutes of Health (NIH) assesses changes in funding for overall biomedical research annually. However, no comparable yearly assessment of such trends has been undertaken for mental illness and substance abuse research funding. In 1978, the Research Task Panel of the President's Commission on Mental Health (PCMH), with a much broader mandate and approach, conducted a one-time assessment of research support in "mental health" (President's Commission on Mental Health 1978). Yet, the task panel's findings are not fully comparable with the present study, given the differences in approach and definition. Regular assessment of research funding, like the present study, can identify and illuminate the sources of research funding for the field as a whole, providing insight into previously untapped or underutilized resources. It also can serve as a basis for assessing the trends and changes in funding patterns over time.

◆ Methods

Process of Inquiry

Funding entities were contacted directly by the study team and inquiry was made regarding agency support for research related to mental illness and substance abuse. In some cases, the study team interviewed specific program staff; in other cases, budget officers were the initial contact. In all cases, study definitions were explained to the respondent. While some agencies maintained data in a manner consistent with the study definitions and provided a response based solely on the study definitions, other agencies' record-keeping methods were not compatible with the study's data needs. In those instances, the study team set forth a series of "key words" relevant to the study definitions and in keeping with concepts employed in that agency's data-based management system.

Some responding agencies provided either oral or written summary information. In other cases, the agency forwarded a compendium of all fiscal 1988 awards made by that agency that described the grants made, the principal investigators, and the funds awarded. The study team then evaluated which grants and awards were relevant to the study topic. This procedure was based on the use of key words and concepts in mental illness and substance abuse. In most cases, summaries prepared by the study team were returned to agency personnel for review and comment.

The study team also relied on secondary analysis of reports, publications, and previously gathered data as another means of identifying support for mental illness and substance abuse research. This method was employed primarily in the areas of state, industry, and foundation support.

When data for fiscal 1988 were not available, the study team used data from the year most proximate to the study year and adjusted the final dollar amount to fiscal 1988 dollars using the PHS biomedical research price index.

A detailed listing of methods used to identify mental illness and addictive disorder research and a brief description of the areas of research interest for each of the sources examined are available from the authors.

Definitions and Their Application

To identify the sources of funding for substance abuse and mental illness research, we developed definitions that were applied consistently across funding sectors. The definition of mental illness research conforms to the NIMH definition of its research mission (NIH 1989a), crosscutting basic, clinical health services, and epidemiologic research. Research on mental disorders and mental illnesses is distinguished by an emphasis on mental disease or mental pathologic characteristics, whether at the level of basic science or of clinical investigation of the person, health service system, or epidemiologic population. Mental illness research subsumes all DSM-III-R disorders, with the exception of substance use disorders (American Psychiatric Association 1987). Research may involve clinical, subclinical, and normal subjects as well as animal models and tissue, as long as they are relevant to the disorder or system under investigation.

Substance abuse research includes that inquiry undertaken in the areas of alcoholism and/or alcohol abuse and drug abuse. The definition, to the extent possible, conforms to the mission statements of the NIAAA and NIDA (NIH 1989a). As in the case of mental illness research, the nature of research crosscuts basic, clinical health services, and epidemiologic inquiry. The definition includes the range of behaviors from dependence or addiction (e.g., cocaine or heroin addiction) to instances of inappropriate substance use (e.g., hazardous use of alcohol before driving).

The NIH Division of Research Grants (DRG) serves as the central clearinghouse for the vast majority of PHS extramural research divisions. Since this process applied definitions similar to ours and routes applications meeting the criteria for mental illness and substance abuse research to the NIMH, the NIAAA, or NIDA, all research supported by these institutes was included in the study. All PHS-supported extramural research distributed by the DRG that falls outside the purview of the NIMH, the NIAAA, and NIDA grant referral guidelines established by the DRG was *excluded* from the study. However, research supported or conducted by other PHS agencies *outside* the DRG process was included, assuming it met the definitional tests above. In some sectors, a "pure" match to the definition was difficult; proxy measures were required.

Research includes intramural and extramural support. Instrumentation and facility development (or improvement) support was included insofar as it was possible to ascertain that the instrumentation or facilities were intended specifically for the use of scientists engaged in research meeting the definitions. Estimates of research administration support for all sectors were included if the data were reliable and consistent. Indirect costs were also included for all sectors.

◆ Study Limitations

Notwithstanding these definitional strictures, precision may have been compromised when the definition was applied to various federal and private sources of research support. To a great extent, the study relied on self-reports from funding agencies; therefore, accuracy depends on the degree of effort by agency personnel. In some cases, agency data were not maintained with sufficient detail to tease mental illness and substance abuse research from broader areas of biomedical or behavioral inquiry. Assumptions made by the study team in the development of proxy measures were discussed with and corroborated by agency personnel and others knowledgeable in the field. In other cases, definitions were translated into key words to facilitate data retrieval. For example, while the National Aeronautics and Space Administration (NASA) personnel initially were unable to identify any awards in the areas of relevant research, inquiry about circadian rhythm disturbances and stress-related research yielded funding data relevant to the field. In the case of foundation support, reliance was placed on Internal Revenue Service reports submitted by the foundations. In some instances, additional materials in the Foundation Center were consulted and foundation officials contacted.

A specific problem arose regarding support for basic research. Once beyond the PHS grant referral process, the distribution of basic science dollars to the research fields of mental illness and substance abuse became increasingly difficult to determine. For example, the prominent federal agency and the major private medical research organization supporting only basic research, the National Science Foundation (NSF) and the Howard Hughes Medical Institute (HHMI), respectively, are unable to specify those portions of the budget that support mental illness or substance abuse research per se. A proxy measure was developed, based on the ratio of NIMH, NIAAA, and NIDA research to the overall PHS research expenditures in the area of neuroscience research. Corroboration of these measures as well as further suggestions were provided by the NIMH, the NSF, and the HHMI personnel.

◆ Results

The three institutes of the [former] ADAMHA are the preeminent source of support for research on mental illness or addictive disorders. In fiscal 1988, all public and private support for substance abuse and mental illness research totaled $858,958,063 (Table 1–1).

Table 1–1.   Substance abuse and mental illness research funding in fiscal 1988

Source	Dollars	Percentage of total
National Institute of Mental Health	317,315,000	37
National Institute on Drug Abuse	144,724,000	17
National Institute on Alcohol Abuse and Alcoholism	88,317,000	10
Other Departments of Health and Human Services	**7,976,636**	0.9
Centers for Disease Control	3,716,542	
Health Care Financing Administration	0	
Health Resources and Services Administration	1,109,210	
Social Security Administration	1,781,687	
Assistant Secretary for Planning and Evaluation	105,554	
Office of Human Development Services	1,263,643	
Department of Education	2,191,305	0.3
Department of Veterans Affairs	17,698,262	2.1
Department of Defense	9,780,800	1.1
National Science Foundation	14,797,457	1.7
Department of Justice	9,237,464	1.1
National Aeronautics and Space Administration	730,000	0.1
Department of Transportation	138,000	0.02
Department of Agriculture	1,456,300	0.2
State government	66,530,160	8
Industry	**148,026,931**	17
Pharmaceutical	145,676,931	
Hospitals/health care organizations	2,350,000	
Private nonprofit	**30,038,748**	3.5
Foundations	16,038,748	
Medical research organizations	14,000,000	
Total	**858,958,063**	

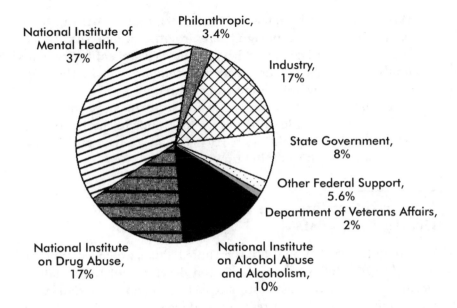

Figure 1–1.   Sources of financial support for mental illness and substance abuse research.

Of the total, 64% ($550,356,000) is derived from only the NIMH, the NIAAA, and NIDA. Industry research and development (pharmaceutical and hospital and/or health care organizations) account for another 17% of the total. All other sources of research support for mental illness and substance abuse research totaled 19%.

State funding represented only 8% of all mental illness and substance abuse research support; foundation support represented 1.9% of fiscal 1988 funding. Inclusion of medical research organizations, essentially the HHMI, with foundation funding brings philanthropic funding to 3.4% (Figure 1–1).

◆ Comment

Findings from this study suggest the following three points:

1. Overall research support for mental illness and substance abuse is extremely limited and disproportionate to the overall costs to society represented by these disorders.

2. While the research budgets of the NIMH, the NIAAA, and NIDA have experienced recent significant growth, the diversification of sources of research support beyond these federal entities remains limited. This is particularly evident in comparison with the range of support for overall biomedical research.
3. Examination of the currently existing segments of research support for mental and substance abuse outside the NIMH, the NIAAA, and NIDA identifies barriers to and strategies for further expanding and diversifying funding sources.

Research Funding as a Percentage of Health Care Costs

According to the NIH, in 1988 the United States expended approximately $126.1 billion on research and development (NIH 1989b). Health research, totaling an estimated $18.7 billion in the same year, represented 14.8% of total research and development (NIH 1989b). This study has found that support for mental illness and substance abuse research represented only 0.7% of total national research and development. The $858,958,063 expended on mental illness and substance abuse research represents only 4.7% of *health* research support. In contrast, the health costs associated with these disorders, $66.8 billion in 1988 (Rice 1990), account for 12% of total health costs in the same year (NIH 1989b). Put another way, approximately 1.3% of mental health and substance abuse direct costs are invested by society in research on these disorders compared with society's investment of 3.4% of overall health care costs in general biomedical research.

Comparison With Overall Biomedical Research Funding

The extent to which mental illness and substance abuse research depends on the institutes of the [former] ADAMHA becomes evident when one contrasts these institutes with the other institutes of the NIH as a source of research and development funding. In this comparison, methods and definitional difficulties must be considered.

The NIH compiles information about national biomedical research expenditures annually in its *Data Book* series (NIH 1989b). Based on this information provided by the NIH staff, it appears that the method employed in the aggregation of the NIH data is generally comparable with that used in the preparation of this report's data set. Questions of accuracy in reporting by agency contacts used by the NIH approximate those in this study; concerns about definitions of research are similar.

However, the NIH amasses information about all health research (including mental illness and addictive disorders research) and does not apply definitional distinctions within that category. Our methods for estimating subsets of health research related to mental illness and substance abuse could have introduced some difficulties in the comparison. The present study likely represents an undercounting of basic research relevant to the mental illness and substance abuse field given the reliance on the DRG referral process and removal of NIH research from the analysis.

Notwithstanding these differences, some interesting comparisons are found. The NIH represents a source of 34% of support for health research and institutes of the [former] ADAMHA, 64% of all support for substance abuse and mental illness research. While industry is estimated to have contributed 17% to the support for mental illness and substance abuse research in fiscal 1988, it accounted for 44% of all health research in the same year (Table 1–2). Given the extensive state responsibilities for service delivery in mental illness and substance abuse, the finding of so small a difference between

Table 1–2.   Health research and development in fiscal 1988

Source of funding	Source of support (%)	
	All biomedical	Mental illness/ substance abuse
National Institutes of Health	34	
Alcohol, Drug Abuse, and Mental Health Administration	2.1	64
Other federal	9	7.3
Industry	44	17
State	7	8
Private nonprofit[*]	4	3.4

[*]Includes foundations, voluntary health agencies, and medical research organizations (e.g., Howard Hughes Medical Institute).

state support of research in these areas, and in health research generally, is surprising.

Although a small segment of the whole, overall health research receives nearly a 20% greater proportion of funds from philanthropic sources than do the fields of mental illness and substance abuse. One interesting finding not reflected in Table 1–2, but found in a comparison of NIH data and study data, is within the category of private nonprofit support. The largest share of support in this area for overall biomedical research comes from voluntary health organizations such as the American Cancer Society and the American Diabetes Association. In fiscal 1988, research funding for mental illness and substance abuse research derived from voluntary organizations was extremely limited. The new voluntary organization that has grown up in the field since that time, the National Association for Research on Schizophrenia and Depression (NARSAD) represents a promising new potential area of support for the field.

Research Support Over Time

The single recent study that examined issues related to funding for mental illness and substance abuse research is found in the report of the Research Task Panel of the PCMH, published more than 12 years ago (President's Commission on Mental Health 1978). However, their definition of mental health research spanned a broader and somewhat different spectrum, encompassing the study of not only mental disorders but also research on mental health beyond the NIH definition of its mission. The study did not include a significant focus on addictive disorders or an analysis of industry support for the conduct of research.

Support for "mental health" research, as defined by the PCMH, totaled $317 million in fiscal 1976. Federal support, including all sectors of the government, comprised 88% of that total, with the NIMH, the NIAAA, and NIDA accounting for 47% (President's Commission on Mental Health 1978).

Bearing in mind the definitional distinctions between the present study and the PCMH, overall research support appears to have risen substantially since that time. However, the increase appears to be restricted largely to the NIMH, the NIAAA, and NIDA. The apparent failure to diversify funding sources leaves the field highly vulnerable to shifts in these primary funding sources. It further suggests that greater effort should be made to expand funding from other sectors.

Sector Issues

We examined the sources of current research support and identified barriers that limit expansion of funding and approaches that may increase the level and diversification of research resources.

National Institute on Alcohol Abuse and Alcoholism (NIAAA), National Institute on Drug Abuse (NIDA), and National Institute of Mental Health (NIMH). Funding by these institutes has grown significantly during the past decade as a result of organized advocacy effort from the field and citizens groups such as the National Alliance for the Mentally Ill, the National Depressive and Manic Depressive Association, and the National Mental Health Association. This also reflects broad societal changes in attitudes about mental illness and the importance of research. In the past several years, the NIH, the NIAAA, and NIDA have successively received greater increases than at any other time in their histories. Not withstanding this progress, the lost buying power resulting from funding curtailments in the 1970s and early 1980s has only recently been recouped (Figure 1–2), and real increases are quite modest, particularly in comparison with the growth of the NIH during the same period (Freedman 1985).

Importantly, the focus and locale for this research have shifted considerably since the 1970s, when the Research Panel of the PCMH noted that the modal type of sponsoring institution for NIMH research grants was schools of arts and sciences (President's Commission on Mental Health 1978). Only 32% of grants were awarded to medical schools. Since that time, the locales of research funding by the NIH have shifted to those with access to patients with mental disorders. In 1989, university medical schools and hospitals were the recipients of almost 57% of all NIMH extramural grant funding, with other hospitals and clinics receiving another 11% (NIMH 1989).

Other Department of Health and Human Services agencies. Elsewhere in the Department of Health and Human Services, small but important contributions can be made, particularly in the areas of health services and epidemiologic research from such agencies as the Agency for Health Care Policy and Research and the Centers for Disease Control. Both the Social Security Administration and the Health Care Financing Administration support different priorities each year. In fiscal 1988, disability and the mentally impaired were of particular interest to the Social Security Administration; the

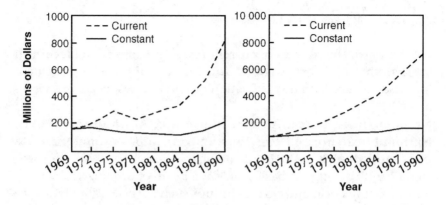

Figure 1–2. Funds received. Increase in funds received by the National Institute of Mental Health, the National Institute on Drug Abuse, and the National Institute on Alcohol Abuse and Alcoholism for research between fiscal 1969 and 1990 *(left)* compared with that received by the institutes of the National Institutes of Health during the same period *(right)*. Data include institute funding for extramural research grants and contracts, direct operations, research training, and intramural research. Note the difference in scale of *y* axes between the two charts.

Health Care Financing Administration supported limited work in diagnosis related groups and the mentally ill. Future years may yield additional research opportunities.

Department of Veterans Affairs (VA).   Department of Veterans Affairs funding for research through its merit review program, cooperative studies program, career development program, and high-priority research program is substantial. In fiscal 1988, while the VA's research commitment exceeded $190 million and supported more than 2,500 researchers, of whom 70% were physicians, only 10% of the medical research budget supported the work of 202 investigators in the fields of mental illness and substance abuse. This level of funding is of particular concern, given the fact that mental disorders alone account for more than 40% of all admissions to VA facilities. Included in VA research support are special initiatives undertaken in the area of rehabilitation research in both Alzheimer's disease and schizophrenia. We hope that a recent task force report on VA medical research will spur expansion of resources in this area (Veterans Affairs Advisory Committee for Health Research Policy 1991).

National Science Foundation (NSF). Basic behavioral and biological research is the focus of the NSF. The NSF's Biological Sciences Directorate and the Social, Behavioral, and Economic Sciences Directorate provide basic research grants in such areas as developmental neurosciences, cellular neurosciences, neural mechanisms of behavior, social and developmental psychology, human cognition and memory, and animal learning and behavior. An estimated $14.7 million was available in fiscal 1988 to support research related to mental illness and substance abuse.

Other federal agencies. Funding within the Department of Education focuses on rehabilitation research under the National Institute on Disability and Rehabilitation Research and on learning disabilities and "serious emotional disturbances" within its Office of Special Education's Division of Innovation and Development. In fiscal 1988, the National Institute for Disability and Rehabilitation Research supported mental illness research at a level of slightly more than $1 million; the Division of Innovation and Development supported research on severe emotional disturbances, learning disabilities, or a combination of emotional and physical disorders at the level of approximately $1 million. Substance abuse research is of secondary consideration in Department of Education research.

However, the Department of Justice maintains substantial interest in issues of substance abuse as well as mental disorders through both its Office of Juvenile Justice and Delinquency Prevention and the National Institute of Justice. The former office has played a limited and focused role in research related to mental disorders and a somewhat more involved role in substance abuse research, totaling nearly $5 million in fiscal 1988. The National Institute of Justice granted more than $4.2 million for research in such areas as violent behavior of abusing spouses; victimization, mental disorders, and violent crimes; psychological factors involved in and predisposition to violent behavior; and assessing linkages among drugs, alcohol, and crime. Both the Department of Defense, through its three major services, and NASA support some research in human performance, stress, and circadian rhythms. In fiscal 1988, the Office of Naval Research made grants in the amount of $1.7 million in the area of stress and the immune system and another $1.3 million in the area of stress and performance. NASA granted some $730,000 for research in neural networking, issues of stress and interpersonal psychodynamics, and psychiatric aspects of crew behavior.

State research support.   State support for mental illness and sub-stance abuse research is highly variable and, in most states, is quite limited. An American Psychiatric Association Office of Research study sought to identify funding resources and determine patterns of that funding (Ridge et al. 1989). Of the 49 states responding to a 50-state survey in 1987–1988, 28 (57%) funded mental health research and 14 (29%) supported research on substance abuse. Funds for research represented about 0.3% of total state expenditures for mental health. Some research was supported indirectly through appropriations to medical schools from the state department of education, not from the state mental health or substance abuse authority (e.g., California). However, such funds were not included because it was impossible to tease the research support from institutional, clinical, or educational support.

   Four types of funding mechanisms were prevalent: 1) joint state-university research units, 2) research grants, 3) state in-house re-search, and 4) contracts to outside agencies. We also found that the presence of state research funding was not related to the size of the state or its overall budget. Rather, state funding was associated with the presence of existing research resources—personnel and facilities. The most critical factors determining a state's involvement in mental illness or substance abuse research were the leadership and receptiv-ity of the state mental health authority and the level of activism by the academic community and citizens groups (Fine et al. 1989). A number of innovative programs are operating in states with lim-ited resources; some states have effectively marshaled efforts through political channels (Fine et al. 1989). Since publication of those data, the NIMH has encouraged greater partnership with states to assist in obtaining additional support for research (Bevilacqua 1991). In addition, the Pew Foundation has underwritten an effort by the American Psychiatric Association and a consortium of other organizations to improve academic and state collaborations.

Philanthropic research support.   Another American Psychiatric Association Office of Research study (Kim et al. 1988) attempted to determine the extent to which foundations support mental health research and the characteristics of such foundations. Of the 4,402 most active foundations during 1983–1985, 44 actually supported mental health research. While 63 foundations with an identified in-terest in mental health research were found, only 15 of those foun-dations actually made grants in mental health research. It is important that an additional 29 foundations that did not state a specific interest in mental health research actually made grants in the field. When compared with demographic and financial features of other foundations, these 44 were more likely to have substantially greater assets and more likely to be nationally oriented in giving patterns. Support for mental health research was related to the presence of 1) a specialized program in mental health (e.g., MacArthur, van Ameringen, Scottish Rite, Hogg, Della Martin, Seeley); 2) the relevance of mental health research to major areas of the foundation's stated interest (e.g., W. T. Grant [children], Florence Burden [aging]); 3) a general interest in biomedical and related research (e.g., W. M. Keck, Metropolitan Life, McGraw, HHMI); or 4) an open funding agenda (e.g., Starr, Doheny, McInerny, New York Community Trust).

With regard to substance abuse, of the 4,402 major foundations that contributed more than 97% of all grant giving between 1983 and 1987, 337 made grants in the general field of substance abuse. These grants totaled $87 million; research grants represented only 0.7% of that total (Foundation Center 1989).

Thus, while general interest in mental illness and substance abuse issues among foundations is significant, support for research in these two fields is relatively limited. Foundations with a stated interest in either substance abuse or mental illness issues are more likely to support model programs and other service delivery mechanisms than research. Foundations that do not specify an interest in either mental illness or substance abuse, nonetheless, may support research in these areas because of an ongoing history of support for overall biomedical research. Thus, a fairly wide net must be cast to ensure the identification of the full range of potential support for the field.

In mental illness research, exciting new directions are promised with the establishment of such entities as NARSAD and the National Alliance for the Mentally Ill Stanley Awards program. While not yet as significant a source of single-purpose research support as the American Cancer Society, the American Diabetes Association, or the Cystic Fibrosis Foundation, they represent a start for the field. For example, NARSAD has funded 299 research grants totaling $11 million in its 5 years of existence.

Industry research funding.   This sector required the most indirect assessment technique of all funding sectors. However, as noted above, the method employed was discussed with pharmaceutical and federal personnel, who concurred in its efficacy as a proxy measure of pharmaceutical industry support.

Although substantial in comparison with most other sectors, industry support for mental illness and substance abuse research appears to lag behind that support associated with overall biomedical research and development. This funding disparity likely results from a number of specific barriers. Regulatory impediments with respect to the issue of abuse potential of psychoactive drugs have restricted interest in new drug development for mental illnesses and substance abuse. The lengthy and expensive drug approval process itself poses yet another barrier. This is coupled with a perception of limited marketing potential for drugs in this field that is associated with both the stigma attached to mental illness and drug abuse as well as the reimbursement limitations for psychiatric conditions. Research in psychopharmacology is exceptionally expensive and requires the cooperation of clinical populations that are difficult to recruit and maintain compliance in clinical trial protocols. In addition, there are particular problems with regard to the clinical costs of conducting research on severely disabled patients who might require in-hospital drug washout periods or placebo control conditions (Pincus et al. 1985).

Sectors outside the scope of the study. Important potential sources for research funding in mental illness and substance abuse not detailed in the study are other PHS agencies that are within the DRG referral system. While there is no reliable method to assess mental illness and substance abuse related research in such agencies, an examination of NIH funding to departments of psychiatry is informative. (Similar analyses could be performed with regard to departments of psychology, neuroscience, etc.) A substantial amount of funding, totaling $31,251,916 in 1988, supported research in departments of psychiatry from the various institutes of the NIH. The National Institute of Neurological Disorders and Stroke and the National Institute on Aging, for example, respectively provided approximately $8.6 million and $8.3 million to departments of psychiatry. Smaller sums from the institutes of the NIH, such as the National Institute of Child Health and Human Development, the National Heart, Lung, and Blood Institute, and the National Institute of Diabetes and Digestive and Kidney Diseases, also fund research in these departments. For the sake of comparison, while NIH support to departments of psychiatry represents less than 0.5% of its overall research budget, this funding equals almost 16% of overall [former] ADAMHA research funding to departments of psychiatry.

◆ Conclusion

In the final analysis, support for research into the mental illness and substance abuse fields is neither broad nor deep. Despite the significant gains in research funding of the NIMH, the NIAAA, and NIDA during the past 5 years, research funding support for these two fields represents less than 5% of all health research dollars. While the economic consequences of these disorders are comparable with those of heart disease and cancer, the NIMH, the NIAAA, and NIDA research funding for these disorders represents only 38% of the National Cancer Institute research commitment to cancer and three-quarters of the support from the National Heart, Lung, and Blood Institute for heart disease research (Board on Mental Health and Behavioral Medicine 1984). Given the tremendous societal costs of these disorders and the disproportionate funding compared with other areas of biomedical research, continued efforts are necessary to expand research support.

Furthermore, the study findings underscore the preeminence of the NIMH, the NIAAA, and NIDA in the conduct of mental illness, substance abuse, and psychiatric research, providing some 64% of all sources of research support. They are the overwhelming sources of research funding for clinical and health services research in mental illness and substance abuse, i.e., research directly involving patients with these disorders. The NIMH, the NIAAA, and NIDA bear nearly twice as much of the cost as the NIH for the conduct of scientific inquiry. As a whole, the federal government contributes more than 72% of all dollars to mental illness and addictive disorders research.

Further expansion of the research resource will require continued coalition building to undertake organized and assertive political advocacy. This strategy has been effective in increasing the research budgets of the NIMH, the NIAAA, and NIDA. The recent establishment and growth of philanthropic organizations such as the NARSAD and the development of the American Psychiatric Association and van Ameringen Foundation Psychiatric Research Resource Center to aid investigators in identifying potential funding sources are auspicious signs. Investigators should cast a wider net and actively participate in broadening the diversification of sources of support for mental illness and substance abuse research as well as play an active role in advocacy on behalf of congressional efforts to increase research funding at the NIMH, the NIAAA, and NIDA.

◆ References

American Psychiatric Association: Diagnostic and Statistical Manual of Mental Disorders, 3rd Edition, Revised. Washington, DC, American Psychiatric Association, 1987

American Psychiatric Association Office of Research: Opening Windows Into the Brain: Mental Illness, Drug Abuse, and Alcoholism Research: Fiscal Year 1989. Washington, DC, American Psychiatric Association, 1988

Bevilacqua J: The NIMH public-academic liaison initiative: an update. Hosp Community Psychiatry 42:71, 1991

Board on Mental Health and Behavioral Medicine, Institute of Medicine: Research on Mental Illness and Addictive Disorders: Progress and Prospects. Washington, DC, National Academy Press, 1984

Fine T, Pincus HA, Ridge B, et al: Models of state funding for mental health research. Hosp Community Psychiatry 40:383–387, 1989

Foundation Center: Alcohol and Drug Abuse Funding: An Analysis of Foundation Grants. Washington, DC, The Foundation Center, 1989

Freedman DX: Research funds are down: take heart! Arch Gen Psychiatry 42:518–522, 1985

Institute of Medicine: Personnel Needs and Training for Biomedical and Behavioral Research. Washington, DC, National Research Council, 1983

Institute of Medicine: Research on Children and Adolescents with Mental, Behavioral, and Developmental Disorders. Washington, DC, National Research Council, 1989

Kim D, Pincus HA, Fine T: Foundation funding and psychiatric research. Am J Psychiatry 145:830–835, 1988

National Institutes of Health (NIH), Division of Research Grants: Referral Guidelines for Funding Components of PHS. Washington, DC, Public Health Service, 1989a

National Institutes of Health (NIH), Office of Science Policy and Legislation: NIH Data Book 1989. Bethesda, MD, National Institutes of Health, 1989b

National Institute of Mental Health (NIMH), Information Management and Analysis Branch: Research Information Source Book: Extramural Programs: Fiscal Year 1988. Rockville, MD, Alcohol, Drug Abuse, and Mental Health Administration, 1989

Pincus HA, West J, Goldman H: Diagnosis-related groups and clinical research in psychiatry. Arch Gen Psychiatry 42:627–629, 1985

President's Commission on Mental Health, Research Task Panel: Report of the Research Task Panel: Task Panel Reports Submitted to the President's Commission on Mental Health, IV:1517–1821, 1978

Rice D: Economic Costs of Alcohol and Drug Abuse and Mental Illness. Rockville, MD, Alcohol, Drug Abuse, and Mental Health Administration, 1990

Ridge R, Pincus HA, Blalock R, et al: Factors that influence state funding for mental health research. Hosp Community Psychiatry 40:377–382, 1989

Veterans Affairs Advisory Committee for Health Research Policy: Final report of the Department of Veterans Affairs Committee for Health Research Policy: January 1990–January 1991. Washington, DC, Department of Veterans Affairs, January 1991 (internal document)

Successful Research Grant Applications

Jane Steinberg, Ph.D., and Cille Kennedy, Ph.D.

W riting a successful grant application is a formidable undertaking. The goal of this chapter is to demystify the research grant application and review process. More specifically, we want to enable new and experienced researchers to compete more successfully for federal funds. This chapter provides a complete road map of the grant application process, from start to finish. Examples are drawn from the National Institute of Mental Health (NIMH), an institute within the National Institutes of Health (NIH), but the advice is sound for approaching most federal, and many private, funding agencies. In addition, a glossary of grant terms and a description of various federal grant mechanisms (Resources 2–1) are provided to ease communication between the applicant and the federal staff.

◆ How to Begin

Begin with a research idea that excites you and is rich enough to keep your interest over the long haul. An application may take 6 months to fully plan, write, and submit; 6 months to receive the review results; and 1–5 years to actually conduct. This is a significant amount of professional time, and the research idea should warrant such a long-term commitment. Another reason to wait until you have an outstanding research idea is that few granting agencies have the resources to fund research without significant methodological, conceptual, or applied interest. Federal agencies and private organizations may not have enough money to fund applications that offer only slight refinements of existing research paradigms, even if the proposed research is technically sound. Ask yourself if the study's results will stir the imagination of the field. If so, you have an idea worth developing.

◆ Identifying Funding Sources

The next step in the process is to identify all the possible funding sources for your project. Why identify *all* possible sources of funds instead of the best source? The answer is simple. You can maximize your probability of success by working up the same research idea for different funding sources. Each federal or private agency has identified specific goals for its research grant funds. If your research idea fits—or can reasonably be made to fit—the goals of several agencies, you can increase the likelihood of obtaining funding with little additional work.

It is important to be clear that applying to multiple agencies or organizations (e.g., the NIMH and the National Science Foundation) with the same idea is fine. Taking money from more than one source to conduct the same work is not. Neither is it acceptable to apply with the same idea to two programs within a federal organization (e.g., two programs within the NIMH) or within the same review structure (e.g., National Institute of Child Health and Human Development and the NIMH).

Many books describe the programs of research available through foundations and agencies, as well as the names and telephone numbers of contact people for each. For example, research interests of private foundations are contained in the *Foundation Directory*. Federal resources are listed in the *Catalog of Federal Domestic Assistance*. Both the directory and the catalog may be found in your library and Office of Sponsored Research. In addition, the American Psychiatric Association's *Psychiatric Research Report* is an excellent, timely source of grant opportunities. Yet another promising source of potential funding for your research ideas is your colleagues. With whom have they had success? From these leads, you will generate a list of potential funding sources for your project with the names and telephone numbers of staff.

◆ Making Contact

Once a list of possible funding sources is developed, you can begin to make telephone calls to each contact person. As a warning, you should know that contact persons frequently change between the time the directory or catalog compiles the information and your call. Do not be concerned by this. Simply ask to speak to the professional staff member who now handles your area.

Be prepared with a three-sentence description of your project. This brief abstract will allow the contact person to determine how best to help you. Do not launch into a lengthy explanation of your proposal unless asked. Be ready to describe your study questions, your sample, and study methodology if asked. Take notes during the call and be sure to ask for a decoding of acronyms you do not understand. Ask each potential grantor the following questions.

Is this research idea fundable? Does it fit within the scope of the granting institution? If not, can it be made to fit the institution's needs?

By fundable we mean whether the agency supports your type of research. This can refer to the content of the research (e.g., depression or tardive dyskinesia) or style of research. For example, some grantors are less likely to fund qualitative research. Others prefer to fund small-scale pilot studies or only support full clinical trials. A research question being asked about adults might not be fundable from a particular grantor while the same question asked about children might.

Will the contact send any special announcements, applications, and the review and funding criteria?

For example, researchers interested in conducting applied research on persons with severe mental disorders might be interested in one or more of the following NIMH program announcements: Research on

Disabilities and Rehabilitation Services for Persons with Severe Mental Disorders; Research on Services for Severely Mentally Ill Persons; Research on Effectiveness and Outcomes of Mental Health Services; Implementation of the National Plan for Research on Child and Adolescent Disorders; Anorexia Nervosa and Bulimia Nervosa: Basic Brain, Behavioral, and Clinical Studies; and Psychotherapeutic Drug Discovery Program. All of these program announcements—and more—are available through the NIMH. Each program announcement outlines the receipt dates, review criteria, and eligibility requirements.

In contrast to an ongoing program announcement, some federal organizations offer a time-limited Request for Applications (RFA). The RFA has a single receipt date and set-aside funds for projects. One should ask that these be sent as well. Also, the contact person should be asked about the various funding mechanisms (i.e., type of award programs) that might be suitable for your application. For instance, in addition to the regular research grants, two other commonly used research mechanisms at the NIMH are small grants and First Independent Research and Support Transition (FIRST) awards. Small grants are for newer, less experienced researchers, investigators at institutions without a well-developed research tradition, or for more experienced investigators who wish to study a new area of investigation or apply a new methodology. A small grant is limited to 2 years of funding at $50,000 per year in direct costs. Small grants are not renewable. FIRST awards are for newly independent researchers who have not been principal investigators on any Public Health Service (PHS)-supported research excepting a small grant (and certain career grant mechanisms). Applicants must provide a 5-year research plan, devote at least 50% effort to the project, and request no more than $350,000 for the grant period. FIRST awards may not be renewed. Regular research grants have no limit on the amount of funding, may be awarded for up to 5 years, and may be extended if a competing continuation application is successful. Additional funding mechanisms exist within the NIMH and within other federal and private funding sources. Ask your contact person.

How much money is available for new applications?

This question is important because some research programs may have committed all of their funds to continuing applications. There

is no point competing for new money that does not exist. Some programs, due to the vagaries of the budget process, may not be able to
tell you an exact dollar amount. Get their best guess on whether new
money will be available after they meet their commitment base (i.e.,
paid their current grantees).

Will the contact person critique a draft of the application?

Preapplication consultation is frequently available and encouraged.
For example, at the NIMH many staff members request prospective
applicants to send a four- or five-page concept paper for critique and
then at least one draft of the application sufficiently prior to submission to incorporate feedback. Staff comments can be helpful since
they are based on years of observing the review process. Staff comments are, of course, only advisory, and the applicant must decide
whether or not to incorporate the suggestions.

Will the contact send a list of the reviewers who may review the application?

In some funding agencies, standing review committees exist, and
their members' names are available. The applicant, however, will remain blind to the specific individuals who are assigned as reviewers
of his or her application. When one reviews the names, one should
check to see if the committee has sufficient expertise in the important
areas of one's research. If not, the applicant may wish to call the
individual organizing the review (a scientific review administrator at
the NIH) and discuss his or her concern. One may find that an ad hoc
reviewer can be added to the standing committee or that another
standing review group is appropriate. The applicant may also look
over the names and find an individual who has a conflict of interest
(e.g., past mentor or an individual who has taken public issue with
the applicant's work or genre of research). Let the person organizing
the review know this **before** the review takes place.

Can the contact think of other funding agencies that might be interested in this idea?

Grantors attempt to keep abreast of funding priorities in other granting sources with similar areas of research interest. They may be the

best source of knowledge on whom to contact in another agency. For example, with the return of the NIMH to the NIH, the mental health service grants, formerly under the NIMH, are now sponsored by the Center for Mental Health Services within the Substance Abuse and Mental Health Services Administration (SAMHSA). With this reorganization, contact persons are invaluable to assist you with appropriate referrals for service demonstration grants versus research and research demonstration grants.

After you have made all of the telephone calls, you should cull through the information you have collected and identify the most promising organizations and programs. Be certain that your research interest truly meets the eligibility criteria for the particular program of a funding agency. Do not fight a losing battle. If the program's area of interest is rural mental health services research, do not try to convince the funder that a study conducted in Manhattan would be a suitable research site for the agency to sponsor. Your contact person will advise you as to the flexibility of the program's stated eligibility criteria.

The next step is to follow up and provide the concept papers and draft applications to program staff who have offered to read them. Another good idea is to call the program person 4 or 5 days after you have submitted the draft document to be sure it arrived and to arrange a telephone call for feedback. Be sure to take notes during the feedback call. The federal program staff often call this type of help "technical assistance" or preapplication consultation. You might find these phrases helpful when making your calls.

◆ Preparing the Application

Before turning on your computer, **read the application instructions thoroughly**. Most experienced funding officials can tell you that very few people do this. Failure to follow the instructions may mean a delay in the application process and may result in your being considered ineligible for one-time-only RFAs. Applications that exceed page or appendix limitations may be automatically returned to the investigator without review. Even experienced grant-getters should read the application instructions since they are frequently revised. For instance, the most widely used Public Health Service application kit for NIMH grants, known as PHS 398, was revised late in 1991. It contains sufficiently important changes to its predecessor as to warrant a thorough review by both new and experienced applicants. The good news is that the study narrative (i.e., the specific aims, background and significance, progress report/preliminary studies, and research design and methodology), which formerly had a 20-page limit, is now allotted 25 pages, including tables and figures. Limitations have been placed on the number and type of materials that may be included in the appendix. For studies that include human subjects, a discussion of the gender and racial/ethnic composition of the sample must be presented. A clear rationale must be given if women or members of minority groups are to be excluded.

Another important point in effective preparation of an application is to allow sufficient time for all of the necessary steps in the application process. Remember to plan for the time associated with proofreading and departmental, college, university, or institutional sign-offs, as well as approval for human or animal subjects.

Elements of a Competitive Application

Significance. Be sure that your literature review provides a crisp synthesis of the crucial literature and justifies your hypotheses. Explain how your results (whether the hypotheses are confirmed or not) will significantly advance or integrate the field.

Feasibility. If there is space for a progress report, insert material that demonstrates the feasibility of the project such as pilot data. Be sure that your pilot data do support your case. If you have no pilot data and have not conducted a preliminary study, you may want to pause and consider whether you have another way to demonstrate: 1) the reliability and validity of procedures; 2) the feasibility of the project; and 3) your ability to oversee a project of this scope.

Strategy. Page limits can be difficult to observe if you are describing a series of experiments. Sometimes applicants offer brief snapshots of designs for 10 to 20 studies. This can be inadequate and confusing. Another approach is to fully describe one prototypical study and then discuss the conceptual and methodological permutations in the other studies as space permits.

Another difficulty is proposing a series of studies in which each study is predicated on confirming the expected hypotheses of the previous study. The applicant must make the reviewers understand that if the expected hypotheses are not confirmed, equally exciting directions will emerge. Alternatively, you may want to scale down the scope of this application and consider a series of grant applications that builds upon your accumulated findings.

Sampling.   A clear, succinct description of your sample size, sample characteristics, selection procedure, and assignment to study condition must be presented. Increasing numbers of granting agencies expect a statistical power analysis to be conducted to determine the adequacy of your sample size. If you are not familiar with estimating power, ask your biostatistician or statistical consultant to conduct the power analysis at the outset of your study planning.

As noted above, you will need to address the inclusion of women and minority group members if you are employing human subjects in an NIH application. Supply as many demographic characteristics as possible: it will assist the reviewer to understand the generalizability of your study. Describe where you will find your sample. Are those sites likely to cooperate with you? Document their support. Will you be able to obtain your sample size in the time allotted? Portray the estimated flow of subjects into the study.

You must describe how you will obtain informed voluntary consent from participants. Decide how you will handle refusals and dropouts and how these may bias your sample. Incorporate the projected refusal rate when you calculate the time frame for collecting your sample.

If you cannot randomly assign your subjects to study conditions, as in some kinds of applied research, justify your assignment procedures and identify the type of quasi-experimental design you will employ.

Methods.   The current literature will assist you in identifying the most recent instruments for your study. Be aware of the psychometric properties of the instruments. Your contact person may be aware of other instruments or modifications to instruments that are being used in ongoing research that has not yet appeared in the literature. Ask the contact person for the names and numbers of other investigators currently using instruments that may be appropriate for your study. Connecting your study to others via instrumentation assists in the generalizability of your study results and your contribution to the field.

Analytic plan.   In preparing an analytic plan, it is mandatory to show how the hypotheses will be tested. A laundry list of high-tech procedures is irrelevant if you have a chi-square question. Other problems to avoid are an uncritical use of change scores, unspecified data reduction plans, and designs with inadequate statistical power.

You may find that adequately testing the proposed hypotheses is beyond your level of statistical proficiency. Consider adding a statistical consultant to your staffing plan. Ask this individual to assist in designing the research and drafting the application. Asking for consultation after the data are collected is much less useful than prior consultation.

Budget plan.   The budget should reflect the ebb and flow of the work. For instance, if all data coding takes place in years two through three of a project, do not ask for a data coder's salary in year one. A task analysis can be a helpful exercise in planning your budget. That is, identify every task that needs to be done, who needs to do it, how long it should take, and when it should get done. Further, if the type of grant you are seeking has a budget limit, be sure that you can effectively complete your project within these limits.

In justifying equipment purchases, the object is to explain why a particular piece is needed for the proposed studies, not why it is the finest available. For instance, although the graphics capability of a particular software package is clearly better than anything else on the market, why is it necessary for the completion of the project?

One of the new mandates for NIMH grants is that any recurring costs must not exceed 104% of the cost in the previous year. For example, the cost of data collection (e.g., a survey interview) over a 2-year period should not cost 4% more in the second year than it did in the first. If a new type of data, such as a clinical interview of a subset of the sample to validate interview diagnoses, is to be collected in the second year, then this cost is considered an expansion and is not part of the recurring cost.

Investigate whether your campus provides assistance in preparing budgets for grants. Typically, staff in the Office of Grants Management or Sponsored Programs are available to advise grant applicants on the financial aspects of an application. A department chairperson can also be helpful.

Final check.   Ask a colleague to read the application for clarity. Pick a researcher you trust, someone who is not familiar with your research plan and who is outside of your specific field. If this person understands the application, you can be sure that the reviewers will.

◆ Application Review

Review procedures vary dramatically across federal agencies. Be sure that you understand the review criteria that will be used to evaluate your application. Many federal agencies use some form of peer review to evaluate applications. That is, outside experts are asked to review your application and discuss its strengths and weaknesses to determine the application's scientific or applied merit. The process of voting and assigning an index of merit for an application is specific to an agency or organization.

Reviewers may decide that no determination of merit can be made without a site visit. Their willingness to come indicates significant interest in the project, but they do have important questions. A dry run with colleagues role-playing the visitors can be helpful preparation.

One of the best ways to learn about the peer review process is to accept invitations to serve as a reviewer when asked. Anecdotally, first-time reviewers report surprise over the high degree of consensus among reviewers and over the huge amount of work that peer review requires.

◆ After the Review

Many agencies and some private foundations have a routine feedback process for grant applications. Ask your contact person what to expect following the review. At the NIMH, for instance, you will receive your priority score and percentile ranking via a letter from the scientific review administrator within 10 days after the review. You will also receive a summary statement of the review after approximately 6 weeks.

If it is apparent that your application will not be funded, review the agency feedback and decide whether or not it is reasonable to revise your application and resubmit. Review committees appreciate thoughtful amended applications, and resubmissions often are successful. For example, at the NIMH during fiscal year 1990, 20% of initial applications were funded, whereas 30% of amended applications received funding.

If you learn that your application received an outstanding ranking and is likely to be funded, you may wish to prepare for budget
negotiations with the agency and establish a possible start-up date.
Many applications need a final review by an advisory board. You will
need to work closely with your contact person, who will provide
guidance through this aspect of the process as well.

◆ Finally

The best bit of advice in this chapter is to make contact with the
various funding sources. Many opportunities exist for meeting federal and private funding officials. Some federal agencies offer technical assistance workshops on grant writing. Many of the specialty
research societies also offer intensive workshops on grant writing
that involve federal and private funding officials.

Resources 2–1
Glossary of Grant Terms and Federal Grant Mechanisms

◆ Glossary of Grant Terms

applicant organization   The one organization that will be legally and financially responsible for the conduct of activities supported by the award. Upon award the applicant organization becomes the grantee.

application   A request for financial support via a grant or cooperative agreement of a project/activity submitted on specified forms and in accordance with instructions provided by the PHS awarding office.

budget period   The interval of time (usually 12 months) into which the project period is divided for budgetary and funding purposes.

Commerce Business Daily   A daily publication that lists the U.S. government procurement invitations, subcontracting leads, and contracts awarded.

competing continuation application   A request for financial or direct assistance to extend for one or more additional budget periods a project period that would otherwise expire. Competing continuation applications compete with other competing continuation, competing supplemental, and new applications for funds.

cooperative agreement   Financial assistance mechanism used in lieu of a grant when substantial federal programmatic involvement with the recipient during performance is anticipated by the awarding program office.

direct costs   Costs that can be specifically identified with a particular project or program.

Division of Research Grants, NIH   Central receipt and referral point for NIH grant applications.

executive secretary Previous position title of the individual responsible for the initial review of an application. Now called a scientific review administrator.

Federal Register A daily publication that provides a uniform system for making available to the public the regulations and legal notices issued by federal agencies, including the announcements of the availability of funds for financial assistance programs.

grant A financial assistance mechanism whereby money and/or direct assistance is provided to carry out approved activities. A grant (as opposed to a cooperative agreement) is to be used whenever the PHS awarding office anticipates no substantial programmatic involvement with the recipient during performance of the financially assisted activities.

grantee The institution, organization, or other legally accountable entity that receives a grant.

indirect costs Costs incurred for common or joint objectives that cannot be identified specifically with a particular project, e.g., facilities operation and maintenance, depreciation, and administrative expenses.

National Institute of Mental Health (NIMH) Administrative entity within the NIH that supports research and research training programs to increase knowledge and improve research methods on mental and behavioral disorders; to generate information regarding basic biological and behavioral processes underlying these disorders and the maintenance of mental health; and to develop and improve mental health service, including prevention and treatment.

initial review group (IRG) Peer review panel that rates the scientific and technical merit of grant applications.

National Institutes of Health (NIH) Administrative entity that houses the National Institute of Mental Health (NIMH) within the Public Health Service (PHS) as of October 1, 1992. The mission of the NIH is to improve the health of the people of the United States by increasing the understanding of the process underlying human health and by acquiring new knowledge to help prevent, detect, diagnose, and treat disease.

new application   A request for financial or direct assistance for a project or program not currently receiving PHS financial assistance.

NIH Guide to Grants and Contracts   All NIH Requests for Proposals, Requests for Applications, and program announcements are published in this document, which is available electronically and in hard copy.

noncompeting continuation application   A request for financial or direct assistance for a second or subsequent budget period within a previously approved project period.

Notice of Grant Award   The legally binding document that serves as a notification to the recipient and others that a grant or cooperative agreement has been made, contains or references all terms of the award, and documents the obligation of federal funds in the Department of Health and Human Services system.

peer review   A system of review that uses experts who are the professional equals of the applicants to evaluate the scientific and technical merit of an application.

percentile score   The percentile score represents the relative position or rank of each priority score among the scores assigned by a particular review panel. The percentile rank of priority scores guides funding decisions.

pink sheet   Old terminology for summary statement.

preapplication   A statement in summary form of the intent of the applicant to request federal funds. It is used to determine the applicant's eligibility; determine how well the proposed application can compete with other similar applications; and eliminate any applications for which there is little or no chance for federal funding before applicants incur significant expenditures for preparing an application.

priority score   The numerical value assigned to each application by each voting review group member that reflects his or her own opinion of the scientific merit of the proposed research relative to the "state of the art." After the meeting, these scores are averaged by the scientific review administrator, providing a three-digit rating. These scores appear on the summary statement.

program announcement   Gives notice of a new or ongoing grant program and invites applications for support.

program officer   Individual who is responsible for a program area within some granting institution. Develops the area through activities such as providing help to potential applicants, making award decisions, identifying program initiatives, holding workshops and conferences, issuing monographs, and monitoring grants, contracts, and cooperative agreements.

project officer   Individual who represents the government for the purpose of technical monitoring of contractor performance.

project period   The total time for which support of a discretionary project has been programmatically approved. A project period may consist of one or more budget periods. The total project period comprises the original project period and any extensions.

recommendation   Decision an NIH initial review group makes if an application is not recommended for further consideration or to defer the application done by majority vote.

referral officer   The individual responsible for determining the relevance of each application to the NIH mission and assigning acceptable applications to an appropriate review group and institute.

Request for Applications (RFA)   Invites grant applications to accomplish a specific purpose in a well-defined scientific area of study with one receipt date.

Request for Proposals (RFP)   The government's solicitation of a contract to prospective offerors to submit a proposal based on the terms and conditions set forth in the RFP.

R01   Regular research grant, traditional research project.

scientific review administrator   Performs administrative and technical review of grant applications at the NIH, including such responsibilities as selecting reviewers, managing study sections, writing summary statements, and conducting site visits.

scientific review group   Peer review panel that reviews both contract proposals and grant applications.

site visit   Conducted when an application requires additional information that can be gained only at the site before a recommendation can be made by the review panel. During the site visit, the site visitors meet with the principal investigator and any other relevant personnel to discuss the areas in question.

stipend   A payment made to an individual under a fellowship or training grant in accordance with preestablished levels to provide the individual's living expenses during the period of training.

summary statement   Document written by the scientific review administrator following the peer review meeting. Based on the combination of the reviewer's written comments and the review panel's discussion during the meeting. The summary statement is sent to the principal investigator.

supplemental application   A request for an increase in support during a current budget period for expansion of the project's scope or research protocol or to meet increased administrative costs unforeseen at the time of the new noncompeting continuation or competing continuation application.

terms of award   All legal requirements imposed by the federal government, whether by statute, regulation(s), or terms in the grant award document. The terms of award may include both standard and government's interests.

◆ Federal Grant Mechanisms

R01

The Research Project Grant is a research grant. These grants are the traditional investigator-initiated research grants awarded by the NIMH. Eligibility to become a principal investigator is training in research and experience showing capability in conducting the proposed work. Awards may be given for up to 5 years of support. After 5 years (or the time period of support), the principal investigator can submit a competing continuation request. R01s have no specific budget limitations. The review criteria for all R01s are technical and scientific merit. R01s are extremely competitive.

Small Grants

Small grants are research grants that provide support for research in four categories: 1) newer, less experienced researchers; 2) investigators at institutions without well-developed research traditions; 3) experienced researchers either doing exploratory studies or proposing research that represents a change in their research direction; and 4) experienced researchers teaching new methods or new techniques. The conditions for the small grant are that the applicant may not use it to supplement an existing grant or as interim support between grants. The grant may not be used to support work on a thesis. The small grant awards offer up to 2 years of support at $50,000 in direct costs per year and are not renewable. The review criteria include an assessment of the ability of the principal investigator to do the proposed work; the innovativeness or promise of the research idea; the potential for future research when pilot studies are being proposed; the basis of the project in the relevant literature; the reasonableness of the methodology; the resources; and the budget.

First Independent Research Support and Transition (FIRST) Awards (R29)

The FIRST award is a research grant with the purpose of providing a sufficient period of research support to highly promising, newly independent researchers in behavioral, psychosocial, and biomedical areas of research. They are intended to help effect the transition to traditional NIMH research grants (R01s). In order to be eligible, the applicant must have no more than 5 years of research experience since completion of postdoctoral training or its equivalent. The applicant must be eligible to be the principal investigator of an R01, and not have been a principal investigator on a PHS grant with the exception of small grants and some K awards. Among the conditions and terms of support is that the proposed research be a 5-year project. In total, the direct costs over the 5 years may not exceed $350,000 and no more than $100,000 in any given year. The principal investigator must devote 50% of his or her time to the study, may not have another PHS grant simultaneously, and may not have an award pending for the same research. The review criteria include that the principal investigator has the potential to carry out the research and is committed to a research career.

Research Scientist Development Awards (RSDA) (K02)

The RSDA is a career development award that enhances the development of outstanding scientists and enables them to expand their potential for making contributions to research. The grant provides salary support to release the awardee from teaching, administration, clinical, and other responsibilities in order to devote at least 80% of his or her time to research and related activities. To be eligible, candidates must have the capacity to carry out independent research, have the potential to become outstanding scientists, have past and present research productivity and funding, and be able to conceptualize and organize long-term research. Awards are made for up to 5 years of support at up to $75,000 per year plus fringes. Awards are renewable only once. Applications must include a career enhancement plan, a research plan, and describe the institutional environment.

CHAPTER 3

Federal Funding and Psychiatric Research

Christopher Dykton

Research provides extraordinary benefits to society through the creation of new knowledge and the training of scientists to provide future contributions. The research and higher education system in the United States has a long history of advancing the state of scientific knowledge. These advances have addressed such goals as enhancing the nation's public health, educational achievement, work force, technological development, environmental quality, and economic competitiveness. Underlying the relationship between government and the scientific community was a social contract or "trusteeship," developed after the scientific breakthroughs spurred by World War II, that delegated much judgment regarding federal research choices to scientific experts. This scientific peer analysis helped spur increases in research support. The principal element of this new relationship between research scientists and the federal government was the research grant, which created a new social contract between the two participants. This social contract implied that in return for the privilege of receiving federal support, the researcher was obligated to produce and freely share knowledge that would benefit—in mostly unspecified and long-term ways—the public good (Meredith et al. 1991)

Over the past 50 years, federal funding for research has not grown unabated. Increases have not been at a constant rate; fluctuations in funding levels have occurred regularly. Funding increased quickly in the 1950s and in the early 1960s during the "golden years" for research during the Kennedy administration and the social policies of Johnson's "Great Society." But it first decreased and then leveled off from the late 1960s until the mid-1970s (Dusek et al. 1984). From 1975 onward overall federal research funding again increased, initially with expansions in health and life sciences research (e.g., the "War on Cancer") and an infusion of funding for defense-related research during the Reagan administration.

Funding of biomedical research has generally mirrored this overall growth pattern. For example, support from the National Institutes of Health (NIH), the federal institution primarily responsible for health-related research support that annually funds over 70% of the federal government's health research awards, expanded from around $81 million in 1955 to $1.4 billion in 1970 in actual dollars (Table 3–1 in Resources 3–1). Throughout the 1970s, funding grew steadily but at a somewhat slower pace. Recent years have witnessed a leveling off of NIH funding in constant dollars (i.e., adjusted for inflation), with slight increases, due in large measure to AIDS funding, in the latter part of the decade to a projected 1995 appropriation totaling $11.5 billion in actual dollars.

As noted by Pincus and Fine (Chapter 1, this volume), the National Institute of Mental Health (NIMH), the National Institute on Drug Abuse (NIDA), and the National Institute on Alcohol Abuse and Alcoholism (NIAAA), the former institutes of the Alcohol, Drug Abuse, and Mental Health Administration (ADAMHA), had more limited research growth than the NIH during the late 1960s and 1970s; more attention was paid in those years to the development of community health service programs. However, research programs have grown significantly during the past decade, reflecting changes in attitudes about mental illness and expanded mental health advocacy. Nevertheless, during this time real increases in buying power have been modest (Pincus and Fine 1991).

Regardless of the pace of overall federal research support, the federal government remains a principal supporter of biomedical research, having annually provided between 39% and 50% of all national support for health research and development from 1983 to

1993 (projected) (Figure 3–1 and Table 3–2 in Resources 3–1). In the early 1980s, the federal share of national health research and development (R&D) was 54%, compared to an industry share of 37% and an "other" (nonprofit) share of 11%. As the 1980s progressed, the federal share of national health R&D actually decreased to the 1992 level of 41%, whereas the industry share grew to 48%; nonprofit health R&D remains stable at 11%.

Despite the overall growth in research funding, the competition for research health funds has remained keen and, in fact, has increased. The NIH reports that applications rose from 16,798 in 1983 to 20,142 in 1992, with 5,389 awards given in 1983 compared to 6,039 in 1992. Thus, the success rate for competing research projects has fallen in recent years (32%–34% funded during 1983–1987 compared to 24%–29.7% in 1989–1992) (NIH 1993).

The intense competition for federally funded grants demonstrates that the scientific community is capable of undertaking far more investigations into all areas of biomedical research, including psychiatry, than the federal government is able to support. Policymakers and sponsors of research must continuously choose between competing "goods." Controversies over the support of younger scientists and established researchers, "have" and "have-not" institutions, and tradeoffs among fields are manifestations of the consequences of choices perceived by various segments of the scientific community (Meredith et al. 1991), as well as the research issues emphasized by the federal political process. Ideally, as Daniel X. Freedman, M.D., suggested, funding should flow from a sophisticated attempt to triangulate among 1) perceived health need, 2) scientific opportunity, and 3) available resources (Freedman 1985).

The Committee on Policies for Allocating Health Sciences Research of the Institute of Medicine (IOM) noted in its report, *Funding Health Science Research: A Strategy to Restore Balance*, that federal support for basic research has been based on 1) stable federal support in order to undertake long-range research, 2) peer review for evaluating scientific merit, 3) academically based scientific investigation, 4) flexible scientific management policies, and 5) accountability to the Congress, the president, and the American public (Bloom and Randolph 1990). This approach has led to the present diverse research infrastructure of federal, state, industry, nonprofit, and voluntary research sponsors; such a broad system of support is essential to continue a vigorous health sciences research program (Meredith et al. 1991).

◆ Creating the Federal Budget

Ultimately, federal research support is determined by the annual Congressional budgetary process in response to the president's goals for his administration as articulated in the budget he presents to Congress. This process and the roles of the varied participants inside and outside the scene are central to understanding, tracking, and advocating future funding for mental health research. The federal budget process, as it relates to research, is the means by which researchers, the president acting through the federal research agencies, Congress, and outside constituencies negotiate budget figures and therefore the goals and direction of research support. This process is time-consuming, complex, and spread over several institutions.

Each annual budget goes through three stages: 1) preparation of a budget request for each agency, to be submitted by the administration to Congress; 2) congressional review of the administration's request, where adjustments may be made according to the current fiscal and political influences; and 3) implementation by federal agencies, including research programs, of the final budget as approved by Congress and signed by the president.

There is limited formal opportunity for direct input from the research community during the preparation of the administration's budget requests because requests are developed through internal processes (Dusek et al. 1984). Congress actually considers the budgets of federal government agencies, including the research agencies, on three concurrent tracks: authorizations, appropriations, and budget reconciliation. For more specific information on the budget processes and the role of advocacy, consult Cutler and Cohen (Chapter 13, this volume).

At the conclusion of these budget processes, funds are appropriated to the individual government agencies for operational, intramural, and extramural funding. Budgetary changes are reflected in the funding of agency programs, redirection or development of new initiatives for research, or elimination. Certain federal agencies, for example, the Department of Veterans Affairs (VA), generally fund scientific investigations primarily within their own institutions. Other agencies have some intramural programs but primarily act as a conduit for congressional appropriations and directives, thereby funding scientists at private institutions for certain research. To understand the implementation of appropriations and extramural research funding process, refer to Steinberg and Kennedy (Chapter 2, this volume).

◆ Profiles of Federal Agency Funding Sources

Mental health and psychiatric research funding is not the exclusive domain of a single agency but is provided by a range of different agencies. Research issues and topics may crosscut the missions of federal organizations, often with overlapping programs and sometimes with multidisciplinary and multiagency collaboration. An overview of federal institutions and their potential areas of psychiatric research interest illustrates that there is a select group of agencies supporting psychiatric research and collaborating, through multidisciplinary, crosscutting fields, with psychiatric investigators. To assist the investigator with federal psychiatric research information, Resources 3–2 provides profiles of federal institutions with an interest or history of funding research in areas related to psychiatry.

◆ References

Bloom FE, Randolph MA (eds): Funding Health Sciences Research: A Strategy to Restore Balance. Washington, DC, National Academy Press, 1990

Dusek ER, Holt VE, Burke ME, et al: American Psychological Association's Guide to Research Support, 2nd Edition. Washington, DC, American Psychological Association, 1984

Freedman DX: Research funds are down: take heart! Arch Gen Psychiatry 42:518–522, 1985

Meredith MA, Nelson SD, Teich AH (eds): Science and Technology Policy Yearbook. Washington, DC, American Association for the Advancement of Science, 1991

National Institutes of Health: NIH Data Book 1993. Bethesda, MD, National Institutes of Health, 1993

Pincus HA, Fine T: The "anatomy" of research funding of mental illness and addictive disorders. Arch Gen Psychiatry 49:573–579, 1991

Resources 3–1
Tables of NIH Extramural Funding

The following tables and figure provide current extramural research funding information from the institutes and centers of the NIH.

Table 3–1. NIH and the former ADAMHA appropriations in current and constant 1988 dollars, 1945–1991 (dollars in millions)

Year	NIH Current	NIH Constant	ADAMHA Current	ADAMHA Constant
1945	3	26	—**	—
1950	59	369	—	—
1955	81	439	—	—
1960	381	1,826	—	—
1965	958	4,063	—	—
1970	1,444	4,828	—	—
1975	2,109	5,146	—	—
1976	2,238	4,971	—	—
1977	2,544	5,350	886	1,863
1978	2,842	5,568	939	1,838
1979	3,190	5,772	1,025	1,854
1980	3,429	5,652	1,019	1,676
1981	3,569	5,328	923	1,377
1982	3,642	5,531	758	1,041
1983	4,024	5,207	808	1,045
1984	4,476	5,468	845	1,031
1985	5,145	5,950	919	1,062
1986	5,494	6,087	927	1,026
1987	6,181	6,505	1,317	1,386
1988	6,667	6,667	1,374	1,374
1989	7,144	6,744	1,867	1,775
1990*	7,576	6,749	2,643	2,377
1991*	7,930	6,741	2,844	2,417

Note. Constant 1988 dollars are calculated using the Biomedical Research and Development Price Index (BRDPI). The values for 1988–1990 are estimates based on Office of Management and Budget projections of the implicit price deflator for GNP and its historical relationship with changes in the BRDPI.
*Estimates. **Data not available.
Sources. U.S. Department of Health and Human Services; Public Health Service. *1989 NIH Almanac.* Publication No. 89-5. Bethesda, MD, National Institutes of Health. U.S. Department of Health and Human Services; Public Health Service. 1989. *ADAMHA Data Source Book 1988.* Rockville, MD, Alcohol, Drug Abuse, and Mental Health Administration.

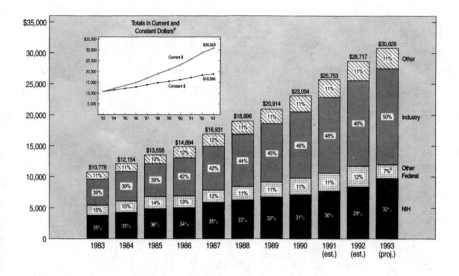

Figure 3–1. National support for health R&D by source, 1983–1993 (dollars in millions).

[a]FY 1983 = 100. Constant dollars based on Biomedical Research and Development Price Index.

[b]Decrease in 1993 reflects transfer of NIAAA, NIDA, and NIMH from ADAMHA into NIH.

Source. Office of Strategic Planning and Evaluation, OSPTT.

Table 3–2. National support for health R&D by source or performer, 1983–1993[a] (millions of dollars)

A. BY SOURCE OF FUNDS

Sector	1983	1984	1985	1986	1987	1988	1989	1990	1991 (est.)	1992 (est.)	1993 (proj.)
Total of A or B	$10,778	$12,154	$13,558	$14,894	$16,931	$18,996	$20,914	$23,094	$25,753	$28,717	$30,828
Government	6,117	6,883	7,669	7,924	9,028	9,725	10,628	11,418	12,429	13,626	14,017
Federal	5,399	6,087	6,791	6,895	7,847	8,431	9,163	9,791	10,602	11,727	11,978
NIH	(3,789)	(4,257)	(4,828)	(5,005)	(5,852)	(6,292)	(6,778)	(7,136)	(7,696)	(8,407)	(9,769)
State & local	718	796	878	1,028	1,182	1,294	1,465	1,628	1,828	1,900	2,040
Industry	4,205	4,765	5,352	6,188	7,104	8,433	9,405	10,717	12,234	13,870	15,562
Private nonprofit	456	506	538	782	799	838	881	959	1,091	1,221	1,248
Foundations	89	111	122	129	161	155	129	155	178	236	211
Voluntary health agencies	206	205	233	260	285	323	354	363	393	420	447
Howard Hughes Medical Institute[b]	54	79	51[c]	247	183	179	197	215	250	273	268
Other	107	112	133	146	170	181	201	226	270	293	322

B. BY PERFORMER

Government	1,813	1,997	2,139	2,155	2,388	2,590	2,576	2,862	2,991	3,382	3,479
Federal[d]	1,577	1,741	1,869	1,848	2,042	2,214	2,162	2,403	2,480	2,837	2,898
State & local	236	256	270	307	346	376	415	460	511	544	581
Industry[e]	3,668	4,216	4,660	5,293	6,003	6,929	7,901	8,877	10,101	11,370	12,620
Private nonprofit	4,665	5,245	5,954	6,471	7,400	8,035	8,977	9,575	10,729	11,760	12,254
Higher education[e]	3,779	4,269	4,839	5,314	6,048	6,573	7,201	7,699	8,684	9,279	9,668
Other[e]	887	976	1,115	1,157	1,352	1,462	1,777	1,877	2,044	2,481	2,586
Foreign	631	697	805	975	1,140	1,443	1,459	1,779	1,932	2,205	2,475

[a] Revised.
[b] These figures report support for the direct conduct of biomedical research. In addition, HHMI's Office of Grants and Special Programs provides support for scientific career development, which is not included here.
[c] Total includes only 8 months of operations due to change in fiscal year.
[d] In addition to in-house research, includes program management and direct operations attributable to health R&D.
[e] Includes federally funded R&D centers.
Source. Office of Strategic Planning and Evaluation, OSPTT.

Table 3–3. Federal obligations for health R&D by source or performer, fiscal years 1983–1992 (millions of dollars)

	1983	1984	1985	1986	1987	1988	1989	1990	1991	1992 (est.)
Total of A or B	$5,399.3	$6,087.1	$6,790.8	$6,895.3	$7,846.5	$8,430.6	$9,163.2	$9,790.6	$10,601.6	$11,726.5
A. BY SOURCE OF FUNDS										
HHS	4,317.0	4,800.3	5,411.4	5,593.6	6,539.5	7,090.3	7,778.1	8,341.2	9,089.5	10,058.6
NIH	3,789.2	4,257.5	4,827.7	5,005.0	5,852.2	6,291.7	6,778.3	7,136.5	7,695.5	8,406.6
Other PHS	484.4	499.0	545.5	556.8	656.9	765.6	948.9	1,152.1	1,324.1	1,575.2
ADAMHA	302.2	316.4	377.6	396.1	475.9	554.8	695.7	891.7	973.5	1,158.9
CDC	78.2	76.4	47.6	52.2	66.2	88.7	117.8	95.6	113.4	146.9
FDA	74.2	72.5	82.1	79.4	84.4	91.0	97.8	99.0	125.0	135.7
HRSA	13.3	16.2	19.7	12.0	9.2	10.0	10.5	10.0	11.0	10.2
OASH/AHCPR	16.6	17.5	18.6	17.1	21.2	21.0	27.2	55.8	101.1	123.5
Other HHS	43.3	43.8	38.2	31.8	30.4	33.0	50.9	52.6	69.9	76.9
Other agencies	1,082.3	1,286.8	1,379.4	1,301.7	1,307.0	1,340.3	1,385.1	1,449.4	1,512.1	1,667.8
Agriculture	147.2	147.9	142.6	77.6	99.3	107.4	114.9	109.8	109.1	119.4
Defense	307.4	414.2	439.9	496.4	407.1	431.0	384.6	429.9	404.2	482.9
Education	29.3	41.0	38.2	44.0	49.0	55.0	57.6	59.3	41.6	48.5
Energy	168.5	182.7	177.5	164.3	177.1	202.0	223.8	272.0	350.6	348.8

Environmental Protection	39.9	43.5	53.3	32.2	49.3	27.5	53.7	32.4	50.1	37.9
International Development (AID)	31.1	17.7	38.5	29.4	33.7	28.9	29.0	16.7	18.7	25.9
Aeronautics and Space	76.0	110.2	116.6	129.9	131.6	131.9	136.2	150.3	160.4	163.6
National Science Foundation	77.0	86.8	89.3	81.4	89.9	86.3	88.1	82.3	79.8	76.2
Veterans	161.4	190.3	226.6	186.2	209.5	215.3	235.3	237.7	217.2	270.4
Other	44.5	52.4	56.9	60.2	60.5	55.1	62.0	59.0	80.4	94.2
B. BY PERFORMER										
Intramural (federal)	**1,574.9**	**1,739.0**	**1,867.3**	**1,845.3**	**2,039.2**	**2,211.2**	**2,158.3**	**2,399.4**	**2,476.8**	**2,833.8**
Extramural (nonfederal)	**3,824.4**	**4,348.0**	**4,923.5**	**5,050.0**	**5,807.3**	**6,219.3**	**7,004.9**	**7,391.2**	**8,124.7**	**8,892.7**
State & local government	60.4	65.6	61.6	63.4	71.6	77.8	82.0	93.6	107.3	116.9
Industry[a]	276.4	361.9	363.5	376.5	429.4	436.9	528.5	601.5	595.9	631.8
Private nonprofit	3,450.8	3,875.9	4,450.4	4,564.2	5,242.9	5,646.1	6,324.5	6,623.0	7,365.1	8,080.6
Higher education[a]	2,760.4	3,124.9	3,587.6	3,685.3	4,226.8	4,564.0	4,975.7	5,216.1	5,857.3	6,182.4
Medical schools	(1,718.9)	(1,906.2)	(2,246.7)	(2,327.5)	(2,573.2)	(2,740.3)	(3,214.6)	(3,290.8)	(3,639.6)	(3,822.6)
Other[a]	690.4	750.9	862.8	878.8	1,016.1	1,082.2	1,348.8	1,406.9	1,507.8	1,898.2
Foreign	36.9	44.7	47.9	46.0	63.4	58.4	69.9	73.1	56.4	63.4

[a]Includes FFRDCs.
Source. Office of Strategic Planning and Evaluation, OSPTT

Table 3–4.   NIH appropriations by NIH component, fiscal years

NIH component	1983	1984	1985	1986	1987[a]	1988
Total	$4,320,255	$4,810,345	$5,520,191	$5,886,170	$6,691,128	$7,243,222
Former ADAMHA components[d]						
Subtotal	296,286	334,204	375,541	391,772	510,468	576,529
NIAAA	43,038	54,827	61,677	66,395	83,357	92,763
NIDA	61,704	71,098	81,130	83,311	139,307	156,252
NIMH	191,544	208,279	232,734	242,066	287,804	327,514
Other NIH components						
Subtotal	4,023,969	4,476,141	5,144,650	5,494,398	6,180,660	6,666,693
NIA	93,996	114,921	144,444	156,352	176,931	194,746
NIAID	279,129	314,117	370,779	383,231	545,523	638,800
NIADDK	413,492	462,578	542,937	568,724	—	—
NIAMS	—	—	—	—	138,713	147,679
NCI	987,642	1,077,303	1,181,949	1,256,147	1,402,837	1,469,327
NICHD	254,324	275,179	313,150	321,581	366,780	396,811
NIDCD	—	—	—	—	—	—
NIDR	79,292	88,163	100,633	103,207	117,945	126,297
NIDDK	—	—	—	—	511,124	534,733
NIEHS	164,867	179,806	194,553	197,379	209,294	215,666
NEI	141,901	154,683	181,586	194,993	216,637	224,947
NIGMS	369,813	415,644	482,168	514,528	570,916	632,676
NHLBI	624,259	703,197	804,456	858,570	930,001	965,536
NINCDS	297,064	335,205	396,683	433,094	490,233	534,692
NINDS	—	—	—	—	—	—
DRR/NCRR	213,917	242,636	303,854	305,553	322,860	368,153
FIC	10,147	11,336	11,578	11,390	11,420	15,651
NCHGR	—	—	—	—	—	—
NCNR/NINR	—	—	—	—	19,000	23,380
NLM	51,943	49,613	55,848	57,759	61,838	67,910
OD	24,683	26,720	38,302	116,990[e]	56,708	61,819
Buildings & facilities	17,500	25,040	21,730	14,900	31,900	47,870

[a]In 1987, NIAMS, NIDDK, and NCNR appropriations were new.
[b]In 1989, NIDCD and NINDS appropriations were new.
[c]In 1990, NCHGR appropriation was new, and DRR was reorganized and renamed NCRR.
[d]In 1993, ADAMHA was reorganized and renamed SAMHSA, and its three research institutes were transferred to NIH. Also, NCNR was made an institute and renamed NINR.
[e]Includes AIDS funds appropriated to OD but transferred out to be awarded and administered. Also includes funds for NCNR, which were administered under OD in 1986.
Source.   Division of Financial Management.

1983–1993 (dollars in thousands)

1989[b]	1990[c]	1991	1992	1993[d]	Percentage change 1983–93	Percentage change 1992–93
$7,885,357	$8,495,328	$9,330,503	$10,065,684	$10,326,603	139.0%	2.6%
733,150	918,976	1,053,764	1,130,866	1,164,076	292.9	2.9
120,051	149,194	158,141	171,481	176,619	310.4	3.0
228,171	329,560	383,656	399,100	403,806	554.4	1.2
384,928	440,222	511,967	560,285	583,651	204.7	4.2
7,152,207	7,576,352	8,276,739	8,934,818	9,162,527	127.7	2.5
222,643	239,455	323,752	383,611	399,924	325.5	4.3
744,152	832,977	906,251	960,914	979,471	250.9	1.9
—	—	—	—	—	—	—
159,897	168,930	193,247	203,913	212,456	—	4.2
1,571,879	1,634,332	1,714,784	1,951,541	1,981,350	100.6	1.5
425,649	442,914	478,956	519,724	527,788	107.5	1.6
91,677	117,583	134,935	149,102	154,814	—	3.8
130,752	135,749	148,918	159,240	161,301	103.4	1.3
559,538	581,477	615,272	662,678	681,342	—	2.8
223,454	229,234	241,028	252,031	251,187	52.4	−0.3
231,230	236,533	253,241	270,300	276,188	94.6	2.2
682,349	681,782	760,010	815,134	832,581	125.1	2.1
1,045,985	1,072,354	1,126,942	1,191,500	1,214,793	94.6	2.0
—	—	—	—	—	—	—
474,943	490,409	541,743	581,847	600,078	—	3.1
358,608	353,734	335,255	314,551	312,468	46.1	−0.7
15,848	15,516	17,519	19,609	19,733	94.5	0.6
—	59,538	87,418	104,878	106,239	—	1.3
29,139	33,513	39,722	44,970	48,119	—	7.0
73,731	81,861	91,408	103,323	103,639	99.5	0.3
72,201	107,419	97,651	142,112	190,325	671.1	33.9
38,532	61,042	168,687	103,840	108,731	521.3	4.7

Table 3–5. PHS grant support of research activities by agency and component, fiscal year 1993 (dollars in thousands)

Agency/component	Total	Traditional research & program projects	Research centers	Other research
Total	$7,769,045	$4,618,875	$912,208	$2,237,961
National Institutes of Health	7,262,315	4,548,143	912,208	1,801,964
National Institute on Aging (NIA)	304,549	183,326	51,542	69,681
National Institute on Alcohol Abuse and Alcoholism (NIAAA)	132,861	87,466	17,342	28,053
National Institute of Allergy and Infectious Diseases (NIAID)	668,566	386,020	7,722	274,824
National Institute of Arthritis and Musculoskeletal and Skin Diseases (NIAMS)	175,666	118,948	23,634	33,084
National Cancer Institute (NCI)	1,201,139	699,252	145,042	356,846
National Institute on Deafness and Other Communication Disorders (NIDCD)	130,336	96,565	17,065	16,706
National Institute of Dental Research (NIDR)	108,759	64,663	18,138	25,958
National Institute of Diabetes and Digestive and Kidney Diseases (NIDDK)	539,292	362,174	47,671	129,447
National Institute on Drug Abuse (NIDA)	296,359	162,735	26,612	107,012
National Institute of Environmental Health Sciences (NIEHS)	136,779	78,054	48,333	10,393
National Eye Institute (NEI)	226,408	165,350	7,639	53,419
National Institute of General Medical Sciences (NIGMS)	738,539	564,014	7,784	166,741

National Institute of Child Health and Human Development (NICHD)	384,119	247,166	50,314	86,640
National Center for Human Genome Research (NCHGR)	95,731	57,463	31,427	6,841
National Heart, Lung, and Blood Institute (NHLBI)	896,181	613,367	96,768	186,046
National Library of Medicine (NLM)	12,033	6,368	4,293	1,373
National Institute of Mental Health (NIMH)	410,152	218,390	65,337	126,425
National Institute for Nursing Research (NINR)	42,847	32,915	1,762	8,170
National Institute of Neurological Disorders and Stroke (NINDS)	465,516	390,810	32,080	42,627
National Center for Research Resources (NCRR)	292,814	13,099	211,705	68,012
Fogarty International Center (FIC)	3,667	—	—	3,667
Health Resources and Services Administration	13,465	1,667	—	11,797
Bureau of Health Professions (BHP)	1,667	1,667	—	—
Bureau of Primary Health Care (BPHC)	2,226	—	—	2,226
Maternal and Child Health Bureau (MCHB)	9,571	—	—	9,571
Centers for Disease Control and Prevention	393,044	6,180	—	386,864
Agency for Toxic Substances and Disease Registry	14,057	—	—	14,057
Office of the Assistant Secretary for Health	1,970	—	—	1,970
Administrative Services Center (ASC)	627	—	—	627
Office of Population Affairs (OPA)	1,343	—	—	1,343
Agency for Health Care Policy and Research	67,223	53,905	—	13,318
Food and Drug Administration	15,170	8,980	—	6,190
Indian Health Service	1,801	—	—	1,801

Table 3–6. PHS grant support of training activities by agency and component, fiscal year 1993 (dollars in thousands)

Agency/component	Total	Training education	Loans & scholarships	Fellowships	General educational support
Total	$803,758	$614,868	$74,872	$74,447	$39,571
National Institutes of Health	397,581	335,079	—	62,501	—
National Institute on Aging (NIA)	11,287	10,443	—	844	—
National Institute on Alcohol Abuse and Alcoholism (NIAAA)	3,348	2,979	—	369	—
National Institute of Allergy and Infectious Diseases (NIAID)	21,884	18,277	—	3,607	—
National Institute of Arthritis and Musculoskeletal and Skin Diseases (NIAMS)	6,437	5,480	—	957	—
National Cancer Institute (NCI)	36,386	32,066	—	4,320	—
National Institute on Deafness and Other Communication Disorders (NIDCD)	4,874	4,038	—	836	—
National Institute of Dental Research (NIDR)	5,704	5,077	—	627	—
National Institute of Diabetes and Digestive and Kidney Diseases (NIDDK)	24,980	20,584	—	4,396	—
National Institute on Drug Abuse (NIDA)	7,054	5,784	—	1,270	—
National Institute of Environmental Health Sciences (NIEHS)	42,110	40,848	—	1,262	—

National Eye Institute (NEI)	7,058	4,394	—	2,664	—
National Institute of General Medical Sciences (NIGMS)	97,691	82,383	—	15,308	—
National Institute of Child Health and Human Development (NICHD)	17,098	13,962	—	3,136	—
National Center for Human Genome Research (NCHGR)	1,928	1,231	—	697	—
National Heart, Lung, and Blood Institute (NHLBI)	43,406	37,224	—	6,181	—
National Library of Medicine (NLM)	4,238	4,023	—	215	—
National Institute of Mental Health (NIMH)	28,646	24,650	—	3,996	—
National Institute for Nursing Research (NINR)	4,017	2,392	—	1,625	—
National Institute of Neurological Disorders and Stroke (NINDS)	13,015	8,761	—	4,254	—
National Center for Research Resources (NCRR)	2,659	2,569	—	90	—
Fogarty International Center (FIC)	13,761	7,915	—	5,846	—
Health Resources and Services Administration	340,516	226,863	74,872	—	38,780
Bureau of Health Professions (BHP)	271,639	191,660	41,199	—	38,780
Bureau of Primary Health Care (BPHC)	33,673	—	33,673	—	—
Maternal and Child Health Bureau (MCHB)	35,203	35,203	—	—	—
Indian Health Service	17,101	5,641	—	11,460	—
Centers for Disease Control and Prevention	21,746	21,746	—	—	—

(continued)

Table 3–6. PHS grant support of training activities by agency and component, fiscal year 1993 (dollars in thousands) (*continued*)

Agency/component	Total	Training education	Loans & scholarships	Fellowships	General educational support
Office of the Assistant Secretary for Health	8,216	7,425	—	—	791
Office of Minority Health (OMH)	791	—	—	—	791
Office of Population Affairs (OPA)	6,082	6,082	—	—	—
Office of Disease Prevention and Health Promotion (ODPHP)	1,343	1,343	—	—	—
Agency for Health Care Policy and Research	3,616	3,131	—	486	—
Food and Drug Administration	1,900	1,900	—	—	—
Substance Abuse and Mental Health Services Administration	13,082	13,082	—	—	—
Center for Mental Health Services (CMHS)	5,557	5,557	—	—	—
Center for Substance Abuse Prevention (CSAP)	2,086	2,086	—	—	—
Center for Substance Abuse Treatment (CSAT)	5,418	5,418	—	—	—

Resources 3–2
Profiles of Federal Agency Funding Sources

◆ Section 1: How to Use the Federal Profiles: Format

This resource section provides the profiles of the federal institutions associated with psychiatric research funding. These profiles are organized by federal department (e.g., Department of Health and Human Services [HHS]) or independent agency (e.g., National Science Foundation [NSF]), and, in general, by significance of funding that is provided for psychiatric research and research training. The first entries, for example, are within the HHS and, within the HHS, the National Institutes of Health (NIH), which is the Public Health Service (PHS) agency with the greatest concentration of research funding. Within the NIH, the entries start with the National Institute of Mental Health (NIMH), the National Institute on Drug Abuse (NIDA), and the National Institute on Alcohol Abuse and Alcoholism (NIAAA), which provide the greatest extramural funding for psychiatric research.

Within the basic format of the federal institutional profile is the title of the federal institution and a description of its mission and its specific interests in psychiatric research-related funding areas. In most cases where a department and its psychiatric research funding are specifically sponsored by specific agencies, divisions, directorates, or some other institutional subset, these groupings are listed and described in further detail under the name "First-level division." In some cases, particularly with NIDA, the NIMH, and the NIAAA, delineation of the next tier within the organizational structure is given when the branch levels are listed and described. These groupings are entitled "Second-level division." Note that although we have made every effort to ensure that the information contained in these profiles is the most current, continuous changes in personnel, program emphasis, location, and agency structure are a standard occurrence within the federal government.

The following categories and definitions are used in the profiles:

Title.   Each profile begins with the name of the federal agency and its recognized acronym.

Contacts.   In most cases, the name of the federal institution's director and phone number for the office of the director are provided. If available, names and phone numbers of the assistant director and contacts at the extramural and public affairs offices may also be provided. All contacts who are acting are noted. Also note that, although we have attempted to maintain accurate, current information, turnover in these positions is common; therefore the specific individuals listed may no longer be in those positions. This caveat also applies to contacts in first- and second-level listings, if present.

Address.   This category provides the street address, building, city, state, and zip code.

Description.   The description of the institution, its mission, organizational structure, and areas of psychiatric research interest are provided. If an institution is further broken down to agency and division levels, this information will be included within this section. Although we have attempted to maintain accurate current information, agency reorganization is common in the federal government.
     If applicable, the following fields appear next:

First-level division.   If the federal institution has a subdivision or agency with a specific directive within its organization, it is listed in this field.

First-level division description.   The subdivision description.

Head.   The subdivision's director and phone number.

Second-level division.   If the subdivision or agency has a further breakdown of divisions or branches with specific missions of psychiatric research interest, they are listed in this field.

Second-level division description.   The second subdivision's description.

Head.   The second subdivision's director and phone number.

Sample program announcements.   If information on program announcements published by the institution is available, the title of the announcement is in this category. All announcements listed were published after September 1991.

◆ Section 2: Listing of Federal Institutional Profiles

Department of Health and Human Services (HHS)
  Public Health Service (PHS):
    National Institutes of Health (NIH)
      National Institute of Mental Health (NIMH)
      National Institute on Drug Abuse (NIDA)
      National Institute of Alcohol Abuse and Alcoholism (NIAAA)
      National Institute on Aging (NIA)
      National Institute of Child Health and Human Development (NICHD)
      National Institute of Neurological Disorders and Stroke (NINDS)
      National Cancer Institute (NCI)
      National Heart, Lung, and Blood Institute (NHLBI)
      National Institute on Deafness and Other Communication Disorders (NIDCD)
      National Institute for Nursing Research (NINR)
      National Institute of Allergy and Infectious Diseases (NIAID)
      National Institute of Arthritis and Musculoskeletal and Skin Diseases (NIAMS)
      National Institute of Dental Research (NIDR)
      National Institute of Diabetes and Digestive and Kidney Diseases (NIDDK)
      National Institute of Environmental Health Sciences (NIEHS)
      National Eye Institute (NEI)
      National Institute of General Medical Sciences (NIGMS)
      National Library of Medicine (NLM)
      National Center for Human Genome Research (NCHGR)
      National Center for Research Resources (NCRR)
      Fogarty International Center (FIC) for the Advanced Study in the Health Sciences
    Substance Abuse and Mental Health Services Administration (SAMHSA)
      Center for Mental Health Services (CMHS)
      Center for Substance Abuse Prevention (CSAP)
      Center for Substance Abuse Treatment (CSAT)

Other Public Health Service Programs:
    Agency for Health Care Policy and Research (AHCPR)
    Centers for Disease Control and Prevention (CDC)
    Food and Drug Administration (FDA)
    Health Resources and Services Administration (HRSA)
Other Health and Human Services Programs:
    Administration for Children and Families (ACF)
    Administration on Aging (AOA)
    Health Care Financing Administration (HCFA)
    Social Security Administration (SSA)

Department of Veterans Affairs (VA)
Medical Research Service (MRS)
Health Services Research and Development Service (HSR&D)
Rehabilitation Research and Development Service (Rehab R&D)

Department of Education (ED)
National Institute on Disability and Rehabilitation Research (NIDRR)

National Science Foundation (NSF)
Directorate for Social, Behavioral, and Economic Sciences (SBE)
Directorate of Biological Sciences (BIO)

Department of Justice (DOJ)
Office for Victims of Crime
National Institute of Justice
Office of Juvenile Justice and Delinquency Prevention

Department of Defense (DOD) and Related Organizations
Air Force Office of Scientific Research (AFOSR)
Army Research Office (ARO)
    Army Research Institute for the Behavioral and Social Sciences (ARI)
Office of Naval Research (ONR)
    Life Sciences Programs Directorate
    Navy Personnel Research and Development Center
    Naval Medical Research and Development Command
North Atlantic Treaty Organization (NATO)

National Aeronautics and Space Administration (NASA)
Department of Agriculture (AG)

Department of Energy (DOE)
Department of Transportation (DOT)

◆ Section 3: Federal Profiles
DEPARTMENT OF HEALTH AND HUMAN SERVICES (HHS)

Public Health Service (PHS)

◆ National Institutes of Health (NIH)
Point of contact:
Harold Varmus, M.D., Director
(301) 496-2433
Ruth Kirchstein, M.D., Deputy Director
(301) 496-7322
Office of Communication
(301) 496-4461
Address:
Building 1
31 Center Drive
Bethesda, MD 20892

Description. The National Institutes of Health is the research arm of the Public Health Service and the Department of Health and Human Services. It serves as primary liaison on health-related research and is composed of 17 institutes with specific health missions, four centers, and main administrative divisions. Although the Office of the Director and supporting offices, which are part of the Office of the Director, generally do not directly fund grant proposals, they help coordinate research in their areas and are explicit sources of information for investigators. Offices within the NIH Office of the Director of particular interest to psychiatric researchers include AIDS Research, Alternative Medicine, Extramural Activities, Protection of Research Risks, Research on Women's Health, and Research and Minority Health. The newly established Office of Behavioral and Social Sciences Research will also be a valuable resource.

First-level division.   Office of AIDS Research
Description.   This office formulates scientific policy and recommends allocation of resources for AIDS research.
Head.   Jack Whitescarver, Ph.D., (301) 496-0357

First-level division.   Office of Alternative Medicine
Description.   Established in 1992, this office facilitates research on the evaluation of various alternative treatment modalities by the institutes within the NIH. It also provides technical assistance to potential grantees who have had little experience with the NIH grants process. It sponsors a fellowship program in complementary medicine. 1994 budget increased to $3.5 million.
Head.   Allen Trachtenberg, M.D. (Acting), (301) 402-2467

First-level division.   Office of Behavioral and Social Sciences Research
Description.   This office, established by law in 1993, is intended to coordinate activities across the NIH on issues related to health and behavior. It also coordinates research in the behavioral and social sciences conducted or supported by the NIH, identifies areas deserving expansion, and develops new research projects.
Head.   Louis Sibal, Ph.D. (Acting), (301) 402-1058

First-level division.   Office of Extramural Activities
Description.   This office is responsible for the planning, review, execution, and direction of the NIH extramural research and research training programs. It provides guidance to the NIH components on extramural research policies and develops new and revised research training programs as needed.
Head.   Wendy Baldwin, Ph.D., (301) 496-1096

First-level division.   Office of Protection From Research Risks
Description.   This office coordinates appropriate regulations and policies within HHS and assists in establishing criteria for both HHS-conducted and -supported research involving human subjects or using animals.
Head.   Gary Ellis, Ph.D., (301) 496-7005

First-level division.   Office of Research on Women's Health
Description.   Established in 1990, this office is responsible for developing an integrated strategy for increasing research into diseases, disorders, and conditions that are unique to, prevalent among, or

more serious in women or for which there are different risk factors or interventions. It also ensures women's representation in biomedical and biobehavioral research studies and aims to increase the number of women in biomedical research careers.

Head.   Vivian Pinn, M.D., (301) 402-1770

First-level division.   Office of Research on Minority Health
Description.   In order to improve the health of minority Americans, this office coordinates the development of NIH policies, goals, and objectives related to minority research and research training programs. It seeks to increase the number of minorities in biomedical research and assures that appropriate minority representation exists in clinical research programs and studies.

Head.   John Ruffin, Ph.D., (301) 402-1366

NIH selected program announcements:
   Research Supplements for Underrepresented Minorities
   Minority Health Initiative
   Women's Health Initiative
   Postdoctoral Training in Alternative Medicine

◆ **National Institute of Mental Health (NIMH)**
Point of contact:
   Rex Cowdry III, M.D., Acting Director
   (301) 443-3673
   Hugh Stamper, Ph.D., Extramural Activities
   (301) 443-3367
   Marsha Corbett, Scientific Information
   (301) 443-3600
Address:
   Parklawn Building
   5600 Fishers Lane
   Rockville, MD 20857

Description.   The NIMH provides the national focus for the federal effort to increase knowledge through research and research training so as to advance effective strategies for dealing with mental illness and related issues. The NIMH accomplishes this mission by developing and assessing innovative approaches to diagnosis, treatment, and prevention of mental illnesses and by exchanging information nationally and internationally.

The NIMH supports research and research training on the biological, neuroscientific, psychological, behavioral, epidemiological, and social science aspects of mental health and illness, as well as the development, improvement, management, and financing of mental health services and service systems. Research studies may take the form of theoretical, laboratory, epidemiologic, clinical, methodological and field research on well and mentally ill human subjects and populations of all ages and on animals where appropriate.

The NIMH consists of five divisions and nine offices. The nine offices are the Office of Prevention, Rural Mental Health Research, Special Populations, AIDS, Legislative Analysis and Coordination, Scientific Information, Resource Management, EEO, and Science Policy and Program Planning. The divisions within the NIMH are the Divisions of Intramural Research Programs, Extramural Activities, Neuroscience and Behavioral Science, Clinical and Treatment Research, and Epidemiology and Services Research, of which the latter three fund extramural research grants and are profiled below.

First-level division.   Division of Clinical and Treatment Research
Description.   This division conducts and supports research, research training, and development in psychopathology, classification, assessment, etiology, genetics, clinical course, outcome, and treatment of mental disorders, with emphasis on schizophrenic disorders, affective and anxiety disorders, and mental disorders of children/adolescents, the elderly, minorities, and other special populations. It also coordinates NIMH's medications development program areas. This division is composed of five branches: Child and Adolescent Disorders Research; Clinical Treatment Research; Mental Disorders of the Aging Research; Mood, Anxiety, and Personality Disorders Research; Schizophrenia Research; and Research Projects and Publications, each of which is described below.
Head.   Jane Steinberg, Ph.D. (Acting), (301) 443-3683

Second-level division.   Mood, Anxiety, and Personality Disorders Research Branch
Description.   This branch supports research and research training in the classification, assessment, etiology, genetics, and clinical course of mood, anxiety, and personality disorders, including eating disorders and suicidal behavior in adults.
Head.   Mary Blehar, Ph.D. (Acting), (301) 443-1636

Second-level division.   Clinical Treatment Research Branch
Description.   This branch plans, supports, and conducts programs of research, research training, and therapeutic medications and development for the pharmacologic, biological, and psychosocial treatment and rehabilitation of mental disorders in adults, specifically schizophrenia and mood, anxiety, sleep, sexual, and personality disorders.
Head.   Robert Prien, Ph.D., (301) 443-4527

Second-level division.   Schizophrenia Research Branch
Description.   This branch plans, supports, and conducts research, research training, and development in the classification, assessment, etiology, genetics, clinical course, outcome, biological markers, electrophysiology, neuroimaging, neurodevelopment, psychosocial factors, and pathophysiology of schizophrenic and related disorders.
Head.   Kate Berg, Ph.D. (Acting), (301) 443-4707

Second-level division.   Child and Adolescent Disorders Research Branch
Description.   This branch conducts research and research training programs in the classification, assessment, etiology, genetics, clinical course, outcome, and the pharmacologic, somatic, and psychosocial treatment and rehabilitation of disorders affecting children and adolescents. Areas of research concern include autism, attention deficit disorder, eating disorders, depression, suicide, learning disorders, sleep, and learning disorders.
Head.   Peter Jensen, M.D., (301) 443-5944

Second-level division.   Mental Disorders of the Aging Research Branch
Description.   The focus of this branch is the support of research and research training in the classification, assessment, etiology, genetics, clinical course, outcome, and the pharmacologic, somatic, and psychosocial treatment/rehabilitation of dementia, delirium, and other mental disorders affecting the elderly, with particular emphasis on Alzheimer's disease.
Head.   Barry Lebowitz, Ph.D., (301) 443-1185

Second-level division.   Research Projects and Publications Branch
Description.   This branch provides technical and administrative support by producing, publishing, or distributing scientific publications

for the lay public and scientific community.
Head.   Joanne Severe, M.S., (301) 443-9772

First-level division.   Division of Epidemiology and Services Research
Description.   This division supports research and research training in prevention, services research, epidemiology, psychopathology, assessment, classification, violence and traumatic stress, and health and behavior. This division is composed of five branches, which are described below: Basic Prevention and Behavioral Medicine Research, Epidemiology and Psychopathology Research, Prevention Research, Services Research, and Violence and Traumatic Stress Research.
Head.   Darrel Regier, M.D., M.P.H., (301) 443-3648

Second-level division.   Violence and Traumatic Stress Research Branch
Description.   This branch supports research and research training on antisocial behavior, violent behavior, rape, sexual assaults, and interactions between mental health and the law. Studies include the development, maintenance, and cessation of antisocial and violent behaviors among children, adolescents, adults, and the mentally ill; rape and other sexual assaults, its effect on mental health, and the social service/criminal justice system; treatment models for dealing with violence; and interaction with the law.
Head.   Susan Solomon, Ph.D., (301) 443-3728

Second-level division.   Prevention Research Branch
Description.   This branch concentrates on research and research training in the creation and assessment of preventive interventions for mental disorders, with particular emphasis on psychosocial interventions, and on promoting mental health in populations at risk.
Head.   Eve Moscicki, Sc.D., (301) 443-4283

Second-level division.   Basic Prevention and Behavioral Medicine Research Branch
Description.   This branch supports research and research training related to basic prevention, behavioral medicine, and behavioral change, with an emphasis on populations at risk. The goal of this branch is to accomplish better understanding of the relationships among behavior, general medicine, and emotional dysfunction.
Head.   Fred Altman, Ph.D. (Acting), (301) 443-4337

Second-level division. Epidemiology and Psychopathology Research Branch

Description. This branch stresses the research programs on epidemiology of mental disorders, including risk factors and population genetics; classification, assessment, etiology, genetics, clinical course, outcome, and treatment of general psychopathology; and other mental disorders.

Head. Charles Kaelber, M.D., (301) 443-3774

Second-level division. Services Research Branch

Description. This branch supports research and research training programs on service delivery/health economics at the clinical and program levels for the mental health field and interventions to improve the quality of care in services delivery, and encourages development of more sophisticated methods for conducting services research.

Head. Thomas Lalley, (301) 443-3364

First-level division. Division of Neuroscience and Behavioral Science Research

Description. This division provides research and research training in the neurosciences, behavioral sciences, and behavior and health. Program areas include molecular biology; neurobiology; psychopharmacology; cognitive processes, personality, emotion, and psychosocial processes; behavioral development; biological, psychological, and social aspects of stress; behavioral medicine; psychoimmunology; and AIDS. This division consists of three branches, which are described below: Behavioral, Cognitive, and Social Processes Research; Behavioral and Integrative Neuroscience Research; and Molecular and Cellular Neuroscience Research.

Head. Stephen Koslow, Ph.D., (301) 443-3563

Second-level division. Molecular and Cellular Neuroscience Research Branch

Description. This branch supports research and research training in developmental neurosciences, neurogenetics, neuroimmunology/ neurovirology, and neurotransmission/neuroregulations.

Head. Steven Zalcman, M.D., (301) 443-3948

Second-level division. Behavioral, Cognitive, and Social Processes Research Branch

Description. This branch focuses its research and research training

on interpersonal and family processes, personality and emotions, and sociocultural and environmental processes. Research emphasizes genetic and experiential factors in explaining individual differences in mental health, developmental changes, lifetime continuities, and interactions among psychological, social, and biological processes.
Head.   Mary Ellen Oliveri, Ph.D., (301) 443-3942

Second-level division.   Behavioral and Integrative Neuroscience Research Branch
Description.   This branch conducts research and research training in cognitive neurosciences and basic behavioral processes, with emphasis on learning, memory, and cognition; behavioral neurosciences, with focus on fundamental, noncognitive behaviors; and theoretical neurosciences, which stresses mathematical and computational needs. It also researches integrated neuronal functions in the understanding of abnormal and normal brain function and behavior and investigations on neural systems. Fostering integration between basic and clinical research is of importance.
Head.   Richard Nakamura, Ph.D., (301) 443-1576

NIMH selected program announcements:
   Bipolar Disorder: Clinical, Biological, and Treatment Research
   Behavioral and Biomedical Studies on Obesity
   Basic Brain, Behavioral, and Clinical Studies on Anorexia
      Nervosa and Bulimia
   Rapid Assessment Post–Impact of Disaster (RAPID)
   Research on Perpetrators of Violence
   Research on Victims of Traumatic Stress
   Studies of Suicide and Suicidal Behavior
   HIV-1 Infection and the Nervous System
   Comparative Approaches to Brain and Behavior
   Behavioral and Neural Approaches to Cognition in Mental
      Health and Mental Disorders
   Neural, Endocrine, Immune, and Viral Interactions, Behavior,
      and Mental Health
   Behavior Change and Prevention Strategies Reducing
      Transmission of HIV-1
   Mental Health Promotion and Prevention Research
   Prevention Intervention Research Centers
   Services Research for Persons With Mental Disorders That
      Co-occur With Alcohol and/or Drug Abuse Disorders

Epidemiologic/Services Research on Mental Disorders That
   Co-occur With Drug and/or Alcohol Disorders Among
   American Indians, Alaska Natives, and Hawaiians
Exploratory Grants for Psychosocial Treatment Research
Psychosocial and Pharmacologic Treatments Research
General and Specialized Mental Health Clinical Research Centers
Children With HIV Infection and AIDS
Child and Adolescent Development Research Centers
National Plan on Child and Adolescent Mental Disorder
Child and Adolescent Disorders Centers for Research on Mental
   Health Services for Children and Adolescents
Research on Emergency Mental Health Services for Children
   and Adolescents
Research on Hospitalization of Adolescents for Mental
   Disorders Depression in Late Life
Mental Disorder and Physical Illness in Later Life
Special Issues in Women's Mental Health Over the Life Cycle
Minority Mental Health Research Centers
American Indian, Alaska Native, and Native Hawaiian Mental
   Health Research
Mental Health Research on Homeless Persons
Research on Mental Disorders in Rural Populations
Research on Disabilities and Rehabilitation Services for Persons
   With Severe Mental Disorders
Caring for People With Severe Mental Disorders: A National Plan
Research on Integrating Mental Health and Related Services for
   Persons With Severe Mental Disorders
Research on Mental Health Care for People With Severe Mental
   Disorders
Research on Severely Mentally Ill Persons at Risk for
   HIV Infections
Centers for Research on Services for People With Severe Mental
   Disorders
Persons With Mental Retardation and Mental Illness
Psychopathology and Mental Retardation
Research on Law and Mental Health
Public-Academic Liaison for Research
Research on Mental Health Economics
Research on Managed Mental Health Care
Research on Mental Health Services in General Health Care
   Sector

Research on Reimbursement Issues in Mental Health Services
   Delivery
Research Infrastucture Support
Social Work Research Development Centers
Mental Health Small Business Innovation Research (SBIR)
National Research Service Awards for Institutional Grants
Behavioral Science Track Award for Rapid Transition

◆ National Institute on Drug Abuse (NIDA)

Point of contact:
   Alan Leshner, Ph.D., Director
   (301) 443-6480
   Richard Millstein, Deputy Director
   (301) 443-6480
   Eleanor Friedenberg, Ph.D., Extramural Program
   (301) 443-2755
   Susan David, Public Information
   (301) 443-6245
Address:
   Parklawn Building
   5600 Fishers Lane
   Rockville, MD 20857

Description. NIDA is the lead federal agency for the conduct of basic, clinical, and epidemiological research to improve the understanding, treatment, and prevention of drug abuse and addiction and the health consequences of these behaviors. It supports research ranging from molecular biology to large-scale population studies, including research and research training on 1) the underlying neurobiological, biomedical, psychological, and social mechanisms of drug abuse and addiction; 2) specific biomedical and behavioral effects of abused substances; 3) neuroscientific research on the effects of abused drugs on the structure and function of the central nervous system; 4) effective prevention and treatment approaches, including research designed to develop new treatment medications; 5) the causes and consequences of drug abuse, including morbidity and mortality in selected populations such as rural, ethnic minorities, and youth; 6) the relationship of drug use to other problem behaviors including unemployment and psychopathology; 7) factors associated with vulnerability/invulnerability to drug abuse; 8) the role of drug use during pregnancy and on human development; 9) the role of drug abuse as a factor in the spread of infectious diseases like AIDS and tuberculosis; and 10) the effectiveness of drug abuse treatment programs and modalities on the organization, financing, and management of treatment services.

The Office of the Director manages the entire range of NIDA's activities, including research programs, administrative and financial activity, the Office on AIDS, the Women's Health Issues Group, and the Office on Special Populations. NIDA is divided into five divisions and four offices. The four offices are the Offices of Science Policy and Communications, Planning and Resource Management, Extramural Program Review, and AIDS. The five divisions are the Divisions of Intramural Research, Basic Research, Clinical and Services Research, Epidemiology and Prevention Research, and Medications Development. The latter four divisions and their branch components are described in further detail.

First-level division.   Medications Development Division
Description.   This division is responsible for conducting studies to develop and obtain FDA marketing approval for new medications for the treatment of drug addiction. It administers a national program of basic and clinical pharmaceutical research designed to develop pharmacological treatment for addiction treatment. It also coordinates legal and regulatory issues for NIDA concerning medications development.
Head.   Charles Grudzinskas, Ph.D., (301) 443-6173

Second-level division.   Pharmacology and Toxicology Branch
Description.   This branch coordinates the extramural studies program in evaluating the efficacy of potential medications in preclinical pharmacological models. It determines the safety of potential medications and interactive effects, offers recommendations for further testing, stores these specific data, and works with the FDA and the pharmaceutical industry as a liaison on preclinical models of drug abuse issues.
Head.   Frank Vocci, Ph.D. (Acting), (301) 443-6173

Second-level division.   Chemistry and Pharmaceutics Branch
Description.   This branch oversees a national research development program in synthetic and medicinal chemistry to discover new chemicals of therapeutic value, pharmacokinetics and drug metabolism research, and bulk chemical preparation and dosage form. This

branch also manages a data base on compound development, screening projects on pharmacological research, distribution of controlled substances, and consultation services/technical support for urine testing for division clinical trials.
Head. Richard Hawks, Ph.D., (301) 443-5280

Second-level division. Clinical Trials Branch
Description. The Clinical Trials Branch plans, designs, and implements programs of extramural clinical studies and performs administrative functions for clinical projects relating to medications development. Besides providing consultation and research training to clinicians, this branch also operates as liaison to the NIMH and the NIAAA on issues of medications development, patient recruitment, and site selection.
Head. Peter Bridge, M.D., (301) 443-3318

Second-level division. Regulatory Affairs Branch
Description. The Regulatory Affairs Branch provides regulatory and legal advice to NIDA medication development activities. It coordinates technology transfer and development and maintains close legal contact with the FDA and the NIH.
Head. Betty Tai, Ph.D. (Acting), (301) 443-1428

First-level division. Division of Clinical and Services Research
Description. The Division of Clinical and Services Research supports a broad extramural program of applied, services, and outcome research and research training focusing on drug abuse treatment. It supports studies designed to understand drug-abusing behavior, the human conditions, and origin; the efficacy of new/existing prevention; evaluating methodology for drug abuse treatment and retention; medical maintenance; intervention treatments; and alternative organizational and financing issues.
Head. Robert Battjes, D.S.W. (Acting), (301) 443-6697

Second-level division. Clinical Medicine Branch
Description. This branch administers an interdisciplinary national program of research focusing on clinical and medical aspects of infectious diseases that occur among drug abusers. Areas of support include modes of transmission, natural history, and risk factors related to infectious diseases; identification of health conditions, including psychiatric, associated with drug use; pathophysiology,

measurement, and nosology/diagnosis; and the effects of prenatal exposure to drugs.
Head. Sander Genser, M.D., M.P.H. (Acting), (301) 443-1801

Second-level division. Treatment Research Branch
Description. This branch plans, develops, and administers research on therapies for drug abuse and addiction, including behavioral therapies, studies on approved pharmacotherapies and its integration with behavioral therapies, diagnosis and treatment of drug abuse and comorbid mental disorders, therapeutic outcome predictors, and studies on the impact of therapies on reducing HIV/AIDS high-risk drug use and sexual behaviors.
Head. Jack D. Blaine, M.D., (301) 443-4060

Second-level division. Services Research Branch
Description. This branch focuses on the effectiveness of drug treatment programs and modalities and on the organization, financing, and management of services. Areas of research include the effectiveness of existing treatments, effectiveness of services for populations at risk or infected with HIV, treatment careers, and evaluation methods for drug treatment.
Head. Frank Tims, Ph.D., (301) 443-4060

Second-level division. Etiology and Clinical Neurobiology Branch
Description. This branch focuses on research associated with etiology and clinical neurobiology, including studies in humans of neurobiological and behavioral correlates of etiology of drug abuse. Areas of neurobiological research include the diagnosis of drug abuse in various stages of the disorder, HIV in drug abusers, and the effects of treatment.
Head. Joseph Frascella, Ph.D. (Acting), (301) 443-4877

First-level division. Division of Epidemiology and Prevention Research
Description. The Division of Epidemiology and Prevention Research supports field studies, population-based research, and surveys on the nature and extent of drug abuse, its consequences, and emerging trends. This division also supports broad-based research and research training in epidemiology, prevention, early intervention, and evaluation and conducts ongoing surveys. It cooperates with other government agencies on the federal and local levels and private

organizations to share information and technical assistance.
Head.   Zili Sloboda, Sc.D., (301) 443-6504

Second-level division.   Community Research Branch
Description.   This branch provides leadership on community-based studies of interventions (treatment and prevention) for drug abuse and related problems (AIDS) and evaluates the efficacy of these intervention programs. Other work of this branch includes working with researchers and organizations to improve community research efforts. Support for conferences, grants, and scientific/technical reports is also given.
Head.   Richard Needle, Ph.D., (301) 443-6702

Second-level division.   Epidemiology Research Branch
Description.   The Epidemiology Research Branch's emphasis is a national extramural program for epidemiologic research on drug abuse. (History, incidence, prevalence, etiology, economic factors, crime, longitudinal studies, women, statistical modeling, and methodology are areas of this research.) Support is given for research and research training, conferences, technical reports, and advisory/consultative services.
Head.   Arthur Hughes, (301) 443-6637

Second-level division.   Prevention Research Branch
Description.   This branch administers a national program of prevention and early intervention research and research training in drug abuse, focusing on drug use practices and problems; motivations/perceptions in drug users; psychosocial functioning, institutional responses; psychological and economic correlates of drug abuse; group behaviors' effects on drug use; effective prevention models; and impact of legal changes on drug use.
Head.   William Bukoski, Ph.D., (301) 443-1514

First-level division.   Division of Basic Research
Description.   The Division of Basic Research administers extramural programs in biomedical and behavioral research and research training that develop knowledge on the mechanisms and sites of action underlying drug abuse. It supports development of methodologies on testing new compounds; studies neurological, behavioral, and biochemical effects of new pharmacological agents; develops research into quota levels of new substances; and manages the distribution of

controlled substances, research drugs, and chemicals.
Head. James Dingell, Ph.D., (301) 443-1887

Second-level division. Behavioral Neurobiology Research Branch
Description. This branch supports research and research training focused on the effects of acute and chronic administration of abused drugs on the structure and functions of the central nervous system; the neurobiology of pain; the neurobiology of drugs' reinforcing properties; and studies of the interaction between brain environment and abused drugs.
Head. Roger W. Brown, Ph.D., (301) 443-6975

Second-level division. Basic Neurobiology and Biological Systems Research Branch
Description. This branch supports research and research training on tolerance, dependence, and metabolism of drug taking; the chemical/toxic effects of developing drugs for treating addiction; effects of drugs on pregnancy, offspring, and genetics; short- and long-term drug abuse effects; and medical consideration and testing in drug scheduling.
Head. Vacant, (301) 443-6300

Second-level division. Behavioral Sciences Research Branch
Description. Developing and implementing a program to evaluate new and existing compounds targeted for their potential therapeutic use, this branch administers an interdisciplinary national program of research and research training on the behavioral, physiological, and cognitive factors contributing to the development, maintenance, and elimination of drug abuse.
Head. Jaylan Turkkan, Ph.D., (301) 443-1263

NIDA selected program announcements:
    Basic, Applied, and Clinical Research on Drug Abuse Issues
    Studies on the Medical and Health Consequences of Drug Abuse
    Psychotherapy, Behavioral Therapy, and Psychosocial
        Intervention on Drug Abuse
    Development of Theoretically Based Psychosocial Therapies for
        Drug Dependence
    Drug Abuse Health Services Research
    Strategies to Reduce HIV Sexual Risk Practices in Drug Users
    HIV-Related Therapeutics on Drug Users
    Research on Needle Hygiene and Needle Exchange Program

Science Education Drug Abuse Partnership Award

Research on the Abuse of Anabolic Steroids

Research on Hair Testing for Drug Abuse

Research on Community-Based Initiatives to Reduce Drug-Taking Behaviors

Research on the Prevalence and Impact of Drug Use in the Workplace

Development of Interventions for Drug Abusers in the Criminal Justice System

Novel Drug Delivery Systems for Treatment of Drug Abuse

Drug Abuse Treatment for Women and Their Children

Entry, Retention, and Compliance in Drug Treatment

Drug Abuse Prevention Research Centers

Comprehensive Prevention Research in Drug Abuse

Neuroscience Research on Drug Addiction

Inhalant Abuse Research

Drug Abuse Aspects of AIDS

Spread and Prevention of Tuberculosis Among Drug Users

Survey Research on Drug Use and Associated Behaviors

Biomedical Factors in Drug Abuse Etiology and Consequences

Drug Abuse in Ethnic and Racial Minority Groups and Underserved Populations

Clinical Research on Human Development and Drug Abuse

Molecular Approaches to Drug Abuse Research

Drug Abuse Treatment Agents

Development of Immunological and Molecular Biological Approaches to Effect Reduction of Cocaine Use

Etiology, Consequences, and Behavioral Pharmacology of Female Drug Abuse

◆ National Institute on Alcohol Abuse and Alcoholism (NIAAA)

Point of contact:

Enoch Gordis, M.D., Director
(301) 443-3885
Loran D. Archer, Deputy Director
(301) 443-3851
Kenneth Warren, Ph.D., Scientific Affairs
(301) 443-4703
Diane Miller, Scientific Communications
(301) 443-3860

Address:
  Willco Building
  6000 Executive Boulevard
  Rockville, MD 20892

Description. The National Institute on Alcohol Abuse and Alcohol-ism is the lead federal agency for research on the causes, conse-quences, treatment, and prevention of alcohol-related problems. It conducts and supports basic and applied research on the multiple determinants and processes of alcoholism and other alcohol-related health problems. The long-range goals are to develop new knowledge that will facilitate the achievement of two broad objectives of reduc-ing both the incidence and prevalence of alcohol abuse and alcohol-ism and the morbidity and mortality associated with alcohol abuse and alcoholism.

The NIAAA consists of four divisions: Intramural Clinical and Biological Research, Basic Research, Biometry and Epidemiology, and Clinical and Prevention Research. The latter three divisions, along with their branch components, are described in further detail below.

First-level division. Division of Basic Research
Description. This division supports studies on the etiologic mecha-nisms associated with alcohol-related disorders, with the long-range goal of identifying specific genes responsible for alcoholic vulner-ability. Genetics and neurobiology, behavioral, environmental, and sociocultural factors relative to alcoholism and its etiology are of importance.
Head. William Lands, Ph.D., (301) 443-2530

Second-level division. Biomedical Research Branch
Description. Biomedical research funded through this branch in-cludes the genetics and molecular biology of alcohol metabolism, al-cohol and pregnancy, immunology and alcoholism with certain emphasis on AIDS transmission, and other alcohol-related medical disorders.
Head. Samir Zakhari, Ph.D., (301) 443-4223

Second-level division. Neurosciences and Behavioral Research Branch
Description. Genetics and molecular biology of neural and behav-ioral responses to alcohol, a wide range of neuroscience issues, and a

wide range of behavioral issues including craving, tolerance, dependence, withdrawal, stress and/or aggression with alcohol consumption constitute major emphases of this branch.
Head. Walter A. Hunt, Ph.D., (301) 443-4223

First-level division. Division of Biometry and Epidemiology
Description. The Division of Biometry and Epidemiology, which primarily supports intramural research, funds broad population studies aimed at understanding the etiology of alcohol abuse. It also develops, analyzes, and maintains national alcohol-related data sets for intramural use and public use.
Head. Thomas C. Harford, Ph.D., (301) 443-3306

Second-level division. Epidemiology Branch
Description. This branch conducts and supports epidemiological studies on occurrence, etiology, natural history, and consequences of alcohol abuse. It analyzes alcohol-related data, collaborates with other scientific organizations, and develops mathematical theory and statistical methodology.
Head. Mary Dufour, M.D., M.P.H., (301) 443-4897

Second-level division. Biometry Branch
Description. The Biometry Branch conducts national surveillance activities to collect and analyze alcohol-related program data, maintains epidemiologic data bases, prepares statistical studies and reports, and collaborates nationally and internationally on alcohol epidemiology.
Head. Bridget F. Grant, Ph.D., (301) 443-3306

First-level division. Division of Clinical and Prevention Research
Description. Research supports studies designed to investigate alcohol treatment and prevention with rigor that is evident in treatment and prevention research for other diseases.
Head. Richard K. Fuller, M.D., (301) 443-1206

Second-level division. Treatment Research Branch
Description. This branch supports research on the treatment of alcoholism and alcohol-related disorders, including treatment methods, effective intervention, and development of new diagnostic tools. The focus of this branch is also on supporting clinical application of biomedical and psychological sciences research, consultation to re-

searchers, and dissemination of research findings.
Head. John P. Allen, Ph.D., (301) 443-0796

Second-level division. Homeless Demonstration and Evaluation Branch
Description. This branch oversees a national demonstration program on the evaluation of recovery modalities for homeless individuals with alcohol and other drug problems. It stimulates applied research on social and demographic characteristics of the homeless, their treatment and rehabilitation, provides consultation, and disseminates research findings.
Head. Robert Huebner, Ph.D., (301) 443-0786

Second-level division. Prevention Research Branch
Description. This branch supports research on the prevention of alcoholism and alcohol-related problems, including assessing the effectiveness of existing preventive strategies, developing new assessment approaches, and developing new methods of prevention. This branch also explores new program directions, disseminates research information, supports increased numbers of research scientists interested in alcoholism prevention topics, and provides consultation.
Head. Jan Howard, Ph.D., (301) 443-1677

NIAAA selected program announcements:
   Linkage Between Alcohol Use and Unprotected Sex
   Research Grants on Alcohol and Immunology Including AIDS
   Mechanisms of Uncontrolled Ethanol Intake
   Research on the Relationships Between Alcohol and Violence
   Research on Job-Related Alcohol Problems
   Research on the Children of Alcoholics
   Research on the Prevention of Alcohol Abuse Among Youth
   Economic and Socioeconomic Aspects of Alcohol Abuse
   Prevention Strategies for Alcohol Abuse in Minorities
   Matching Patients to Alcoholism Treatments
   Process Factors in Alcoholism Treatment
   Exploratory/Developmental Grants for Alcoholism Treatment
      Assessment Research
   Research on Alcohol-Related Trauma
   Research on the Homeless and Alcoholism

◆ **National Institute on Aging (NIA)**
Point of contact:
    Richard Hodes, M.D., Director
    (301) 496-9265
    Miriam Kelty, Ph.D., Extramural Programs
    (301) 496-9322
    Jane Shure, Public Information
    (301) 496-1752
Address:
    Gateway Building
    31 Center Drive
    Bethesda, MD 20892

Description. Authorized by the Congress' 1974 Research on Aging Act and the Public Health Service Act, the NIA is responsible for the conduct and support of biomedical, social, and behavioral research and research training related to the aging process and the diseases and other special problems and needs of the aged. The NIA collaborates with other NIH institutes and federal agencies to carry out this mission by research conducted through trials and interventions. Research priorities include Alzheimer's disease and related dementias; understanding the aging process; frailty, disability, and rehabilitation; health and effective functioning; long-term care; special older populations; career development/training; and international activities.

The NIA is organized into two intramural and four extramural programs. The intramural programs are the Intramural Research Program (Gerontology Research Center), which is composed of NIH laboratories that study the basic mechanisms of the aging process; and the Epidemiology, Demography, and Biometry Program, which supports research in the epidemiology of health and disease and the demographic, social, and economic factors affecting the health of older people. The four extramural programs, which are described below in further detail, are the Behavioral and Social Research Program, Biology of Aging Program, Geriatrics Program, and Neuroscience and Neuropsychology of Aging Program.

First-level division. Behavioral and Social Research Program
Description. The Behavioral and Social Research Program supports research on the aging process and the role of older people in society. Special attention is given to maintenance and enhancement of health

and independence, long-term care, older workers, and the impact of retirement.
Head. Ronald Abeles, Ph.D., (301) 496-3136

First-level division. Biology of Aging Program
Description. The Biology of Aging Program funds research on the basic mechanisms of the aging process and the onset of age-related disease. Areas of research include biochemistry, molecular and cell biology, genetics, and pathobiology.
Head. Richard Sprott, Ph.D., (301) 496-4996

First-level division. Geriatrics Program
Description. The Geriatrics Program sponsors research on the causes, prevention, and treatment of older people's health problems, including frailty, osteoporosis, infections, nutrition, and cardiovascular disorders.
Head. Evan Hadley, Ph.D., (301) 496-6761

First-level division. Neuroscience and Neuropsychology of Aging Program
Description. The Neuroscience and Neuropsychology of Aging Program supports research on the structure and function of the aging nervous system and the behavioral manifestations of the aging brain, such as memory, learning, sleep, and Alzheimer's disease.
Head. Zaven Khachaturian, Ph.D., (301) 496-9350

NIA selected program announcements:
   Special Emphasis Research Career Award (SERCA):
      The Demography and Economics of Aging
   SERCA—Rehabilitation and Aging: Biomedical and Psychosocial
      Perspectives
   Home Health Care and Support Services for Older Adults
   Women's Health Over the Lifecourse
   Social and Behavioral Aspects of Women's Health
   Economics of Aging, Health, and Retirement
   Physiological Role of the Adrenal Androgen, DHEA, in Aging
   Studies of the Failure to Thrive Syndrome in Older Populations
   Behavioral and Social Research
   Perceptual and Cognitive Aging: From Structure to Function
   Health and Effective Functioning in the Middle and Later
      Years

Causes and Effects of Elderly Population Concentrations
Forecasting Life and Health Expectancy in Older Populations
Research on Factors Affecting Aging and Health in Older People
    in Rural Areas
Psychosocial Geriatrics Research: Health Behaviors and
    Immunology of Aging
Demography and Population Epidemiology
Medical Demography of Dementias of Aging
Claude D. Pepper Older Americans Independence Centers
Neural and Behavioral Bases of Cognitive Change With Age

◆ **National Institute of Child Health
   and Human Development (NICHD)**
Point of contact:
   Duane Alexander, M.D., Director
   (301) 496-3454
   F. Haseltine, Extramural Programs
   (301) 496-1101
   Michaela Richardson, Information
   (301) 496-5133
Address:
   6100 Executive Boulevard
   Bethesda, MD 20892

Description. The NICHD provides support for research and research
training in biological and behavioral human development, with a
major research emphasis on the birth of healthy babies, reduction in
unwanted pregnancies, and prevention strategies in early childhood.
Research program areas include population research, contraceptive
development and evaluation, demographic and behavioral sciences,
genetics and teratology, endocrinology and nutrition, human learning and disabilities, adolescent research, rehabilitation, and prevention. Areas of special consideration within these broad research areas
include sudden infant death syndrome, reproductive problems of
the physically disabled, improving demographic research on families and children, biochemical and molecular basis of placental nutri-
ent transport, blastocyst implantation, perinatal research centers,
pediatric drug safety, effects of aftercare, and mitochondrial DNA in
mental retardation.
    The extramural activity of the NICHD is within the institute's
three divisions and three centers. These components are the National

Center for Medical Rehabilitation Research; Center for Population Research; Center for Research for Mothers and Children; Division of Epidemiology, Statistics, and Prevention Research; Division of Scientific Review; and Division of Intramural Research, of which this profile focuses on the first four components.

First-level division. National Center for Medical Rehabilitation Research
Description. This center supports research and research training that develop orthotic and prosthetic devices, dissemination of health information, and other rehabilitation programs that address the needs of individuals with neurological, musculoskeletal, cardiovascular, pulmonary, or other physiological system disorders, including psychosocial treatment. Medical rehabilitation research is directed toward restoration or improvement of functional capability lost because of injury, disease, or congenital disorder.
Head. Marcus Fuhrer, Ph.D., (301) 402-2242

First-level division. Center for Population Research
Description. This center serves as the central federal agency for population research and research training activities related to the biomedical, social, and behavioral sciences. It develops the research program in contraceptive development and its social, psychological, and demographic aspects, and coordinates intramural and foreign population studies.
Head. Florence Haseltine, M.D., Ph.D., (301) 496-1101

First-level division. Center for Research for Mothers and Children
Description. This center coordinates study of health problems of mothers and children in the biomedical, social, and behavioral sciences, particularly in such areas as perinatal biology, developmental disabilities, and mental retardation. Within this center, the Human Learning and Behavior Branch (Norman Krasnegor, Ph.D., Chief, [301] 496-6591) focuses on areas of particular interest to psychiatric investigators, including developmental psychobiology, behavioral pediatrics, social and affective development, and cognitive and communicative processes.
Head. Sumner Yaffe, M.D., (301) 496-5097

First-level division. Division of Epidemiology, Statistics, and Prevention Research

Description. This division develops and coordinates funding and programs for prevention related to health problems associated with reproduction that affect mothers, children, and their families. Areas of psychiatric research include infant mortality, low birth weight, congenital malformations, and mental retardation, among others. It also directs epidemiologic and biometric studies.
Head. Heinz W. Berendes, M.D., (301) 496–5064

NICHD selected program announcements:
    Child Health Small Business Innovation Research (SBIR)
    Basic and Clinical Studies of Normal Development and
      Developmental Defects
    Fertility and Fertility-Related Behavior
    Genetic Disorders Causing Mental Retardation
    Medical Rehabilitation Research

◆ **National Institute of Neurological Disorders and Stroke (NINDS)**
Point of contact:
    Zach W. Hall, Ph.D., Director
    (301) 496–3167
    Edward Donohue, Extramural Activities
    (301) 496–4188
    Marian Emr, Scientific and Health Reports
    (301) 496–5751
Address:
    Building 31A
    31 Center Drive
    Bethesda, MD 20892

Description. NINDS serves as the focal point for basic and clinical research aimed at improving the diagnosis, treatment, and prevention of disorders of the nervous system. NINDS is composed of six divisions, which are the Divisions of Intramural Research; Extramural Activities; Convulsive, Developmental, and Neurosmuscular Disorders; Demyelinating, Atrophic, and Dementing Disorders; Fundamental Neurosciences; and Stroke and Trauma. The latter four extramural research divisions are described in further detail.

First-level division. Division of Convulsive, Developmental, and Neuromuscular Disorders

Description. This division is composed of two branches, Developmental Neurology and Epilepsy, and supports basic and clinical research on disorders early in life, convulsive and paroxysmal disorders, and peripheral neuropathies and neuromuscular disorders.
Head. Floyd J. Brinley Jr., Ph.D., (301) 496-6541

First-level division. Division of Demyelinating, Atrophic, and Dementing Disorders
Description. This division supports basic and clinical research in neurological disorders of adult life, including Alzheimer's disease, Parkinson's disease, and Huntington's disease; demyelinating and sclerosing disorders; infectious diseases of the nervous system; neuroimmunology; neuroendocrinology; and the neurology of pain.
Head. Carl Leventhal, Ph.D., (301) 496-5679

First-level division. Division of Fundamental Neurosciences
Description. This division supports research involving neural structure and function, neuroanatomy, neurochemistry, and neurophysiology, neurobiology of cognition, and the influence of the nervous system on the immune system.
Head. Eugene Streicher, Ph.D., (301) 496-5745

First-level division. Division of Stroke and Trauma
Description. This division supports research on cerebrovascular disease, trauma of the central and peripheral nervous systems including head injury, regeneration of the damaged nervous system, tumors of brain, headaches, chronic and acute pain, and neuroimaging.
Head. Michael Walker, Ph.D., (301) 496-2581

NINDS selected program announcements:
   Neurogenetic Disorders of Infancy and Childhood
   Research Program Projects for the Study of Human
      Neurochronobiology
   Basic and Clinical Research on Narcolepsy
   Selective Cognitive Deficits in Neurodevelopmental Disorders
   Basic and Clinical Research on Movement Disorders
   Surgical Approaches to Epilepsy
   Research on Lyme Disease and the Nervous System
   Viral Interactions and Mental Health and Neurophysiological
      Research

Research Grants on Neural Systems and Mental, Neurological,
and Aging Disorders
Neuroscience Research Aboard Decade of the Brain Neurolab
Space Mission
Research Grants on the Neurological Basis of Cognition
Restitution of Ambulation Following Disability From
Neurological Disorders
Research on Causes and Treatment of Headaches
Mechanisms of Neuronal Regeneration and Plasticity

◆ **National Cancer Institute (NCI)**
Point of contact:
Edward Sondik, Ph.D., Acting Director
(301) 496-5615
Barbara Bynum, Extramural Activities
(301) 496-5147
J. Paul Van Nevel, Communications
(301) 496-6631
Address:
Building 31
31 Center Drive
Bethesda, MD 20892

Description. The NCI, the largest of the institutes comprising the
NIH, coordinates a national research program on cancer cause, prevention, detection, diagnosis, treatment, rehabilitation, and control.
Through its grant program, the NCI supports scientists all over the
world in a broad spectrum of research activities. The NCI also maintains its own laboratories and clinics through which its laboratory
researchers and practicing physicians form a unique partnership by
working side by side to develop knowledge about the basic biology
of cancer and to apply that knowledge to develop new prevention
techniques and therapies for cancer patients.

The NCI has five divisions: the Divisions of Cancer Treatment;
Cancer Etiology; Cancer Prevention and Control; Cancer Biology, Diagnosis, and Centers; and Extramural Activities. The Division of Cancer Prevention and Control is of particular significance in psychiatric
research funding ([301] 496-6616). Areas of research that overlap
with psychiatric research issues include behavioral cancer intervention and prevention strategies, pain management, and issues related
to women's health and cancer.

NCI selected program announcements:
   Culturally Sensitive Intervention Strategies for Promoting or
      Implementing Compliance with NCI Dietary Guidelines
      Among African Americans
   Cancer Prevention and Control Research Small Grant Program
   Cancer Pain Management in Outpatient Settings
   Studies on Breast, Prostate, Ovarian, and Cervical Cancer

◆ **National Heart, Lung, and Blood Institute (NHLBI)**
Point of contact:
   Claude Lenfant, M.D., Director
   (301) 496-5166
   Peter Frommer, M.D., Deputy Director
   (301) 496-1078
   Ronald Geller, Ph.D., Extramural Affairs
   (301) 496-7416
   Ellen Summer, Communications
   (301) 496-4236
Address:
   Building 31
   31 Center Drive
   Bethesda, MD 20892

Description.   The NHLBI conducts and supports research relating
to the causes, prevention, diagnosis, and treatment of heart, blood
vessel, lung, and blood diseases and resources. Extramural support
includes research in arteriosclerosis, hypertension, cardiology, developmental biology, behavioral medicine, lung diseases, thrombosis
and hemostasis, sickle cell anemia, and epidemiology. The NHLBI's
six divisions are the Divisions of Extramural Affairs, Intramural Research, Heart and Vascular Diseases, Lung Diseases, Blood Diseases
and Resources, and Epidemiology and Clinical Applications; also,
newly established in February 1994 is the National Center on Sleep
Disorders Research.
   Areas of interest to psychiatric researchers include behavioral
neuroscience and clinical applications of behavioral research in the
detection and treatment of and recovery from cardiovascular diseases. Funding has focused on the neuroactive peptide mediation of
stress impact in cardiovascular diseases, cardiovascular hyperreac-
tivity, behavioral interventions for hypertension, psychological
factors in coronary artery bypass graft patients, and methods to

improve patient adherence to clinical trial interventions. Information on this funding is available from Peter Kaufmann, Ph.D., Chief, Behavioral Medicine Branch, Division of Epidemiology and Clinical Applications, (301) 496-9380.

The Division of Lung Diseases also supports research of interest to psychiatric investigators, including investigations into behavioral medicine as related to lung diseases, such as smoking-related health problems and asthma. The National Center on Sleep Disorders Research supports basic and applied research related to sleep and circadian rhythms. For further information on the activity of these NHLBI programs, contact James Kiley, Ph.D., Acting Chief, Prevention, Education, and Research Training Branch, Division of Lung Diseases, who is also the Acting Director of the National Center on Sleep Disorders Research, at (301) 496-7443.

NHLBI selected program announcements:
 Collaborative Projects on Women's Health
 Physical Activity Intervention in Health-Care Settings for High
  Risk Sedentary Behavior

◆ **National Institute on Deafness and
 Other Communication Disorders (NIDCD)**
Point of contact:
 James Snow, M.D., Director
 (301) 402-0900
 Jay Moscowitz, Ph.D., Deputy Director
 (301) 402-0495
 John Dalton, Ph.D., Extramural Programs
 (301) 496-8693
 Marin Allen, Public Affairs
 (301) 496-7243
Address:
 Executive Plaza South
 6120 Executive Boulevard
 Bethesda, MD 20892

Description. The NIDCD supports research and research training on the normal mechanisms and disorders associated with hearing and other communication processes, including diseases affecting hearing, balance, smell, taste, voice, speech, and language. The NIDCD is composed of three major divisions: Intramural Research, Extramural Activities, and Communication Science and Disorders (Judith Cooper, Ph.D., Director, [301] 496-5061). This last division is broken down into the Hearing and Balance Vestibular Sciences Branch and the Voice, Speech, Language, Smell, and Taste Branch. Areas of psychiatric research interest at the NIDCD include special biomedical and behavioral problems that are found in people with communication impairments.

NIDCD selected program announcements:
Deafness and Communications Disorders Small Grants
Research and Training Centers on Communications Science
Childhood Language Impairment in Multicultural Populations
Research on Literacy in Deaf Individuals
Mechanisms of Voice Disorders
Articulation Disorders in Children

◆ National Institute for Nursing Research (NINR)
Point of contact:
Patricia Grady, Ph.D., Director
(301) 496-8230
Suzanne Feetham, R.N., Ph.D., Deputy Director
(301) 402-1446
Terry Radebaugh, Extramural Programs
(301) 594-7590
Marianne Duffy, Information and Legislative
(301) 496-0207
Addresses:
Building 31
31 Center Drive
Bethesda, MD 20892
Westwood Building
5333 Westbard Avenue
Bethesda, MD 20892

Description. The NINR, reorganized as an institute in 1993, supports programs focusing on health promotion and disease prevention, understanding and mitigating the effects of acute and chronic illnesses and disabilities, and the delivery of nursing services. Its research programs are complementary to the research activities supported by other components of the NIH, with a major focus of the NINR to develop collaborative intramural research programs with other NIH institutes. Postdoctoral training opportunities exist for qualified nurse researchers and other scientific investigators under regular announcements of NINR.

The institute is divided into the Division of Intramural Programs and the Division of Extramural Programs, which is composed of three branches: Acute and Chronic Illness Branch, Health Promotion and Disease Prevention Branch, and Nursing Systems Branch. Areas of psychiatric interest may include research on intervention and psychosocial adjustment issues associated with chronic and genetic diseases.

NINR selected program announcements:
    Clinical Outcomes of Nursing Practices
    Neonatal Nursing Care of Low Birthweight Infants
    Prevention of Low Birthweight
    Research on Community-Based Interventions for Adolescent
        Health Promotion

◆   **National Institute of Allergy and
    Infectious Diseases (NIAID)**
Point of contact:
    Anthony Fauci, M.D., Director
    (301) 496-2263
    James Hill, Deputy Director
    (301) 496-9118
    John McGowan, Extramural Activities
    (301) 496-7291
    Patricia Randall, Public Affairs
    (301) 496-5717
Address:
    Solar Building
    6003 Executive Boulevard
    Bethesda, MD 20892

Description. The NIAID conducts and supports research for the understanding, treatment, prevention, and diagnosis of allergic, immunologic, and infectious diseases. Divisions supporting extramural activity include Allergy, Immunology, and Transplantation; Microbiology and Infectious Disease; AIDS; and special programs in international collaboration, tropical medicine research, and United States–Japan cooperation in medical science. Areas of specific psychiatric research interest include the interplay between behavioral and biomedical risk factors for sexually transmitted diseases (STD) and intervention-oriented behavioral research for STD prevention, which are under the auspices of the Division of Microbiology and Infectious Diseases, (301) 496-4433. AIDS-related behavioral research and chronic fatigue syndrome research are also of interest.

NIAID selected program announcements:
Behavioral Research in Sexually Transmitted Diseases
International Collaborative AIDS Research and Epidemiology
Exercise-Induced Fatigue in Chronic Fatigue Syndrome (CFS)

◆ **National Institute of Arthritis and Musculoskeletal and Skin Diseases (NIAMS)**
Point of contact:
Michael Lockshin, M.D., Acting Director
(301) 496-4353
Steven Hausman, Deputy Director
(301) 402-1691
Michael Lockshin, M.D., Extramural Programs
(301) 496-0802
Connie Raab, Public Affairs
(301) 496-8188
Address:
Building 31
31 Center Drive
Bethesda, MD 20892

Description. The NIAMS has the primary responsibility for the three disease areas incorporated in its name and for research on the normal structure and functioning of muscles, bones, joints, and skin. Programs providing extramural support include arthritis, muscle biology, bone biology/diseases, skin diseases, and epidemiology. The NIAMS funds extramural research through four branches: Rheumatic Diseases Branch, Musculoskeletal Diseases Branch, Muscle Biology and Training Branch, and Skin Diseases Branch, and supports research centers programs. Areas of psychiatric research may include research on low back pain.

◆ **National Institute of Dental Research (NIDR)**
Point of contact:
> Dushanka Kleinman, D.D.S., Acting Director
> (301) 496-3571
> Lois Cohen, Ph.D., Extramural Programs
> (301) 496-7723
> Susan Johnson, Public Information
> (301) 496-4261

Address:
> Building 31
> 31 Center Drive
> Bethesda, MD 20892

Description. The NIDR fosters research on the causes, treatment, and diagnoses of dental and oral disease and conditions, including AIDS, and dental issues and research on pain and other sensory issues. NIDR is divided into three programs: Intramural Research Program, Extramural Research Program, and the Epidemiology and Oral Disease Prevention Program. Psychiatric research areas may include behavioral and social science research addressing factors influencing oral health status and the impact on the individual and society of oral diseases and disorders. One area of particular interest is behavioral and biomedical research into chronic dental pain.

NIDR selected program announcement:
> Research on Chronic Dental Pain

◆ **National Institute of Diabetes and Digestive and Kidney Diseases (NIDDK)**
Point of contact:
> Phillip Gorden, M.D., Director
> (301) 496-5877
> Earl Laurence, (Acting) Deputy Director
> (301) 496-5741
> Walter Stolz, Ph.D., Extramural Activities
> (301) 594-7527
> Elizabeth Singer, Public Affairs
> (301) 496-3583

Address:
> Westwood Building

5333 Westbard Avenue
Bethesda, MD 20892

Description. The NIDDK supports research and research training on diabetes and other metabolic disorders, gastrointestinal disorders, endocrine disorders, kidney and urological diseases, and diseases of the blood and bone. The NIDDK is divided into four divisions, which support extramural research: the Divisions of Diabetes, Endocrinology, and Metabolic Diseases; Digestive Diseases and Nutrition; Kidney, Urologic, and Hematologic Diseases; and Extramural Activities. Areas of interest to psychiatric researchers include research in neurochemistry and neuroendocrinology; the physiological, psychological, and genetic factors affecting food choices, intake, and eating behavior; and eating disorders (Van Hubbard, M.D., Ph.D., Chief, Obesity, Eating Disorders, and Energy Regulation Program, [301] 594-7573).

◆ National Institute of Environmental Health Sciences (NIEHS)

Point of contact:
Kenneth Olden, Director
(919) 541-3201
Richard Griesemer, Deputy Director
(919) 541-3267
Anne Sassaman, Ph.D, Extramural Programs
(919) 541-7723
Sandy Lange, Communications
(919) 541-2605
Address:
PO Box 12233
Research Triangle Park, NC 27709

Description. The mission of the NIEHS is to identify the chemical, physical, and biologic factors in the environment that can adversely affect people, to contribute to an understanding of the mechanisms and manifestations of human diseases produced by these agents, and to provide the scientific basis for the development of control measures by other agencies. The NIEHS is particularly concerned with the effects of agents at low concentrations acting over a long period, the interaction of multiple agents resulting in enhanced effects, and the modifying effects of variable physical and biologic states within people on the susceptibility to and course of disease induced by these agents.

The NIEHS consists of the Divisions of Intramural Research, Extramural Research and Training, Toxicology Research and Testing, and Biometry and Risk Assessment. Areas of particular interest to psychiatric researchers include biological and behavioral responses to environmental agents and psychosocial research on exposure of humans to toxic substances.

NIEHS selected program announcement:
   Environmental Health Sciences Program Project Grants

◆ **National Eye Institute (NEI)**
Point of contact:
   Carl Kupfer, M.D., Director
   (301) 496-2234
   Edward McManus, Deputy Director
   (301) 496-4583
   Jack McLaughlin, M.D., Extramural Programs
   (301) 496-9110
   Judith Stein, Public Affairs
   (301) 496-5248
Address:
   Building 31
   31 Center Drive
   Bethesda, MD 20892

Description. The NEI conducts and supports research on the cause, natural history, prevention, diagnosis, and treatment of disorders of the eye and visual system. Areas of funding interest include retinal and choroidal diseases, corneal diseases, cataracts, glaucoma, visual processing, and rehabilitation for low vision. The NEI has its clinical and research activity as a part of the Extramural and Collaborative Program, which is composed of six programs: retinal and choroidal diseases; corneal diseases; cataract; glaucoma, strabismus, and amblyopia; visual processing; and collaborative clinical research. Research areas that may incorporate issues of relevance to psychiatric research include neuroscience research, functioning of the neural pathways, visual perception, and processing of visual information.

◆ **National Institute of General Medical Sciences (NIGMS)**
Point of contact:
  Marvin Cassman, Ph.D., Director
  (301) 594-2172
  W. Sue Shafer, Ph.D., Program Activities
  (301) 496-5575
  Ann Diefenbach, Research Activities
  (301) 496-7301
Address:
  Natcher Building
  45 Center Drive
  Bethesda, MD 20892

Description. The NIGMS fosters research in the sciences basic to medicine that form the foundation needed to make advances in understanding diseases studied by the other NIH institutions. This funding advances new knowledge, theories, and concepts for the disease-targeted studies that are supported by other NIH components. The program work of the NIGMS is divided into the following programs: Cellular and Molecular Basis of Disease Program, Biophysics and Physiological Sciences Program, Genetics Program, Pharmacological Sciences Program, and Minority Opportunities in Research Program. These programs provide broad areas of research in the basic sciences by studying genetics, pharmacology and biological molecular interaction, and the foundations of cellular and molecular diseases.

The Pharmacological Sciences Program (Michael Rogers, Ph.D., Acting Chief, [301] 594-7776) supports research on the biological phenomena and related chemical and molecular processes involved in therapeutic drugs, anesthetics, and their metabolites, including psychopharmacological medication.

◆ **National Library of Medicine (NLM)**
Point of contact:
  Donald Linberg, M.D., Director
  (301) 496-3014
  Harold Schoolman, M.D., Deputy Director
  (301) 496-4725

Milton Corn, M.D., Extramural Programs
(301) 496–4621
Robert Mehnert, Public Information
(301) 496–1030
Address:
Building 38A
31 Center Drive
Bethesda, MD 20892

Description. The NLM assists the health community in researching, developing, and implementing improved methods and systems for the organization and access of health science knowledge. Research support is provided for a broad range of areas, such as data acquisition techniques (particularly with computer systems), artificial intelligence, cognitive processes involved in medical decision making, information storage and retrieval and related effects of human-machine interaction, transfer of information technologies to health data base design, medical software development, and medical bibliography research.

Three divisions and two centers compose the NLM. The centers are the National Center for Biomedical Communications and the National Center for Biotechnology Information. The Divisions of Specialized Information Services, Library Operations, and Extramural Programs constitute the divisions within the NLM.

◆ **National Center for Human Genome Research (NCHGR)**
Point of contact:
Francis Collins, M.D., Ph.D., Director
(301) 496–0844
Elke Jordan, Ph.D., Deputy Director
(301) 496–0844
Mark Guyer, Ph.D., Program Coordination
(301) 496–0844
Sharon Durham, Communications
(301) 402–0911
Address:
Building 38A
9000 Rockville Pike
Bethesda, MD 20892

Description. The NCHGR seeks to characterize the structure of the human genome and the genomes of selected "model" organisms. Areas of support include mapping and DNA sequencing, the effects of mapping on information technology, and ethical, legal, and social implications of genetic research.

NCHGR selected program announcements:
Technology Development, Mapping, and DNA Sequencing on the Human Genome Program
Genome Research Centers
Ethical, Legal, and Social Implications of Human Genome Research Program

◆ National Center for Research Resources (NCRR)
Point of contact:
Judith Vaitukaitis, M.D., Director
(301) 496-5793
Louise Ramm, Ph.D., Extramural Activities
(301) 496-6023
Marie Milander, Science and Health Reports
(301) 594-7938
Addresses:
Building 12A
31 Center Drive
Bethesda, MD 20892
Westwood Building
5333 Westbard Avenue
Bethesda, MD 20892

Description. The NCRR develops and supports research technologies for NIH intramural and extramural biomedical research so as to maintain and improve the nation's health. These resources include sophisticated instrumentation and technology, mammalian/non-mammalian models of human disease studies, flexible and innovative research support mechanisms, clinical research center networks, research infrastructure for minority institutions, and state-of-the-art equipment. The NCRR supports multidisciplinary projects and projects that crosscut the NIH institutes. Areas of particular interest to psychiatric researchers may include issues on animal/nonanimal models of research and research infrastructure support; e.g., through the General Clinical Research Center (GCRC) program, the

NCRR supports important psychiatric research in major academic centers.

NCRR selected program announcements:
    Investigations Into Methods That Replace or Reduce Vertebrate
       Animals Used in Research or Lessen Their Pain and Distress
    Comparative Medicine Research Program Projects in
       Biomedical Research

◆ **John E. Fogarty International Center (FIC)**
   for Advanced Study in the Health Sciences
Point of contact:
    Philip Schambra, Ph.D., Director
    (301) 496-1415
    David Wolff, Ph.D., Extramural Programs
    (301) 496-1653
    Robert Eiss, Communications
    (301) 496-1491
Address:
    Building 31
    31 Center Drive
    Bethesda, MD 20892

Description. The FIC fosters international cooperation, consultation, and fellowship support in the biomedical, behavioral, and other related health fields for discussion, study, and research relating to the development of health science internationally. By providing support for fellowships, research conferences, seminars, and other international collaboration, the FIC promotes the exchange of scholars and scientific research findings throughout the world.

FIC selected programs:
    International Research Fellowship (IRF) Program
    Senior International Fellowship (SIF) Program
    Neurosciences Fellowship Program
    International Tropical Disease Research Fellowship Program
    Fogarty International Research Collaboration Awards (FIRCA)

◆ Substance Abuse and Mental Health Services Administration (SAMHSA)

Point of contact:
Nelba R. Chavez, Ph.D., Administrator
(301) 443-4795
Daniel Melnick, Ph.D., Applied Studies
(301) 443-1038
Communications
(301) 443-8956

Address:
Parklawn Building & Rockwall Building
5600 Fishers Lane
Rockville, MD 20857

Description. The SAMHSA, established in 1993 after the reorganization of the Alcohol, Drug Abuse, and Mental Health Administration and the transfer of NIDA, the NIMH, and the NIAAA to the NIH, is focused on efforts to enhance services and prevention related to addictive and mental disorders. Its mandate is to provide a stimulus to advance knowledge about effective programs, recognize the common interests of substance and mental health service providers, provide a voice for the support of substance abuse and mental health treatment services in evolving health care reform, and address areas of special interest such as AIDS/HIV, violence, incarcerated populations with substance abuse problems, and other public health issues related to substance abuse and mental illness. Duties include assisting state and local agencies to expand capacity and access to treatment and prevention programs, evaluate treatment and prevention effectiveness, and develop community-wide approaches.

Support for academic programs may come in several forms. Academic departments may receive funds through the states, direct service providers who receive grants, or (in certain specific programs) as direct grant recipients. Some academic departments gain access to program support through community-based organizations. Grants often include funds for evaluation, consultation on methodology, support for training, and treatment or diagnostic services, in addition to funds for services. In some cases, individual center-supported grants may serve as a comparison group for related ongoing research.

Involvement by academic departments in evaluation activities can complement ongoing research activities and serve as the basis for the development of new research initiatives. Virtually all discretionary SAMHSA programs mandate evaluation. The sophistication of these evaluation activities has increased over the past several years. Evaluation protocols may now include, and sometimes are mandated to include, comparison groups. Many academic departments serve as the evaluator of community-based programs. In some cases, academic departments have assumed statewide responsibility for evaluation of discretionary and block grant-supported programs.

Besides the Office of the Administrator, the SAMHSA was established with three major centers, the Center for Mental Health Services (CMHS), the Center for Substance Abuse Treatment (CSAT), and the Center for Substance Abuse Prevention (CSAP), which are described below.

◆ **Center for Mental Health Services**
Description. This center, established to create a focus for increased federal attention to issues related to mental health service delivery in the United States, helps identify and enable adjustments and modifications in mental health services systems at the state and local levels. The emphasis is to provide improved access to treatment, prevention, and rehabilitation for mental illness while reducing the impact on the family and community.
Head. Bernard Arons, M.D., (301) 443-0001
Extramural. Barbara Silver, Ph.D., (301) 443-7883

◆ **Center for Substance Abuse Prevention**
Description. This center focuses on two funding programs, the Community Partnership and High-Risk Youth programs. The Community Partnership program helps local community coalitions plan substance abuse prevention efforts, and the High-Risk Youth prevention demonstration grants target young people at risk of initiating or increasing drug or alcohol use. Reducing the use of tobacco is also a focus of this program.
Head. Elaine Johnson, Ph.D. (Acting), (301) 443-0365
Extramural. Joel Goldstein, Ph.D., (301) 443-4266

◆ **Center for Substance Abuse Treatment**
Description. This center funds comprehensive residential treatment programs for pregnant and postpartum women, outpatient treatment, state capacity expansion grants, counselor training, substance abuse treatment and criminal justice systems, and block grants.

Head. David Mactas, M.A., (301) 443-2467
Extramural. Ellen Shapiro, (301) 443-5052

Other Public Health Service Programs

◆ **Agency for Health Care Policy and Research (AHCPR)**
Point of contact:
    Clifton R. Gaus, Sc.D., Administrator
    (301) 594-6662
    Division of Communications
    (301) 594-1361
Address:
    Executive Office Center
    2101 East Jefferson Street
    Rockville, MD 20852

Description. The AHCPR serves as the focal point for federal health services research by expanding on the work undertaken by its predecessor, the National Center for Health Services Research. Its mission is to enhance the quality of patient care services through improved knowledge that can be used in meeting society's health care needs. The agency achieves this mission by 1) promoting improvements in clinical practice and patient outcomes through appropriate and effective health care services bases through extramural and intramural research activities; 2) demonstrating/evaluating new ways to organize, finance, and direct health care services to improve delivery, access, and outcomes of services; 3) assessing new technologies that may be federally funded; 4) facilitating practice guidelines development and other standardized measurements of quality care; and 5) promoting the utilization of health services research findings through systematic, broad-based information dissemination.

The AHCPR is divided into six offices and four centers. The offices are the Offices of the Administrator, Forum for Quality and Effectiveness in Health Care, Science and Data Development, Health Technology Assessment, Program Development, and Management. The centers are the Centers for General Health Services Intramural Research, General Health Services Extramural Research, Medical Effectiveness Research, and Research Dissemination and Liaison. Of particular interest to extramural investigators are the activities of the latter three centers, which are described in further detail.

First-level division.   Center for Research Dissemination and Liaison
Description.   This center publishes AHCPR reports and collaborates with NLM to disseminate information. It supports grants studying use and effects of health services research findings and clinical practice guidelines.
Head.   Phyllis Zucker, (301) 594-1360 X145

First-level division.   Center for Medical Effectiveness Research
Description.   This center focuses on funding patient outcomes research, outcomes research methodologies, practice variations, and other medical effectiveness topics.
Head.   Richard J. Greene, M.D., Ph.D., (301) 594-1485

First-level division.   Center for General Health Services Extramural Research
Description.   This center oversees funding on research of health care organization, delivery, and finance by focusing basic research on quality of care, health status measurement, primary care, access, and cost-effectiveness of interventions.
Head.   Norman W. Weissman, Ph.D., (301) 594-1349 X109

AHCPR selected program announcements:
   Rural Health Care Research: Impacting Vulnerable Populations
   Research on Health Care Services and Systems Reform
   Health Services Research on Rural Health
   Short-Term Research on Cost and Finance Reform of the
      U.S. Health Care System
   Health Services Research Related to HIV and AIDS
   Studies on Cost and Services Utilization on HIV-Related Health
      Issues
   Dissemination of Health and Clinical Information and Research
      Findings
   Applied Research and Demonstrations on Effective Dissemination
      of Health-Related Information and Practice Guidelines
   Health Services Research Conference Grants

◆ Centers for Disease Control and Prevention (CDC)
Point of contact:
   David Satcher, M.D., Director
   (404) 639-3291
   Public Inquiries (404) 639-3534

Address:
  255 East Paces Ferry Road, NE
  Atlanta, GA 30305

Description. The CDC supports research aimed at developing effective disease interventions, prevention, and control and promoting health education and health prevention programs. The CDC surveys national disease trends, epidemics, and environmentally related health problems. Coordinating with state and local health departments, the CDC attempts to address research related to sexually transmitted diseases, tuberculosis, immunization, and chronic disease and injury.

One institute and six centers compose the program work within the CDC: National Institute for Occupational Safety and Health (NIOSH) and the National Centers for Chronic Disease Prevention and Health Promotion, Environmental Health, Health Statistics, Infectious Diseases, Injury Prevention and Control, and Prevention Services. The centers support funding for applied research, surveys, data gathering, injury control, HIV and AIDS issues, and conferences. CDC extramural research of interest to psychiatric researchers is primarily centered in NIOSH and the National Centers for Injury Prevention and Control and Infectious Diseases.

First-level division. National Institute for Occupational Safety and Health (NIOSH)
Description. This institute administers research in the field of occupational health and safety, including conduct of health hazard evaluations. The behavioral effects of workplace hazards and behavioral intervention research related to workplace health and safety are areas of interest.
Head. Bryan Hardin, (202) 690-7134; 200 Independence Avenue, SW, Washington, DC 20201

First-level division. Center for Infectious Diseases
Description. This center studies prevention of unnecessary illness, disability, and death caused by infectious diseases within the United States and around the world. Behavioral research in prevention of infectious diseases, including sexually transmitted diseases and AIDS, is included in its funding.
Head. James Hughes, M.D., (404) 639-3401

First-level division.   Center for Injury Prevention and Control
Description.   This center aims to reduce morbidity, disability, mortality, and costs associated with injuries outside the workplace. Areas of research interest include studies in unintentional injury prevention, violence prevention, care and rehabilitation of injured persons, and injury biomechanics.
Head.   Mark Rosenberg, M.D., M.P.P., (404) 488-4690

CDC selected program announcements:
  Public Health Conference Support Grants
  Injury Control Research
  Injury Control Research Centers
  Applied Research on Occupational Safety and Health
  Research and Demonstration Grants Relating to Occupational
    Safety and Health

◆   **Food and Drug Administration (FDA)**
Point of contact:
  David A. Kessler, M.D., Commissioner
  (301) 443-2410
  James A. O'Hara III, Consumer and Public Affairs
  (301) 443-3170
  Marie Moses, Orphan Products Development
  (301) 443-4903
Address:
  5600 Fishers Lane
  Rockville, MD 20857

Description.   The FDA oversees the regulation of food and drugs in the United States. It provides some research support for biotechnology, orphan drug development, and other health issues. It is composed of four major offices: Office of Operations, Policy, External Affairs, and Management and Systems, with specific, limited extramural research programs located in the various centers within the Office of Operations. These centers are the Centers for Drug Evaluation and Research; Food Safety and Applied Nutrition; Toxicological Research, Biologics Evaluation, and Research; Devices and Radiological Health; Veterinary Medicine; and the Office of Orphan Products Development.
    Psychopharmacologic drug research is supported within the Office of Orphan Products Development, which encourages clinical development of products such as drugs, biologics, medical devices, or

foods for use in rare diseases or conditions (those conditions affecting fewer than 200,000). Orphan products research received $9.1 million in fiscal year 1992. Up to $100,000 a year in direct costs may be given for up to 3 years. Funding interests are especially for products for rare diseases or conditions where no therapy exists, where current therapy can be improved, and that are ready for clinical development. For further information on the orphan products development program, contact Carol Wetmore, Grant Program Coordinator, (301) 443-4903.

◆ **Health Resources and Services Administration (HRSA)**
Point of contact:
   Ciro Sumaya, M.D., M.P.H., Administrator
   (301) 443-2216
   Office of Communications
   (301) 443-2086
Address:
   5600 Fishers Lane
   Rockville, MD 20857

Description. HRSA is responsible for primary care health services and resource issues related to access, quality, equity, and cost of health care. It works with state and community efforts on primary health care delivery issues, particularly for underserved areas and groups with special health needs. It also focuses on improving the education, distribution, and utilization of health professionals for the nation's primary health care system. HRSA consists of four major components: the Bureaus of Primary Health Care, Health Professions, Health Resources Development, and Maternal and Child Health; the latter bureau has a research component supporting areas of interest to psychiatric investigators.

The Maternal and Child Health (MCH) Bureau (Audrey H. Nora, M.D., M.P.H., Director, [301] 443-2170) is the federal government's focal point for planning, implementing, and overseeing national maternal and child health activities. Areas of research supported by this bureau include maternal and child health issues; genetic disease testing and screening; health care services research directed at mothers, infants, and children; pediatric AIDS health care research; and information dissemination. For further information on MCH research programs, contact Samuel Kessel, M.D., M.P.H., Director of Systems Education and Science, (301) 443-2340.

Other Health and Human Services Programs

◆ **Administration for Children and Families (ACF)**
Point of contact:
    Mary Jo Bane, Assistant Secretary
    (202) 401-9000
    Office of Public Affairs
    (202) 401-9215
Address:
    370 L'Enfant Promenade, SW
    Washington, DC 20447

Description. The Administration for Children and Families is responsible for federal programs that promote self-sufficiency for disadvantaged Americans. Through providing mostly income support and
social services, although some research funding is available, the ACF
improves the well-being of low-income families, neglected and
abused children, Native Americans, refugees, and people with developmental disabilities and with mental retardation. The ACF is composed of three separate administrations: Administration for Children,
Youth, and Families (ACYF); Administration for Native Americans
(ANA); and the Administration on Developmental Disabilities (ADD).

First-level division. Administration for Native Americans (ANA)
Description. The ANA promotes the goal of social and economic self-
sufficiency through the enhancement of institutions of self-gover-
nance for Indian tribes and organizations and other Native American
communities. In 1993, $34.1 million supported community-based de-
velopment programs. Other programs of interest are enhancement of
local decision making, economic development, and services coordination. Each of these areas supports limited applied research.
Head. Dominic Mastrapasqua (Acting), (202) 690-7776

First-level division. Administration on Developmental Disabilities
(ADD)
Description. The ADD programs assist nearly four million Americans who are severely, chronically disabled either physically or mentally, resulting in substantial limitations in major life activity.
Programs emphasized include coordinated services, advocacy systems, training, information dissemination, and research on pressing

national issues affecting the disabled. Each of these areas supports limited applied research.
Head. Robert Williams, (202) 690-6590

First-level division. Administration on Children, Youth, and Families (ACYF)
Description. The ACYF, the most extensive program within the ACF, provides assistance to at-risk children and families. Programs emphasized in the ACYF include at-risk child care, child abuse and neglect, child support enforcement, child care and development block grants, child welfare services, foster care/adoption, Head Start, runaway and homeless issues, community services, and social services block grants. Each of these areas supports limited applied research.
Head. Olivia Golden, (202) 205-8347

◆ **Administration on Aging (AOA)**
Point of contact:
    Fernando Torres-Gil, Assistant Secretary
    (202) 401-4634
    Jack McCarthy, Office of Program Development
    (202) 619-0441
    Public Affairs
    (202) 619-0724
Address:
    330 Independence Avenue, SW
    Washington, DC 20201

Description. The AOA seeks to strengthen knowledge building, program innovation and development, information dissemination, training, technical assistance, and other efforts focused on elder care service systems for older Americans at risk of losing their independence. The administration focuses its efforts on services and applied research assisting services for adult elder care.

Research inquiries and extramural support are handled by the Office of Program Development ([202] 619-0441). Areas of recent funding interest, including mental health research issues, have focused on long-term care, elder abuse, older women, multipurpose senior centers, elder transportation, housing and supportive services, nutrition services, human resources development, health promotion, income security, and aging and business. The AOA issues its program announcements annually, generally with a July deadline.

◆ Health Care Financing Administration (HCFA)

Point of contact:

Bruce Vladeck, Administrator
(202) 690-6726
Carl Hackerman, Research and Demonstration
(410) 966-6644
Public Affairs
(202) 690-6113

Address:

200 Independence Avenue, SW
Washington, DC 20201

Description. The Health Care Financing Administration supports research demonstration projects that aim to resolve the major financing issues facing the U.S. health care system, particularly issues affecting the Medicare and Medicaid programs and their beneficiaries. In addition, the HCFA oversees the refinement and testing of alternative models for rural health care and health care facilities. The HCFA Office of Research and Demonstration ([410] 966-6644), its chief policy and research component, emphasizes funding programs in areas such as coordinated care systems, hospital payment, physician and ambulatory care payment systems, prevention and access, and acute and long-term care.

Research of interest to psychiatrists in fiscal year 1994–1996 includes feasibility studies of financing systems for different disability groups, including chronic mental illness and mental retardation, studying such factors as the relationship between the quality of care standards for licensing service providers and the quality of community-based services, issues influencing the costs of intermediate care facilities, and the change of venues of care for the chronically mentally ill over time.

HCFA selected program announcement:

Studies on Feasibility of Different Financing Systems for
   Different Disability Groups

◆ Social Security Administration (SSA)

Point of contact:

Louis Enoff, Commissioner
(410) 965-3120
Serge Harrison, Office of Research and Statistics
(410) 965-2843

Allen Shafer, Office on Disability
(410) 965-0091
Larry Pullen, Grants and Acquisitions
(410) 965-9502
Address:
  6401 Security Boulevard
  Baltimore, MD 21235

Description. The SSA has limited research funding; it supports research on economic issues, disability issues, aging, and children. According to the SSA budget office, SSA has not supported research directly related to psychiatric research over the past 3 years but is currently reviewing program support on disability research associated with mental illness issues and children's issues. SSA funded several studies in 1987, including one with the APA, on Social Security Administration standards and methods for evaluating disabilities based on mental impairment.

The SSA research component is the Office of Research Statistics, which compiles statistics on beneficiaries, conducts economic research on recipients and SSA's relationship with the economy, and analyzes the effects of Social Security legislation.

DEPARTMENT OF VETERANS AFFAIRS (VA)

Point of contact:
  Jesse Brown, Secretary
  (202) 535-8900
  Dennis Smith, Chief Medical Officer for R&D
  (202) 535-7155
  Public Affairs
  (202) 535-8300
Address:
  810 Vermont Avenue
  Washington, DC 20420

Description. The Department of Veterans Affairs oversees the benefits, services, and research affecting those who have served in the U.S. military. The health research activities at the VA cover biomedical, rehabilitation, and health services research and development. The VA supports mental illness research projects in these areas in the department's Medical Research Services (MRS), Health Services Research and Development Services (HSR&D), and Rehabilitation Research and Development (Rehab R&D). This research ranges from basic neurobiological studies to clinical studies of the effectiveness of psychosocial and psychopharmacological interventions. Requests for research funding from these programs are subject to a scientific peer review group, which analyzes proposals on evidence of qualifications to do scientific research and of past productivity.

◆ Medical Research Service (MRS)

Description. Five programs compose the research of the MRS, the largest being the Merit Review Program, which supports 1,600 investigators for average periods of 3 years. Researchers must have at least a 5/8-time VA appointment. The Research Advisory Group Program provides start-up funding for research by newly recruited VA medical center clinicians. The Career Development Program, with five levels of award, enables VA clinicians to spend a majority of time in research rather than clinical work. The Cooperative Studies Program supports clinical trials evaluating the effectiveness of diagnostic or therapeutic techniques and has supported trials in pharmacotherapy for schizophrenia, alcohol treatment, and hypertension. The last program is the Special Research Initiatives Program, which solicits research efforts in biomedical and behavioral medicine of particular significance to the veteran population.

Head. Murray Albert, Ph.D., (202) 535-7155

◆ Health Services Research and Development Service (HSR&D)

Description. The HSR&D supports three primary programs for research funding. Investigator-Initiated Research is a competitive program funding large and small grants for individual researchers investigating a specific topic at a single medical center. Services Directed Research focuses on large-scale, multisite studies responding to a congressional, executive, or VA directive. Cooperative Studies in Health Services is a multisite initiative blending health care services and delivery orientation with clinical expertise in MRS. Centers established have focused on alcoholism and drug abuse, schizophrenia, depression, posttraumatic stress disorder, and patients with multiple diagnoses.

Head. Daniel Deykin, M.D., (202) 535-7156

◆ **Rehabilitation Research and Development Service (Rehab R&D)**

Description. This service supports rehabilitation research in prosthetic amputation/orthotics, spinal cord injury and related neurological disorders, communication cognitive and sensory aids, dementia, and schizophrenia. Mental health research is a focus of this program through its research on aging veterans, particularly veterans suffering from Alzheimer's disease, patients who have frequent returns to the hospital with marginal adjustment to their communities, and patients with limited response to standard antipsychotic drugs.

Head. Victoria Mongiardo, (410) 962-2563

DEPARTMENT OF EDUCATION (ED)

Point of contact:
    Richard Riley, Secretary
    (202) 401-3000
    Sharon P. Robinson, Educational Research and Improvement
    (202) 219-2050
    Judith Heumann, Special Education and Rehabilitative Services
    (202) 205-5465
    Joseph Conaty, Office of Research
    (202) 219-2079
    Public Affairs
    (202) 401-1576
Address:
    400 Maryland Avenue, SW
    Washington, DC 20202

Description. The ED establishes and oversees education policy for the federal government and acts as principal adviser to the president on educational matters. It also coordinates most federal assistance programs on education. Its research components, the Office of Educational Research and Improvement and the Office of Special Education and Rehabilitation Services, primarily gather and disseminate statistics and research findings on the condition of American education, the processes of teaching and learning, curriculum, factors contributing to excellence in education, effective drug and AIDS prevention, vocational training, and academic programs.

◆ **National Institute on Disability and Rehabilitation Research (NIDRR)**

Description. The NIDRR, a part of the Office of Special Education and Rehabilitation Services, aims to increase the independence of persons with disabilities and those in rehabilitation, including individuals with spinal cord injury, head injury, and psychosocial rehabilitation and severe mental illness. Its emphasis is on practical, outcome-oriented projects conducted by investigators who practice research with patient participation, with the largest funding being provided for rehabilitation research and training centers that provide behavioral, vocational, or medical rehabilitation, areas of interest to psychiatric research.

Head. Katherine D. Seelman, (202) 205-8134

NATIONAL SCIENCE FOUNDATION (NSF)

Point of contact:
Neal Lane, Ph.D., Director
(703) 306-1000
Public Affairs
(703) 306-1070
Address:
4201 Wilson Boulevard
Arlington, VA 22230

Description. The NSF, established in 1950, is an independent federal agency devoted to the promotion and advancement of science and engineering, including education in these fields. Overseen by a presidentially appointed director and a board of 24 scientists, university officials, and industry leaders, the NSF is responsible for the overall "health" of science and scientific research across all disciplines. It pursues this mission by awarding grants to research institutions; because the NSF operates no in-house laboratories, it supports cooperative research efforts by universities and industry. Secondary interests include boosting the nation's scientific and technical literacy and monitoring human and fiscal resources for science and engineering.

Seven directorates compose the NSF; they are the Directorates for Social, Behavioral, and Economic Sciences; Biological Sciences; Computer and Information Science and Engineering; Education and Human Resources; Engineering; Geosciences; and Mathematical and

Physical Sciences. The first two directorates are of particular interest to psychiatric researchers and are profiled with their division components.

◆ Directorate for Social, Behavioral, and Economic Sciences (SBE)

Description. The SBE seeks to advance science and engineering in social sciences by collecting and analyzing social and behavioral sciences and resources. It develops basic science in human social behavior, interaction, and decision making. The major programs include social and economic science, including research in economics, law, political science, and sociology; behavioral and cognitive sciences, including research in language, cognition, and behavior, science and technology, and anthropology; sciences resources studies; and international cooperative science and engineering research. Initiatives in the SBE include human perception and interactions, research on global political change, economics of manufacturing and intelligence systems, and poverty.

Head. Cora Bagley Marrett, Ph.D., (703) 306-1700

First-level division. Division of Social, Behavioral, and Economic Research

Description. Research support is provided in economics, geography, sociology, social research measurement methods and data improvement, political science, legal issues in social science, decision/risk management, and behavioral issues, including anthropology, language cognition, and social behavior.

Head. Allen Kornberg, Ph.D., (703) 306-1766

First-level division. Division of International Programs

Description. Scientific activities mandating international cooperation are of great interest to this division.

Head. Marcel Bardon, Ph.D., (703) 306-1710

First-level division. Division of Science Resources Studies

Description. This division supports studies of science and engineering resources.

Head. Kenneth Brown, (703) 306-1780

◆ **Directorate of Biological Sciences (BIO)**
Description. The BIO supports research in molecular and cellular biosciences, including cell biology, biochemistry, and genetics; integrative biology and neuroscience, including developmental mechanisms, neuroscience, neural mechanisms of behavior, neuroendocrinology, animal behavior, and integrative plant biology; environmental biology; and biological instrumentation and resources.
Head. Mary Clutter, Ph.D., (703) 306-1400

First-level division. Biological Instrumentation and Resources
Description. Support is provided for instrumentation and instrument development, as well as special projects dealing with technology development.
Head. Susan Stafford, Ph.D., (703) 306-1470

First-level division. Molecular and Cellular Biosciences
Description. Areas of research support include biochemistry and molecular structure and function, cell biology, and genetics and nucleic acids.
Head. James Brown, Ph.D., (703) 306-1440

First-level division. Integrative Biology and Neurosciences
Description. Areas of research include physiology and behavior, neurosciences, and developmental biology.
Head. Thomas Brady, Ph.D. (Acting), (703) 306-1420

First-level division. Environmental Biology
Description. Systematics and population biology, ecological studies, and long-term projects in environmental biology are the main areas of research interest.
Head. James Gosz, Ph.D., (703) 306-1480

NSF selected program announcements:
    Small Grants for Exploratory Research
    Neural Mechanisms of Behavior

DEPARTMENT OF JUSTICE (DOJ)

Point of contact:
    Janet Reno, Attorney General
    (202) 514-2001

Philip B. Heumann, Deputy Attorney General
Public Affairs
(202) 514-2007
Office of Justice Programs
(202) 307-5933
Address:
633 Indiana Avenue, NW
Washington, DC 20531

Description. The Department of Justice serves as the chief legal institution for the federal government and oversees law enforcement functions for the government, providing advice to the president, the cabinet, and federal agencies, and provides federal legal services. The Office of Justice Programs (OJP) is the part of the DOJ that is responsible for program policy and research on crime, criminal behaviors, delinquency, victims, and related technology, and other areas of psychiatric research interest.

◆ Office for Victims of Crime
Description. This office provides leadership to states and localities through grants to balance the system of justice by assisting and compensating victims, including program guidelines, training assistance, and implementation activities. It aims to ensure that crime victims are an integral part of the justice process and are afforded fairness, respect, and courtesy. Research of psychiatric interest sponsored by this office includes topics of victim stress, anxiety, and trauma.
Head. Brenda Meister (Acting), (202) 307-5983

◆ National Institute of Justice (NIJ)
Description. The NIJ is the main research and development agency of DOJ. It was established to prevent and reduce crime and to improve the criminal justice system. As mandated by Congress, its purview includes R&D programs that improve and strengthen the criminal justice system and prevent/reduce crime, national demonstration projects, technology development to fight crime, evaluations of effectiveness of current programs, research on criminal behavior, and new methods of crime prevention and reeducation.
Head. Michael Russell (Acting), (202) 307-2942

◆ **Office of Juvenile Justice and Delinquency Prevention**
Description. This office administers state formula grants for state and local governments designed to assist states in removing juveniles from adult jails, removing status offenders from institutions, and separating adults from juveniles in correctional facilities. It also has a special emphasis discretionary grant program designed to improve the juvenile justice system and prevent delinquency. Most research focuses on prevention and intervention issues associated with juveniles and crime.
Head. John Wilson (Acting), (202) 307-5911

DOJ selected program announcement:
     Annual Discretionary Grant Program at the DOJ

DEPARTMENT OF DEFENSE AND RELATED ORGANIZATIONS

◆ **Air Force Office of Scientific Research (AFOSR)**
Point of contact:
     Helmut Hellwig, Ph.D., Director
     (202) 767-5017
     Daniel L. Collins, Ph.D., Life Sciences
     (202) 767-5021
     Technical Information
     (202) 767-4910
Address:
     AFOSR/NL
     110 Duncan Avenue
     Bolling Air Force Base
     Washington, DC 20332

Description. The AFOSR supports both extramural and intramural basic research on life science issues that are of interest to the Air Force within its Directorate of Life and Environmental Sciences. Areas of interest to psychiatric investigators include research in neuroscience, chronobiology, perception and recognition, spatial orientation, and cognition. Opportunities for collaborative research between Air Force researchers and academic scientists are encouraged, and opportunities for short- and long-term research training exist as well.
     The neuroscience program supports basic research on the neuro-

biology of behavior, with the aim of understanding the neural mechanisms determining the effectiveness of skilled persons performing demanding mental and physical tasks. Research focuses on neuronal responsiveness, learning and memory, fatigue, attention, and arousal, with a particularly strong focus on the psychobiology of stress. For additional information, contact Genevieve M. Haddad, Ph.D., (202) 767-5021. The chronobiology program focuses on the biological mechanisms responsible for circadian rhythms and their influence on behavior and skilled human performance. Research on neurophysiology, pharmacology, and behavior and circadian rhythm regulations are of special interest. For additional information, contact Genevieve M. Haddad, Ph.D., (202) 767-5021.

Research on visual and auditory theory and modeling and psychophysical research aims to discover and quantitatively model featural processing mechanisms underlying sensory patterns, perception, and recognition. For additional information, contact John F. Tangney, Ph.D., (202) 767-5021. Cognition research explores the cognitive processes of individual and small teams, particularly the performance-related aspects of attention, memory, information processing, learning, reasoning, problem solving, and decision making under stress. Research support is given for behavioral methods or a combination of behavioral and biological or computational methods. For additional information, contact John F. Tangney, Ph.D., (202) 767-5021.

AFOSR selected program announcements:
   University Initiative for Academic-AFOSR Collaboration
   Basic Research on Circadian Rhythms and Human
      Chronobiology

Army Research Office (ARO)

◆ **Army Research Institute for the
   Behavioral and Social Sciences (ARI)**
Point of contact:
   Michael Kaplan, Director, Basic Research
   (703) 274-8641
   Michael Drillings, Ph.D., Performance Processes
   (703) 274-5572

Address:
   5001 Eisenhower Avenue
   ATTN: PERI-BR
   Alexandria, VA 22333

Description. ARI is the behavioral research arm of the Army Research Office, with the purpose of researching and developing behavior and behavioral technologies to improve the effectiveness of Army personnel and their units. ARI supports research in its Office of Basic Research, which attempts to add new, fundamental knowledge to behavioral science subdisciplines. It is interested in funding innovative concepts and methodologies that advance new behavioral science discoveries in areas such as language, learning, and cognition; individual and group performance, including issues of motivation, stress, and peer pressure; human chronopsychology; and other innovative methodologies in behavioral and social science.

ARI selected program announcements:
   Behavioral and Social Sciences Technology Research
   Fundamental Research in Behavioral Science

Office of Naval Research (ONR)

Point of contact:
   Bruce B. Robinson, Director
   (703) 696-4101
   Scott A. Sandgathe, Deputy Director
   (703) 696-4102
Address:
   800 North Quincy Street
   Arlington, VA 22217

Description. The ONR was established in 1946 to encourage scientific research programs increasing knowledge that is paramount to the maintenance of future naval power and national security. The ONR focuses this research through its Research Programs Department (RPD), which funds a base research program (70% of funding) and accelerated research initiatives (30%). The RPD also aims to attract and train outstanding students in science and engineering. The RPD base research funding is directed to four directorates: Mathematical and Physical Sciences Programs, Ocean Sciences Programs,

Engineering Sciences Programs, and Life Sciences Programs; this last directorate and its divisions are profiled. Other ONR components of interest to psychiatric investigators include the Navy Personnel Research and Development Center and the Naval Medical Research and Development Command.

◆ **Life Sciences Programs Directorate**
Description. The Life Sciences Programs Directorate encourages basic research in understanding fundamental principles of biological organization and the functioning of human beings in complex environments. The directorate is committed to explorations at the leading edges of biotechnology, molecular and cellular biology, neurobiology, sensory perception, cognition, learning and memory, decision making, and human–machine interactions.
Head.   Steven F. Zornetzer, (703) 696-4501

First-level division.   Biological Sciences Division
Description.   This division supports the development of fundamental knowledge in molecular and cell biology, marine biology, immunophysiology, biochemistry, biophysics, molecular genetics, microbiology, and sensory biology.
Head.   Robert W. Newburgh, (703) 696-4986

First-level division.   Cognitive and Neural Sciences Division
Description.   This division supports the development of fundamental knowledge about human capabilities and performance characteristics in guiding restructuring of naval personnel codes. Understanding neurobiological constraints/computational capabilities/ performance enhancement of the human is central to this division's research. Application to artificial intelligence is also an important research issue.
Head.   Willard S. Vaughan, (703) 696-4505

◆ **Navy Personnel Research and Development Center**
Description.   The Navy Personnel Research and Development Center is responsible for the creation and updating of all testing and training procedures within the Navy. Areas of interest to psychiatric researchers include instructional technology, the design and management of instructional contingencies between teachers, material, and students, personnel testing, and bioelectric and biomagnetic brain wave research.
Head.   Robert Thorpe, (619) 553-0754

◆ Naval Medical Research and Development Command

Description. The Naval Medical Research and Development Command provides the focal point for research and development medical investigations for the Navy. It operates seven laboratories and detachments throughout the United States. Major research topics include combat casualty care, infectious diseases and AIDS, diving and submarine medicine, aviation medicine and human performance, environmental and occupational medicine, and combat dentistry. Major components of the command include the Naval Health Research Center, the Naval Biodynamics Laboratory, the Naval Aerospace Medical Research Laboratory, and the Naval Medical Research Institute.
Head. Anthony Melaragno, (202) 295-1468

ONR selected program announcements:
Functional Consequences of Stress and Traumatic Injury
Behavioral Sciences Research

◆ North Atlantic Treaty Organization (NATO)

Point of contact:
Scientific Affairs Division
Address:
Scientific Affairs Division, B-1110
Brussels, Belgium

Description. The NATO Science Programme was established in 1958 in recognition of the role science and technology play in maintaining economic, political, and military strength in the Atlantic Community. The programs are designed to promote and encourage more effective research in the allied countries by providing the stimulus of constant interaction between scientists and laboratories. These programs include the International Scientific Exchange Programmes, which focus on individual scientists in both the university and private sectors. Support is offered as fellowships for postgraduate training or research in another NATO country and Collaborative Research Grants, given to international research teams in NATO countries to support travel and living expenses of investigators. Other programs include advanced study institutes, advanced research workshops, and other special projects and the Science for Stability Programme, which assists Greece, Portugal, and Turkey in the development of their scientific and technological infrastructures and projects.

National Aeronautics and Space Administration (NASA)

Point of contact:
Daniel Goldin, Administrator
(202) 358-1010
Lennard Fisk, Space Science and Applications
(202) 358-1409
Ronald White, Life Sciences Program Officer
(202) 453-1525
Public Affairs
(202) 358-0000
Address:
Life Sciences Division, Code EB
Office of Space Science and Applications
300 E Street, SW
Washington, DC 20546

Description. The National Aeronautics and Space Administration funds a wide range of research supporting its mission to research flight within and outside the earth's atmosphere, including study in the life sciences and space medicine. The main research component dealing with psychiatric and mental health issues is the Office of Space Science and Applications, which conducts research on the origin, evolution, and components of the universe. Life science issues of interest in this office include cell functioning for disease treatment; pharmaceutical, health care, and agricultural production; and applied research in crystal growth for biotechnology or drug development. Areas of particular interest to psychiatric investigators include studies on environmental human health and performance.

NASA selected program announcements:
Pilot Studies in Space Research
Research in Gravitational Biology

DEPARTMENT OF AGRICULTURE (AG)

Point of contact:
Dan Glickman, Secretary
(202) 720-3631

Charles Hess, Science and Education
(202) 720-5923
R. D. Plowman, Agricultural Research Service
(202) 720-3656
Public Affairs (202) 720-2798
Address:
14th & Independence Avenue, SW
Washington, DC 20250

Description. The AG oversees policy and research related to agriculture and farming within the United States. Its research activities are administered by the Office of Science and Education; although most research focuses on the agricultural sciences, environment, forestry, and animal and plant issues, limited behavioral research has been supported on stress and the farmer, agricultural crisis management, and rural concerns.

DEPARTMENT OF ENERGY (DOE)

Point of contact:
Hazel O'Leary, Secretary
(202) 586-6210
Public Affairs
(202) 586-5575
Address:
1000 Independence Avenue, SW
Washington, DC 20585

Description. The DOE oversees federal energy policy issues, including programs in nuclear energy, conservation, international affairs in energy emergencies, fossil programs, energy research, and other administrative functions. Although most of its research is related to the physical sciences, the DOE does support research concerning the human genome project, including social and ethical concerns. For more information on DOE's human genome research, contact Dan Drell at (301) 903-6488.

DOE selected program announcements:
Ethical, Legal, and Social Implications of Genome Research
Human Genome Technical Advances

DEPARTMENT OF TRANSPORTATION (DOT)

Point of contact:
Frederico Pena, Secretary
(202) 366-1111
Travis P. Dungan, Research and Special Programs
(202) 366-4831
Public Affairs
(202) 366-5580
Address:
400 7th Street, SW
Washington, DC 20590

Description. The DOT deals with policy and issues affecting most areas of transportation within the United States. Composed of a wide range of agencies, such as the Coast Guard, Federal Aviation Administration, Maritime Administration, and Federal Highway Administration, the DOT supports research through its Research and Special Programs Administration, which focuses on R&D to improve safety systems, including pipeline safety and hazardous materials shipment, effective and viable transportation systems, and economic matters affecting the airline industry. The DOT is limited in its support of mental health research; topics of possible psychiatric research interest that have been funded in the past include the relation of stress and accidents, alcohol and drug abuse and travel systems and accidents, and the effects of sleep and its lack on professionals within the travel industry.

CHAPTER

4

Foundations and Nonprofit Research Support

Theodora Fine, M.A.

F ew researchers, particularly those engaged in psychiatric research, venture far beyond the federal government for support
of their basic, clinical, epidemiological, or health services research
activities. After all, the federal government remains the dominant
source of U.S. funds for overall health research and development,
accounting for some $11.3 billion in 1990 alone (Office of Science
Policy and Legislation 1991). When casting the funding net beyond
the federal circle of grant giving, researchers tend to think of the
private nonprofit sector, represented primarily by the nation's more
than 30,000 foundations. Interest in foundation support is not particularly surprising; such organizations are established for the express purpose of distributing private wealth to do public good. The
nature of that "public good" is defined by each foundation, often
phrased in broad terms, enabling it to cast its own wide net for programs worthy of support. Notwithstanding the availability of foundation support and the interest in tapping this resource, few
researchers are well armed to identify and work with a foundation
to receive its support. This chapter offers some insights into the na-

128 Research Funding and Resource Manual

ture and structure of foundations, the extent of current support for mental health research, and the mechanisms available through which access to and funding by foundations may be achieved.

◆ The Nature and Characteristics of Foundations

Defining Foundations

Andrews has described a foundation as a "nongovernmental, nonprofit organization having a principal fund of its own, managed by its own trustees or directors, and established to maintain or aid social, educational, charitable, religious, or other activities serving the common welfare" (Andrews 1956, p. 11). Within this broad definition, foundations range widely in size, organization, orientation, and giving patterns. Four types of foundations have been identified by the philanthropic community and by tax statute:

◆ *Independent foundations* are those private nonprofit entities traditionally associated with the concept of a foundation. The endowment that underwrites the foundation generally is derived from a single source (most often a family, individual, or group of individuals). Funding priorities are determined and awards are made by the donor, the donor's family, a board of trustees, or board of directors. Classic examples of such independent foundations are the MacArthur Foundation, the Pew Charitable Trusts, and the Ford Foundation. Of the foundations identified and catalogued in the *Foundation Directory*, fully 82.6% (or 6,264 foundations) are defined as independent foundations.
◆ *Company-sponsored foundations* are named for and supported by annual donations from parent for-profit corporations. The foundation serves to shelter corporate profits and to render community or national service through giving. Just as the interests of the sponsor of an independent foundation are reflected in the foundation's objectives, the focus of the corporate sponsor generally is reflected in the giving patterns of the company-sponsored foundation. Thus, corporate foundations related to the health care industry may focus grant attention in the areas of health care services and research. The distilling industry often

focuses grants in the area of substance abuse prevention, as a countervailing force to criticisms of the corporate parent. Similarly, foundations connected to heavy industry and energy production may place an emphasis on environmental issues. Grant-making decisions are made most often by a board of directors that may include both corporate and noncorporate officials, providing a diversity of opinion to the grant-giving process. These foundations include such common corporate names as the Westinghouse Foundation, the GTE Foundation, and the Merck Foundation. This growing group of foundations represents nearly a 13% share of the Foundation Center's top 7,581 foundations, with annual giving of $1.3 billion.

◆ *Community foundations*, while functioning in a manner similar to that of independent foundations, depend on support from a multiplicity of sources. Indeed, in order to qualify as "public charities," and not be subject to many of the tax rules and regulations governing other types of foundations, community foundations must meet a "public support" test. A certain proportion of funds is required to be at-large public donations, not coming from major donors or corporate sponsors. While they constitute a growing area of nonprofit support, community foundations as a class represent a much smaller share of annual foundation giving—generally less than 3% of total giving in any single year. Grants generally are made at the local level; decisions are made by a board of directors or trustees that is representative of the community in which the foundation is located. Grants, too, tend to be community-based, focusing more on services than on research. Among the largest of these foundations are the Houston Endowment, the New York Community Trust, and the San Francisco Foundation. While community foundations rank third in both number and total giving, nine of these foundations are ranked in the top 100 of all foundations when ranked by assets (Foundation Center 1991). These include the New York Community Trust ($830 million), the Houston Endowment ($615 million), the Cleveland Foundation ($580 million), the Marin Community Foundation ($457 million), the Chicago Community Trust ($316 million), the Colorado Trust ($233 million), the Northwest Area Foundation ($228 million), and the San Francisco Foundation ($194 million).

◆ *Operating foundations* are single- or special-purpose organizations, designated as foundations for tax purposes, that use their resources to conduct research or to provide a direct service. Grants made by such foundations generally support work related directly to the foundation's purpose. Endowments may be from a single source or from a variety of sources, including public contributions. These include organizations such as the World Wildlife Fund, the United Way, and, in the health field, the March of Dimes, the American Cancer Society, the Cystic Fibrosis Foundation, and the American Foundation for AIDS Research (AFAR). Because grant giving is restricted to the specific field of direct interest, operating foundations provide the smallest share of foundation support, $92.8 million in 1990 (Foundation Center 1991).

However, health care-related operating foundations are the most likely direct source of research support among all types of foundations. At the height of the polio epidemic, for example, the March of Dimes supported considerable research directed toward the cause, cure, and treatment of this disorder. More recently, AFAR has supported a substantial number of AIDS researchers or has supplemented federal support to these researchers. While not yet reaching the stature of the American Cancer Society or the American Lung Association, the National Alliance for Research on Schizophrenia and Depression (NARSAD) has since 1986 grown and flourished as the only operating foundation dedicated to mental illness research. It has done this through donations from large and small contributors, including funds received from independent foundations.

A fifth type of organization, combining features of an independent foundation and an operating foundation, exists in the form of the Medical Research Organization (MRO). The most notable of these organizations is the Howard Hughes Medical Institute (HHMI), now a significant source of support for exceptional biomedical researchers and research facilities. It has grown, through judicious investments, in its 40 years of existence; it began in 1953 with the transfer of the assets of Hughes Aircraft to the HHMI. After a quiescent period, the HHMI emerged in 1985 as the world's richest and perhaps most generous medical philanthropy, outstripping the Ford Foundation by nearly $2 billion in assets and the Robert Wood Johnson Foundation by as much as $4 billion. (For a detailed description of the HHMI, the reader is referred to Resources 4–1, Profiles of Foundation Funding Sources.)

What differentiates MROs from other foundations that support health care is that the MRO itself must be engaged actively in medical research in conjunction with a hospital. Thus, individuals and facilities that receive support from an MRO become part of the MRO itself. In exchange, the MRO is able to avoid many of the tax law burdens imposed on other types of private foundations.

The unique role of foundations in the support of health care and medical education is set forth by another author (Gunzburger 1994), who gives thumbnail sketches of 31 foundations working in these arenas. She concludes that foundations have offered government, medical schools, and other health-promoting institutions an array of innovative options and have thus provided challenges to these institutions to stretch toward better ways of fulfilling their missions.

The Economics of Foundations

In 1990, foundations awarded over $7.5 billion in grants; foundation holdings totaled over $130 billion (extrapolated from Foundation Center data). These figures exclude awards made by the HHMI, since it does not give awards to outside organizations but brings those organizations under the HHMI research umbrella through support of specific identified research scientists of excellence. The Foundation Center identifies the nation's largest and most active foundations in its annual compendium of foundations and grant giving, the *Foundation Directory*. The directory includes only those foundations either with assets of at least $1 million or with annual giving of $100,000 or more. Other resources developed by the Foundation Center and by other nonprofit and for-profit entities detail foundations of smaller size.

The 7,581 foundations identified in the 13th edition of this volume represent approximately one-fourth of all U.S. grant-making foundations. Yet, in the last year for which IRS records are available, this same cadre of foundations actually held all but 4% of all foundation fiscal resources and made 93% of all grant awards (Foundation Center 1991).

However, the sum of foundation support remains small in comparison to that amassed through all sources of funding. The financial base of foundations constitutes less than 5% of the dollars expended by all private sector organizations; foundation grant giving totals under 4% of the private sector's total operating expenditures (Ylvisaker 1987). Indeed, Ylvisaker reports that foundation giving totals less than four cents of every dollar spent by independent-sector (read "private-sector") organizations, and is outmatched by total federal spending at a ratio of approximately 200:1.

While the absolute dollars awarded by foundations pale in comparison to overall independent sector giving and are minuscule when weighed against federal support, they represent a significant portion of this nation's sheltered wealth. Thus "the public cannot afford to regard with indifference how foundation funds are spent, so precious are they . . . in the vital process of social change, and so limited are they in amount" (Reeves 1970, p. 55).

The magnitude of foundation giving and the sheer concentration of wealth represented by these entities have not escaped the watchful eyes of federal legislators who, over the years, concerned about the tax benefits reaped by foundations, have imposed greater restrictions and reporting requirements on the two largest types of foundations: independent and corporate foundations. These reporting requirements, including public disclosure of grant giving, have provided tools through which those seeking foundation support can identify and target sources based on past funding histories detailed in the tax records. In contrast to federal grant-making processes, foundation grant-giving decisions are not made "in the sunshine"; thus, tax records have shed considerable light on foundation decision-making processes, a subject described later in this chapter. As also discussed later, these tax records have enabled the careful investigator to discern potential sources of support that are not evident from reports of particular foundations' specified funding interests.

Range of Activities Supported

Notwithstanding their relatively small contribution to overall national giving, foundations play an important and influential role in the public and private sectors alike. In the aggregate, foundations donate their wealth to many traditional causes: the church, institutions of higher education, social welfare programs, the arts, and the sciences. When viewed collectively, foundations appear to support predominantly mainstream causes, in part as the result of trustee conservatism and in part as the result of tax code strictures imposed over the last 30 years (Ylvisaker 1987).

Global evaluation of these highly individualized and personalized organizations, however, does them a disservice. The very nature of funding from this source varies considerably from that found in the federal or corporate sectors. Foundation interests are as varied as the interests of individual foundation trustees or members of a foundation's board of directors. Foundations may be established for self-interested reasons or for altruistic ones; foundation philosophies may be liberal or conservative. Just as federal program emphases may change from time to time, so too may the interests of foundations. Indeed, foundations often have been on the cutting edge of future public and private sector policy, influencing the direction of that policy by supporting innovative and untried concepts.

Two attributes of foundations, providing considerable flexibility, enable foundations to initiate social change and innovations in a manner distinctly different from and faster than government programs and corporate initiatives. In contrast to the federal sector, foundations are unfettered by congressional mandates limiting their discretion. In contrast to corporate decision making, foundation decisions are not subject to scrutiny of shareholders; they need not be profitable or guaranteed successes. Thus, within identified areas of interest that have been painted with a broad stroke and with a substantial endowment, foundations have both the financial capacity and the freedom to support the experimental and the unconventional. Moreover, because they have uncommitted funds available to them at any given time, foundations are able to move quickly to support particularly unusual or novel projects that come before their boards of directors or their trustees (Kim et al. 1988).

Historically, foundation support and federal support have experienced an interesting and intertwined relationship, particularly in the area of health care research. For example, while the Rockefeller Foundation essentially built today's academic medical education and research centers through the 1940s and 1950s, it subsequently withdrew to other pursuits when the federal government stepped into the biomedical and behavioral research endeavor (Daniel X. Freedman, personal communication). The Pew Charitable Trusts 1987 report, *U.S. Funding for Biomedical Research* (Boniface and Rimel 1987) noted that over the past 30-odd years, foundations generally have adopted the role of the "venture capitalist." Common strategies include support of the first independent efforts of young researchers and initial investment in emerging fields of research. Rather than resenting the federal usurpation of carefully nurtured research initiatives, foundations have come to view this development as a signal of success.

Thus, foundations tend to engage in areas that are either under-funded or not funded at all at the federal level.

While the federal government remains the dominant source of U.S. funds for overall health research and development, foundations as a whole represent an interesting and generally untapped resource. The nature of foundation funding "offer[s] a case where a technically private asset is of such potential value to the nation that it must, perforce, be regarded as a public asset" (Reeves 1970, p. 55).

◆ Foundation Structure and Decision Making

Without regard to its phenotype, foundations generally are structured similarly, with a board that bears ultimate responsibility for decision making and, in the case of the larger active foundations, a staff that undertakes the day-to-day office work necessary to the grant-giving process. The benefactor, a board of directors or trustees, or, in the case of community foundations, a disbursement committee, establishes the goals and mission of the foundation, identifies investment strategies to maintain the fiscal soundness of the foundation's resources, and makes a range of grant-giving decisions. Because few restrictions are placed on foundation giving patterns, a foundation's donors and/or board of directors have wide latitude to determine the fields of endeavor chosen for funding support and the levels of that funding. Within these broad parameters, however, foundations function idiosyncratically, with greater or lesser involvement by the governing board and staff (if present), with greater or lesser specificity in goals, and with greater or lesser presence in the public eye.

The Board

Foundation boards of directors or boards of trustees vary in size and composition. As noted earlier, community foundations are required to maintain boards that reflect the diversity of the community; corporate foundations most frequently include key corporate personnel and, on occasion, scientists or other individuals renowned in the field of the corporation's activities. Thus, pharmacology experts from academia may sit on the boards of various pharmaceutical company foundations; energy experts and environmentalists may serve on the boards of petroleum industry foundations. Such a composition not only provides alternative viewpoints but guards against self-interest, a matter of significant concern in tax law. Independent foundation boards may include the benefactor or family of the benefactor, coupled with distinguished individuals in business, academia, and other walks of life that are related directly to the general goals and missions of the foundation. At least one member of the board generally is expert in the field of investment banking to help direct the investments that maintain the foundation's grant-giving capacity. Indeed, over the past decade, foundations have become increasingly concerned that their beneficent activities and their investment strategies are consonant; ethical issues such as investment in South Africa, in industries that affect the environment or in real estate, pose potential incongruities in the context of grant giving that require resolution (Ylvisaker 1987).

The Staff

Foundation staffing is a relatively new development in the history of foundations and varies widely. Among the 7,581 foundations catalogued in the *Foundation Directory*, the vast majority maintain staffs. Tax law has restricted the administrative costs that may be paid out by a foundation, holding down both the number of staff and the salaries available. The presence of staff is advantageous to the conduct of a foundation's activities; simply, a greater number of proposals can be reviewed and evaluated in greater depth. Indeed, small awards (perhaps under $25,000) may be left to the discretion of the foundation's chief of staff, subject to board monitoring on a regularly scheduled basis. At the same time, however, the presence of staff may create additional tensions. Ylvisaker has noted that staff-board tensions

> may stem from differences among trustees in which staff can easily get caught; differences in personalities and perspectives; conflicting interpretations of board and staff prerogatives; . . . the imperative for trustees to reserve judgment; [and] the inherent subjectivity in analyzing and deciding social issues.

Moreover, in the search for the innovative and untried, staff and board members may reach an impasse, whether because what appears innovative to the staff does not appear novel to the board or because the board's decision making moves too slowly for the often younger and more enthusiastic staff.

Decision-Making Process

Most foundations maintain a series of general areas of interest—health care, social welfare, international relations, environment, among others—that often are dictated by the conditions of the initial foundation bequest or by the corporate sponsor. However, within the stated area or areas of interest, the foundation's directors often sharpen the focus. This greater selectivity of subject allows the foundation to concentrate its influence. Thus, the Retirement Research Foundation has emphasized aging; the Kaiser Family Foundation supports efforts to improve the practice of medicine and delivery of health care; the Spencer Foundation underwrites projects in education. While the Ittleson Foundation's general focus is on health, welfare, and education for health and welfare, it has winnowed this overly broad area down to place special emphasis on mental health, including public education for mental health and psychiatric research. Even within this more narrow focus, its priorities may change from year to year or from funding cycle to funding cycle based on the ebb and flow of unmet needs or shifting opportunities.

Grant-giving decisions are made somewhat differently from foundation to foundation. Over the years, the number of foundations with clearly identified funding interests has grown, in part as the result of codified "Recommended Principles and Practices" established by the Council on Foundations for use predominantly by independent foundations. Government tax regulations, too, have forced greater uniformity and clarity of grant processing and evaluation practices, requiring an extensive paper trail from receipt of the proposal through award of funds to the completion of the funded project or program. However, neither the size of awards nor the nature of the funding cycle is consistent from foundation to foundation. Awards may range from as little as $50 to millions of dollars; grant decisions may be made annually, semiannually, quarterly, or on an ad hoc basis. Here, too, much depends on the size of the foundation, its board, and its staff.

How foundations become known to prospective grantees varies widely. According to Ylvisaker (1987):

Foundations range from being extremely active—assertively promoting their objectives and soliciting proposals—to being extremely
passive, accepting whatever requests come their way. Most operate
somewhere in the middle, leading when they . . . know what they
want to accomplish, but following when they are in a noncommittal and exploratory mode.

Some foundations publish annual reports that detail past
spending and current areas of interest in an effort to solicit grant
applications. These foundations tend to be among the largest and
those with the most extensive portfolios of grant support. Other
foundations are more passive, providing information when requested and reviewing unsolicited applications or proposals when
submitted. The most aggressive and generally larger foundations
become well known by underwriting large-scale, innovative projects with well-recognized project directors or university-based project teams that receive widespread media coverage. This serves both
to enhance the foundation's public image and to boost the number
of likely new grant proposals to be received for the next funding
cycle.

◆ Foundations and Mental Health/ Substance Abuse Research

In 1985, private foundations made grants, gifts, and awards totaling
$4.3 billion, a sum over 4.5 times that of the fiscal year 1992 com-
bined extramural research budgets of the three former Alcohol, Drug
Abuse, and Mental Health Administration institutes. Yet, over the
past three decades, foundations in general have not placed significant
emphasis on mental health as a focus of endowment; even less attention has been paid to grants for mental health research. In 1982,
foundation support for the broadly defined category of mental
health totaled only 1.1% of all grant dollars. Two years later, the
Foundation Center reported that among the 4,402 then most active
foundations, the percentage had risen to only 1.7% of all foundation
grant dollars. In 1978, the President's Commission on Mental Health
reported that private sector support for mental health research was
"shockingly low," accounting for only 3.5% of the total federal and
private support to mental health research (PCMH 1978). By 1985,
that figure had not changed as a proportion of total giving to the
field; it remained at 3.5% (Pincus and Fine 1992). The Institute of

Medicine (IOM) (Board on Mental Health and Behavioral Medicine 1984) found that of the nation's 970 largest foundations (funded on either a national or regional basis), fewer than 30 identified mental health, psychiatry, or psychology as an area of interest or support. The IOM found the results surprisingly low in light of the marked progress being made in basic and clinical mental illness research. Until the establishment of the National Alliance for Research in Schizophrenia and Affective Disorders (NARSAD) in 1986, no single major national operating foundation focused on mental illness. In its first 5 years of existence, NARSAD awarded nearly 300 research grants, spending $11 million, a considerable sum for the field, but only 1% of the National Institute of Mental Health (NIMH) extramural research budgets over the same 5-year period.

A study conducted by the American Psychiatric Association's (APA) Office of Research, assessing the extent of foundation support for mental health research and attempting to determine the characteristics of such foundations, attested to the frustration and potential of foundation support for mental health research. Prospective foundations were identified from a variety of written and database sources provided by the Foundation Center, including the *Foundation Directory*, the *Foundation Grants Index Annual and Database* (listing all foundation grants over $5,000 in any given reporting year), and microfiche copies of foundation-submitted mandatory Internal Revenue Service Form 99-PF, which records detailed information about annual grant giving by individual foundations. (The study defined "mental health research" to include a stated interest in any research on mental illness or illnesses in general, psychiatric research, and behavioral or biomedical research related to mental illness.) When assessing specific grant activities, a number of topic areas were included in the definition: affective, emotional and social development; psychopharmacology; neuropsychiatry; neuropsychology; psychosocial development; geriatric mental disorders; mental disorders of childhood and adolescence; and psychotic disorders (Kim et al. 1988). (Basic, clinical, health services, and epidemiological research were considered within the definition.)

Working from this broad definition, the researchers undertook a close evaluation of the data sources for the period 1983–1985. The annual reports of 63 foundations were found to contain a specific stated interest in the broader area of mental health. The majority supported mental health services, not research, viewing service delivery as a pressing social issue, comparable to health care for AIDS victims, housing the homeless, and feeding the hungry. Only 15 of these 63 foundations actually had made at least one grant for mental health research. Surprisingly, the study found another 29 foundations that had made awards for mental health research despite the fact that mental health in general and mental health research in particular were not identified as areas of foundation focus. Thus, of the 4,402 foundations evaluated, only 44 private foundations actually made at least one grant in the area of mental health research. Of these foundations, only eight appeared highly likely to support future research; six were considered unlikely future sources.

Four general reasons for foundation giving to the mental health research field were identified by the study: identified interest in mental health, receipt of a mental health proposal with a target population or subject relevant to the major area of interest, interest in general medical research, or sufficiently broad interests to encompass mental health research.

In a separate evaluation, the APA's Office of Research found that substance abuse research suffered much the same fate with respect to foundation support. The Foundation Center reported that of the 4,402 foundations responsible for more than 97% of all grant giving between 1983 and 1987, only 337 made awards categorized as pertaining to substance abuse. The $87 million awarded by these 337 foundations supported service programs almost exclusively; only 0.7% (or just over $600,000) of the support was for grants related to substance abuse research (Pincus and Fine 1992).

The results of the study speak to the paucity of private foundation funding sources for mental health research. Moreover, among the foundations with specified interests in mental health, where support for mental health research might be expected to be highest, only 24% made any grants for research. Efforts to reverse these trends have begun. The ever-increasing excitement and vigor of the psychiatric research enterprise itself already have made a difference. Since the time of the APA study, a significant number of other foundation resources that will support mental health research have been identified. Equally, the emergence of NARSAD, both a fund raiser and a grant giver, has begun to make the link between science and mental illness that may enhance the interest of private philanthropy in mental illness research.

◆ Identifying and Working With Foundations

Foundation grantsmanship bears both close relationships to and differences from grantsmanship in the federal sector. In both sectors, it is critical to identify the most likely sources of support for a particular proposal, to determine the appropriate format and materials to be included in a proposal, and to solicit technical assistance to enhance the likelihood of funding. However, foundation grant giving may be even more competitive than that found in federal grant programs. While rigorous design and scientific merit may allow a proposal to clear a federal peer review panel, the same proposal may fail at a foundation review because a trustee does not believe its results will have a sufficiently wide-ranging impact on society. Moreover, federal initial review groups do not compare applications to each other; they judge each based on its scientific merit and potential. In contrast, foundation boards may compare the potential impact of a host of proposals to determine those most likely to have a positive effect on the foundation's various areas of concern. Indeed, while all grants submitted for a particular grant cycle that receive a priority score at or above a particular level will receive funding in any funding cycle, foundations need not disburse funds in all identified areas of interest in any funding cycle. Timing thus becomes an important factor in soliciting and receiving foundation support. However, before determining when to solicit foundation grants, it is necessary to identify the potential sources of support.

Identifying Foundations

In the field of mental health research, the NIMH obviously represents the most significant source of extramural research support. However, other NIH institutes and other federal agencies also serve as potential award-making entities. For example, Alzheimer's disease research is supported not only by the NIMH but also by the National Institute on Aging (NIA) and the National Institute of Neurological Diseases and Stroke (NINDS). Issues of youth violence are supported by the NIMH, the National Institute on Drug Abuse (NIDA), the National Institute on Alcohol Abuse and Alcoholism (NIAAA), the Department of Justice (DOJ), and the Office of Maternal and Child Health of the Department of Health and Human Services.

Similarly, while certain foundations are obvious sources of support for mental health research, others, perhaps apparently further afield, also provide funding opportunities. Competition for support from foundations such as van Ameringen and MacArthur is keen, primarily because they are widely known to engage in support for mental health research activities. However, the knowledge that foundations without a stated interest in mental health do give grants for mental health research raises optimism that a broader range of resources may be available (Kim et al. 1988). Since mental illness issues affect many different populations and the conceptual approaches include attention to the behavioral and biological sciences, foundations generally interested in biomedical research can be approached. The Foundation Center has identified more than 140 foundations that offer some form of support for medical research.

A variety of source materials is available to identify potential foundation funding sources. The most prominent and comprehensive of these are published by the Foundation Center.

The *Foundation Directory* includes the latest information on foundations with assets of at least $1 million or with annual giving of $100,000 or more. Individual entries for over 7,600 foundations in the 1991 edition provide detailed information about application procedures, types of support awarded, range of grant awards, limitations on giving, donors, board members, staff, and foundation publications. Indexes cross-reference the foundations by donors, officers, and trustees; by geographical location; by specific types of support; and by general purposes. The officer and trustee cross-reference is of particular use. It is surprising to discover how many academic colleagues, neighbors, or acquaintances may sit on foundation boards.

The *Foundation Directory, Part 2,* provides similar information on the second largest set of foundations, those with grant programs ranging from $25,000 to $100,000. Subject directories have also been developed, covering funding in aging; AIDS; children, youth, and families; health; and higher education. A separate subject directory profiles corporate foundations. Each directory provides an annual snapshot of individual foundation funding in each of these fields, with detailed information similar to that found in the *Foundation Directory.* The subject directories also list samples of actual grants made by the foundations in the previous year.

The Foundation Center also provides a host of topic-specific computer-based searches, and, for those without the time or access to one of the Foundation Center's offices, an annual program of searches and information tailored to individual needs.

Other organizations in the for-profit sector provide newsletters on giving, directories, and other resources through which potential foundations may be identified. Newspapers, too, are a source of information, particularly with respect to the larger foundations. Academic offices of sponsored affairs may provide insights into potential foundation funding sources.

Colleagues may also have connections to foundations. A number of psychiatric researchers surveyed by the APA have identified foundations, both large and small, as sources of research support. A number of APA members also sit on the boards of foundations, helping to decide which proposals will benefit from the foundation's beneficence.

Developing a Proposal

Once a listing of potentially interested foundations is compiled, still further data gathering is necessary. If the foundation has an annual report that describes its funding interests, it should be requested; similarly, any specific application forms should be obtained. Increasingly, foundation staffs are providing technical assistance to potential grantees, similar to the way in which federal program officers function. Armed with this information, the researcher should develop a proposal or letter of intent. The nature of the submission varies from foundation to foundation. Some request letters prior to the submission of a formal proposal, enabling the foundation to prescreen potential applicants. Others request submission of the full-blown proposal as the first step in the process.

According to the executive director of a foundation with a long history of awarding grants in the area of mental health research,

> Given the number of proposals that even a small foundation will see in any year, the best way to be heard is to provide a convincing case that the "product" of your research has clear application to either a particular population or an acknowledged societal problem. The conduct of research must be placed in a context through which foundations can perceive the work will have some practical consequence. (David Nee, personal communication, September 1988)

It is critical to remember that foundations generally support proposals that will "make a difference," or that will move promptly toward application in the larger community context. Innovation, creativity, and impact are among the most important components of a successful foundation grant proposal.

◆ Conclusions

While foundations, with few exceptions, have not supported mental health research, the fault is probably not restricted solely to the foundations' mission statements or board directives. In part, mental health research has been a small subset of overall biomedical research activity. With the ever-rising federal commitment to biomedical and behavioral investigation, foundations in the main have looked elsewhere for the disbursement of their funds. Yet even today, innovative, cutting-edge research that might not be supported by traditional research resources remains the province of the foundation, particularly if that research could help influence health care or social policy.

> Whether foundations in the past funded or today fund psychiatric research is, in large part, a product of a combination of factors: how psychiatry presents itself, the extent to which research is perceived as an important component of dealing with mental illness, and the extent to which public—including foundation executives'—perception of mental illness is as a disease and not a "social problem." (Daniel X. Freedman, personal communication, September 1988)

Presenting a convincing case—perhaps more political than scientific—for a research project that clearly demonstrates how the foundation's relatively small contribution will reap significant dividends by helping to meet a significant social need poses the best direct means of eliciting the sought-for foundation support.

◆ References

Andrews FE: Philanthropic Foundations. New York, Russell Sage Foundation, 1956

Board on Mental Health and Behavioral Medicine, Institute of Medicine: Research on Mental Illness and Addictive Disorders: Progress and Prospects. Washington, DC, National Academy Press, 1984

Boniface ZE, Rimel RW: U.S. Funding for Biomedical Research: A Report for The Pew Charitable Trusts. Philadelphia, PA, The Pew Charitable Trusts, 1987

Foundation Center: The Foundation Directory, 13th Edition. Washington, DC, Foundation Center, 1991

Gunzburger LK: Foundations that support medical education and health care: their missions, accomplishments, and unique role. Acad Med 69:8–17, 1994

Kim D, Pincus HA, Fine T: Foundation funding and psychiatric research. Am J Psychiatry 145:830–835, 1988

Office of Science Policy and Legislation: NIH Data Book 1990. Bethesda, MD, National Institutes of Health, 1991

Pincus HA, Fine T: The "anatomy" of research funding for mental illness and addictive disorders. Arch Gen Psychiatry 49:573–579, 1992

Reeves TC (ed): Foundations Under Fire. Ithaca, NY, Cornell University Press, 1970

Research Task Panel, President's Commission on Mental Health (PCMH): Report of the Research Task Panel, in Task Panel Reports Submitted to the President's Commission on Mental Health. Washington, DC, Government Printing Office, 4:1517–1821, 1978

Ylvisaker PN: Foundations and nonprofit organizations, in The Nonprofit Sector: A Research Handbook. Edited by Powell WW. New Haven, CT, Yale University Press, 1987, pp 360–379

Resources 4–1
Profiles of Foundation Funding Sources

◆ Section 1: How to Use the Foundation Profiles: Format

This section provides information about the institutional profiles of foundations and other nonprofit institutions that offer varying levels of support for psychiatric researchers. While an attempt has been made to be as comprehensive as possible, there are certainly foundations that have not been included. Also, foundation giving patterns change and some of those listed may no longer fund projects in psychiatric research. The information on the foundations is divided into five sections, related to the nature of the financial support. This *first section* instructs the user in how the profile section is formatted. The *second section* provides descriptive information on foundations that give some indication of specifically funding psychiatric and mental health-related research; accompanying these profiles is the *third section*, which provides an index organized by research topic of these foundations' funding interests. The *fourth section* of profiles lists foundations that fund general biomedical research and research related to specific diseases that may provide support for psychiatric investigations. The point of contact, organization, address, phone number, and specific areas of research funding interest, if any, are provided. The *fifth section* contains information in the same format as the previous section but lists foundations that have funded mental health research in the past at the local level. The locale of interest to the foundation is listed with these entries.

The profiles in the second section provide the most extensive information, supplying points of contact, address, foundation mission and description, and sample grants, if available. The format of the profiles in this section is as follows:

Title.   Each profile begins with a name of the foundation and, if applicable, an acronym.

Subject codes.   These codes are used to delineate areas of psychiatric research in which the foundation has either expressed an interest or has funded projects. The following subject codes are used:

1   Research training funding/Career development
2   Basic biological sciences/Neuroscience
3   Behavioral/Cognitive sciences
4   Social sciences, including cross-cultural issues
5   Clinical psychobiology
6   Diagnosis/Nosology
7   Epidemiology
8   Psychopharmacology
9   Psychosocial treatments
10   Health/mental health services research
11   Consultation-liaison psychiatry/Behavioral medicine
12   Psychotic disorders/Schizophrenia
13   Affective/Mood disorders
14   Anxiety/Stress-related disorders
15   Personality disorders
16   Child/Adolescent mental disorders
17   Geriatric psychiatry/Delirium, dementia, and other cognitive disorders
18   AIDS
19   Alcohol abuse
20   Other drug abuse
21   Sleep, eating, or sexual disorders
22   Movement disorders and other neurologic conditions
23   Forensic/Legal/Violence issues
24   Other

Other subject areas. If code "24" is listed for a profile, this field will be added to describe other areas that the foundation supports that may be of interest to psychiatric researchers.

Point of contact. The foundation's director, executive director, or grants manager is listed, along with his or her phone number. In some cases, more than one contact may be listed.

Address. This category provides street address, room and building if applicable, city, state, and zip code.

Description. The description of the foundation, its mission, pro–grams, and funding priorities are provided.

Sample grants. If information on recent grants awarded by the foundation is available, they are listed in this field. Information may include the awardee, city, state, amount of the award, and the project funded.

For locating those foundations by subject area, a subject index is provided at the end of this first section.

◆ Section 2: Foundation Profiles

AARP Andrus Foundation (AARP)

Subject code(s):
    4 10 17 19 20 24
Other subject areas:
    Older women's issues; geriatric public policy/health issues.
Point of contact:
    Kenneth G. Cook, Ph.D., Administrator
    (202) 443-6190
Address:
    601 E Street, NW
    Washington, DC 20049

Description. The AARP Andrus Foundation focuses its funding on applied research in gerontology, with a particular emphasis on issues involving behavioral, social, and health science policy, planning, or practice. Grant awards are given to those applicants who address the changes and critical needs of people growing older in the late 20th century. Areas of particular interest in the gerontological research program include research related to alcohol and medication use/ misuse in midlife and older women; adult day care; the influence between public policy and health issues; and aging and mental health, especially studies addressing the role of the physician in the delivery of mental health services to older patients, delivery of mental health services to older populations, and the relationship between physical and mental health.
Sample grants:
    Columbia University, New York, NY. Study of predictors and barriers to older adults participating in psychotherapy and counseling. Year of award: 1993

Eastern Michigan University, Ypsilanti, MI. Study on "Confidence Swindles of Older Consumers: A Positive Behavioral Model for Avoiding Victimization." Year of award: 1993

University of North Carolina, Greensboro, NC. $73,888 to study older adult friendship patterns and mental health. Year of award: 1991

Michigan State University, East Lansing, MI. $175,000 to study mood and memory through the dilemmas associated with coping in the aging process. Year of award: 1991

Old Dominion University, Norfolk, VA. $50,005 to study couples' work/retirement pattern and marital relationships. Year of award: 1991

Catholic University of America, Washington, DC. $74,838 to study the factors associated with the discharge of hospitalized dementia patients. Year of award: 1991

Alcoholic Beverage Medical Research Foundation

Subject code(s):
  16 19
Point of contact:
  A. A. Pawlowski, Ph.D., Vice President
  (410) 327-0361
Address:
  2013 East Monument Street
  Baltimore, MD 21205

Description. Established in 1982, the Alcoholic Beverage Medical Research Foundation provides support for scientific studies on the use and prevention of misuse of alcoholic beverages. It is one of the few organizations in the United States and Canada which provides funds for research in the physiological, epidemiological, behavioral, and social sciences in this field. The mission of the foundation is to prevent alcohol misuse and alcohol problems and to disseminate research knowledge about alcohol.

Current areas of research funding interest include the factors influencing the transition from moderate to excessive use of alcohol, effects of moderate alcohol use on health and behavior, mechanisms underlying the biomedical effects of alcohol, alcohol and youth, alcohol and traffic accidents, and alcohol and work-related issues. The foundation does not provide research support in areas of treatment and complications from advanced alcoholism. Likewise, funding for purely nonresearch activities (education projects and public awareness) is not provided. The types of support from the foundation are research support grants, new research awards, data analysis grants, and pilot/preliminary studies. Application deadlines are February 1 and September 15.

Sample grants:

Cheryl Alexandre, The Johns Hopkins School of Hygiene and Public Health, Baltimore, MD. $40,000 to study gender differences in drinking patterns among rural adolescents. Year of award: 1992

Helene Raskin White, Rutgers University, New Brunswick, NJ. $28,000 to study the effects of moderate levels of alcohol use on physical and mental health. Year of award: 1992

Douglas Kenrick, Arizona State University, Tempe, AZ. $47,200 to study alcohol, arousal, and risk. Year of award: 1992

Vicki Pollock, University of California School of Medicine, Los Angeles, CA. $38,000 to study psychological factors in alcoholism development. Year of award: 1993

M. Lynne Cooper, State University of New York, Buffalo, NY. $39,470 to study adolescent alcohol use and abuse: the influences of family history of alcoholism, parent coping, and expectancies. Year of award: 1990

Gary S. Ward, Johns Hopkins University School of Medicine, Baltimore, MD. $30,000 for the study of alterations in the hypothalamic-pituitary-adrenal axis by ethanol. Year of award: 1990

Andrea M. Allan, Washington University, St. Louis, MO. $25,000 for research on genetic selection on differences in neurochemical responses to alcohol. Year of award: 1990

Allied-Signal Foundation

Subject code(s):
   1 17
Point of contact:
   Alan Painter
   (201) 455-5876

Address:
    PO Box 2245 R
    Morristown, NJ 07960

Description. The Allied-Signal Foundation makes contributions to local and national organizations that relate to the interests of its business operations. Substantial support is provided for education grants and scholarships in areas of biomedical research, especially aging research, and a significant portion is given to the United Way or other capital campaigns in its business communities.

It offers a dual approach for funding aging research. It provides a program offering $30,000 grants to experts in biomedical research and public policy, and it offers general grants for the study of diseases that afflict the elderly.

Alzheimer's Disease and Related Disorders Association, Inc. (ADRDA)

Subject code(s):
    1 17
Point of contact:
    Henrietta Kamp
    (312) 335-5779
Address:
    919 North Michigan, Suite 1000
    Chicago, IL 60611

Description. The ADRDA offers support for research on Alzheimer's disease and other related disorders (ADRD). The Association sponsors three research grant and award programs that are available to qualified investigators from nonprofit institutions; decisions for these awards are made on a competitive, peer review basis, and proposals are rated for innovativeness, scientific rigor, and relevance.

These programs are: 1) Investigator-initiated research grants, structured to provide sustained support for individual research projects. Proposals are solicited for degenerative brain disease and must have the potential to add to knowledge of relevant issues. Maximum of $45,000 per year for 2 or 3 years is given. Applications are due in January with funding given in July. 2) Faculty scholar awards provide sustained salary support to experienced junior faculty level or equivalent investigators who are committed to research on ADRD. Applicants must have 2 years of postgraduate experience; a maximum of $45,000 is given per year for 3 years. Applications are due in January, with funding given in January. 3) Pilot research grants are small 1-year grants for worthwhile research supporting investigators who are new to research in ADRD. The objectives are to stimulate interest by new researchers, enable investigators to test the feasibility of new ideas on a small scale, and enable researchers to generate data to support projects with larger grants from other sources. Proposals are solicited for biological, clinical, and social/behavioral research relevant to degenerative diseases research. Applications are due in July, with December funding.

Sample grants:
> Merrill D. Benson, M.D., Indiana University School of Medicine, Indianapolis, IN. Study of a family with inherited AD to determine whether a certain genetic mutation in the APP gene causes B-amyloid to accumulate and AD to develop. Year of award: 1991
>
> Yasuko Nakajima, M.D., Ph.D., University of Illinois, Chicago, IL. Study of cholinergic and noradrenergic cells, two types of nerve cells that degenerate in AD. Year of award: 1991
>
> Sanford P. Markey, Ph.D., NIMH, Bethesda, MD. Study of the limited ability of nerve cells to repair damage to themselves in AD and other age-related brain disorders. Year of award: 1991
>
> Joseph Barbaccia, M.D., University of California, San Francisco, CA. Study of the degree to which support groups help early stage Alzheimer patients cope with their diagnosis. Year of award: 1991
>
> John K. Fink, M.D., University of Michigan Medical Center, Ann Arbor, MI. Studies of genetic factors and their roles in Alzheimer's disease. Year of award: 1992

American Health Assistance Foundation (AHAF)

Subject code(s):
> 10 17

Point of contact:
> Sherry A. Marts, Ph.D.
> (301) 948-3244

Address:
   15825 Shady Grove Road, Suite 140
   Rockville, MD 20850

Description. The American Health Assistance Foundation, founded
in 1973, supports scientific research of age-related and degenerative
diseases, educates the public about these diseases, and provides relief
funds to Alzheimer's disease patients and their caregivers. The foundation administers four separate programs: Alzheimer's disease research, national glaucoma research, coronary heart disease research,
and the Alzheimer's family relief program.
Sample grants:
   Suzanne M. De La Monte, M.D., Harvard Medical School, Cam-
      bridge, MA. Neuronal thread protein assay for Alzheimer's
      disease. Year of award: 1991
   Donald L. Price, M.D., The Johns Hopkins University School of
      Medicine, Baltimore, MD. Cholinergic systems in models of
      Alzheimer's disease. Year of award: 1991
   Bernardino Ghetti, M.D., Indiana University School of Medicine,
      Indianapolis, IN. Hereditary PRP amyloidosis with Alzhei-
      mer's changes. Year of award: 1991
   William C. Mobley, M.D., Ph.D., Department of Neurology, Uni-
      versity of California, San Francisco, CA. Defining NGF do-
      mains which activate its receptor. Year of award: 1991

American Medical Association Education and Research Foundation (AMAERF)

Subject code(s):
   1
Point of contact:
   Percy Wootton, M.D., President
   (312) 464-5000
   Rita Palulonis, Secretary
Address:
   515 North State Street
   Chicago, IL 60610

Description. The AMAERF is dedicated to ensure that medical
schools and medical students receive funds to supplement the cost of

education and training. Over the past 40 years, more than $51 million has been distributed to medical schools. The foundation distributes its awards through four funds: 1) the Medical School Excellence Fund distributes funding to medical schools, is unrestricted, and may be used where it is needed; 2) the Medical Student Assistance Fund provides an average of $500,000/year to financial aid programs of medical schools to defray costs of tuition; 3) the Development Fund supports research, health, or other medical programs as well as educational forums; and 4) the Categorical Research Fund funds grants for research in specific fields such as arthritis, mental health, or cardiovascular disease.

The AMAERF grant program distributes between $100,000 and $150,000 annually. Half of this money is used to support medical student research forums, and the remaining money funds small research projects or provides interim funding for large grant approvals from other sources. Funding is requested by writing the foundation and stating the objectives of the research and requesting total amount needed; other materials should include research protocol, budget, time frame of the project, curricula vitae of investigators, and other sources of funding.

American Paralysis Association

Subject code(s):
    2 11 22
Point of contact:
    Susan P. Howley, Director of Research
    1 (800) 225-0292
Address:
    500 Morris Avenue
    Springfield, NJ 07081

Description. The goal of the American Paralysis Association is to find a cure for paralysis associated with spinal cord injury and other central nervous system (CNS) disorders. Since its founding in 1982, this association has invested over $8 million in its research program by supporting three types of activities: research (supporting well-established and "new" investigators, pilot grants, and clinical trials), symposia and conferences, and distinguished lecture program. Funding is only given to those activities that hold promise toward achieving a cure for paralysis and other sequelae of CNS injury. Recent funding has emphasized research studying natural phenomena promoting neuronal growth, drug efficacy for primary and secondary neuronal damage, approaches improving concomitant function, anatomical characteristics of spinal cord injury, and development of evaluations of recovery after injury.

Sample grants:

> Dana Guilian, M.D., Ph.D., Baylor College of Medicine, Houston, TX. Neuron-killing factors found in spinal cord injury after acute injury. Year of award: 1990
>
> Michael J. Bolesta, M.D., and Dennis Landis, M.D., Case Western University School of Medicine, Cleveland, OH. Astrocyte response in spinal cord injury. Year of award: 1991
>
> Martin Pinter, Ph.D., and Alan Tessler, M.D., Medical College of Pennsylvania, Philadelphia, PA. Electrophysiological investigations of spinal cord transplants. Year of award: 1991

American Suicide Foundation (ASF)

Subject code(s):
> 24

Other subject areas:
> Suicide and related issues

Point of contact:
> Herbert Hendin, M.D., Executive Director
> (212) 410–1111
> Shari Faith Fisch, Executive Assistant

Address:
> 1045 Park Avenue
> New York, NY 10028

Description. Formed in 1982, the American Suicide Foundation funds research, education, and treatment programs that advance knowledge of suicide and assist in its prevention. In creating a coalition of business, community, and professional leaders to combat suicide, the ASF funds research grants through its institutional grants, individual grants, and postdoctoral research fellowship and psychiatric research development awards. In 1993, the institutional grants were awarded to Columbia University, Albert Einstein School of

Medicine, Western Psychiatric Institute, Rush-Presbyterian-St. Luke's Hospital (Chicago, IL), and Harvard Medical School.

Sample grants:

Michael Maes, M.D., Ph.D., Case Western Reserve University, Cleveland, OH. Seasonality in suicide occurrence in relation to depressive phenomenology.

Wayne S. Fenton, M.D., Chestnut Lodge Research Institute, Rockville, MD. Risk factors for suicide in schizophrenia.

Juan Lopez, M.D., University of Michigan, Ann Arbor, MI. Serotonin receptor gene regulation in brains of suicide victims.

Nicolas Sanchez, Albert Einstein College of Medicine, Bronx, NY. Assessment of correlations between suicidal risk and soft neurological signs in a schizophrenic population.

Naveed Iqbal, M.D., Albert Einstein College of Medicine, Bronx, NY. Correlates of suicidality in schizophrenia.

Arca Foundation, The

Subject code(s):

24

Other subject areas:

International issues; human rights abuse

Point of contact:

Janet Shenk, Executive Director

(202) 822-9193

Address:

1425 21st Street, NW

Washington, DC 20036

Description.   The Arca Foundation, founded in 1952, has addressed a variety of issues both domestically and internationally. Its current focus encompasses human rights, national sovereignty, and international law, especially in the area of U.S. policy and democratization and peaceful resolution of conflict. Funding stresses this international interest, and research involving international human rights abuse and psychiatric issues is an area of previous funding. Foundation funding priorities may vary from year to year.

Bristol-Myers Squibb Foundation, Inc., The

Subject code(s):
   2
Point of contact:
   John Skule
   (212) 546-5764
Address:
   345 Park Avenue
   New York, NY 10154

Description. The Bristol-Myers Squibb Foundation, Inc., provides broad support in five areas: Medical Research and Health, Education, Civic and Community Services, Cultural Activities, and International Affairs. The medical research and health program is the largest funding area of the five programs. Activity concentrates primarily on restricted medical research grants to leading institutions throughout the world in support of cancer, neuroscience, nutrition, orthopedic, and pain research.

Since 1977, Bristol-Myers Squibb Co. has committed more than $25 million in unrestricted support of these five disciplines. This program was designed as a "no-strings-attached" program in order to encourage innovative proposals that may not find funding elsewhere.

Burden Foundation, Florence V.

Subject code(s):
   10 16 17 23
Point of contact:
   Barbara R. Greenberg, Executive Director
   (212) 872-1150
   Gail Gershon, Grants Officer
Address:
   630 Fifth Avenue, Suite 2900
   New York, NY 10111

Description. The Florence V. Burden Foundation focuses its funding on the fields of aging and crime and justice. Within aging, the two priority areas are encouraging volunteer and paid employment opportunities for older people and supporting families caring for frail elders. Within the crime and justice program area, there are three priorities: 1) teaching young children how to avoid violence, 2) preventing elder abuse, and 3) maintaining the mother-child bond between imprisoned mothers and their children.

The foundation supports four types of grants. Development grants are given to new or innovative ideas within the fields of interest. Pilot project grants fund start-up of innovative programs with consideration at a later date for replication. Research and demonstration grants test pilot projects to see if test models can bear further funding. Dissemination and replication grants fund actual restructuring of and repeating a successful program.

Burroughs Wellcome Fund, The

Subject code(s):
   1 2 8
Point of contact:
   Martha G. Peck, M.Sc., Executive Director
   (919) 991-5100
Address:
   4709 Creekstone Drive, Suite 100
   Morrisville, NC 27560

Description. The Burroughs Wellcome Fund has encouraged research over the past 35 years with the purpose of advancing medical knowledge through research and education. The foundation uses its funds to support medical research in the United States. Research supported by the fund is selected on the basis of scientific merit and importance through competitive awards in targeted scientific fields.

The fund's programs and 1992 funding percentages were 1) Research (2%)—Support of basic and applied medical research with an emphasis on the support of science faculty and encouraging new lines of research. Continuous deadlines. 2) Scholar Awards (48%). 3) New Investigator Awards (9%). 4) Fellowships (19%)—Support of graduate/postdoctoral training for periods of 1–3 years in 11 disciplines. Many of the fellowships are administered by scientific/professional organizations. 5) Travel Grants (3%)—Established scientists from the United States, Britain, and Ireland may apply for grants to visit one another's countries to learn specific therapies or research techniques; 35 awards are given annually; continuous deadlines. 6) Education (15%)—Educational grants encourage students to pursue careers in biomedical research and support continued training of faculty who shape the next generation of investigators; this funding includes support for National Medical Fellowships, Inc., which assists minority physicians. 7) Visiting Professorships (3%). 8) Special Grants (1%).

In 1993, The Wellcome Trust in Great Britain provided a $400 million gift to the Burroughs Wellcome Fund, boosting future annual giving from $5 million to an anticipated $22 million. With this additional support, it has developed the annual Career Awards in the Biomedical Sciences, which support up to 6 years of research with $500,000 provided for each award.

Sample grants:

> Massachusetts Institute of Technology, Cambridge, MA. $20,000 for the Minority Summer Science Program to attract undergraduate students to science through direct involvement in research projects. Year of award: 1990

> Sharon Perry, Vanderbilt University, Philadelphia, PA. $14,000 to support the Clinical Pharmacology Fellowship Stipend, which assists in the study of the molecular basis of dopamine-beta hydroxylase deficiencies. Year of award: 1990

> Constance Royden, University of California, Berkeley, CA. $35,000 for research on the perception of depth and egomotion from optic flow: a computational and psychophysical approach. Year of award: 1990

> American Psychological Association, Washington, DC. Sponsored annual award to Kathryn Cunningham, Ph.D., University of Texas, to study electrophysiological techniques in rodents; and to Leonard Howell, Ph.D., to study the effects of drugs on respiration. Year of award: 1991

Visiting professorships:

> Royal Society of Medicine, London, England. $5,500 to Paul S. McHugh, M.D., of Johns Hopkins Hospital, Baltimore, MD. Year of award: 1990

> Vanderbilt University School of Medicine. $3,303 to Xandra O. Breakefield, Ph.D., of Harvard Medical School to lecture on monoamine oxidase genes and their role in human disease. Year of award: 1990

Carnegie Corporation of New York

Subject code(s):
  4 16
Point of contact:
  David A. Hamburg, President
  (212) 371-3200
  Vivien Stewart, Chair for Children and Youth Programs
Address:
  437 Madison Avenue
  New York, NY 10022

Description. Created in 1911 by Andrew Carnegie, the Carnegie Corporation of New York "promotes the advancement and diffusion of knowledge and understanding among the people of the U.S." Its charter was amended to include the use of funds for the same purposes in other countries that are or have been members of the British Overseas Commonwealth. The major emphasis of the foundation is on four programs: 1) education and healthy development of children and youth; 2) strengthening human resources in developing countries; 3) avoiding nuclear war; and 4) special projects.
Sample grants:
  Harvard University, Cambridge, MA. $25,000 to the preparation of an international report on mental and behavioral health. Year of award: 1993
  National Academy of Sciences, Washington, DC. $210,000 to study ways of preventing unintended and high-risk pregnancy. Year of award: 1993
  University of Colorado, Denver, CO. $300,000 for a 21-month grant to study the costs and quality of child care programs. Year of award: 1993
  Pennsylvania State University, University Park, PA. $110,000 to fund a year of interdisciplinary research to identify areas of potential research in education, media, prevention, family ties, and international comparative research on adolescents. Year of award: 1990
  George Washington University, Washington, DC. $334,790 to support a training program in human psychological development and international politics for a period of 39 months. Year of award: 1992
  University of Rochester, Rochester, NY. $330,000 for a 3-year

study of the effectiveness of nurse home-visiting programs
for low-income mothers and infants. Year of award: 1991
Harvard University, Cambridge, MA. $490,000 to support a 1-
year fellowship series designed to train African candidates in
an interdisciplinary approach to health care. Year of award:
1990
University of Chicago, Chicago, IL. $212,000 to study the impact
of peer groups and multimedia on children's function and
activity within a family setting. Year of award: 1990
Carnegie Mellon University, Pittsburgh, PA. $150,000 for 1 year
to continue research on the long-term consequences of high-
risk behavior by adolescents. Year of award: 1990

Clark Foundation, The Edna McConnell

Subject code(s):
  16 17 20 23
Point of contact:
  Peter D. Bell, President
  (212) 551-9100
  Susan J. Notkin, Director of Children's Programs
Address:
  250 Park Avenue
  New York, NY 10177

Description.   Founded in 1950, the Edna McConnell Clark Foundation has grown from a small family fund to one of the largest foundations in the country. Since 1970, the foundation has made grants
totaling $295 million in supporting services, research, and other pro-
grams that focus on the needs of the poor, children, elderly, and the
developing world.
Sample grants:
  Vera Institute of Justice, Inc., New York, NY. $45,000 to support
      research that would promote the development of quality
      drug treatment programs for offenders. Year of award: 1992
  Pennsylvania Commission on Sentencing, State College, PA.
      $100,000 to gather and analyze information on the justice
      system in Pennsylvania. Year of award: 1992
  City Limits Community Information Service, Inc., New York, NY.
      $30,000 to continue to study the resettlement of formerly

homeless families and neighborhood revitalization. Year of award: 1992

Children's Defense Fund, Washington, DC. $91,000 to improve family preservation services across the child welfare, mental health, and juvenile justice systems. Year of award: 1992

Commonweal, New York, NY. $20,000 to study exemplary foundation-funded programs for disadvantaged children. Year of award: 1992

University of South Florida, Tampa, FL. $176,000 to support the integration of family preservation into the mental health system, collaborating among mental health, child welfare, and juvenile justice agencies. Year of award: 1992

Commonwealth Fund, The

Subject code(s):
    1 10 16 17 24
Other subject areas:
    Urban issues, particularly in New York City
Point of contact:
    Margaret E. Mahoney, President
    (212) 535-0400
    Karen Davis, Executive Vice President
    Adrienne Fisher, Grants Manager
Address:
    Harkness House
    One East 75th Street
    New York, NY 10021

Description.   The Commonwealth Fund, a philanthropic foundation established by Anna Harkness in 1918, has a broad mandate to enhance the common good. To carry out this mission, the fund has searched for new opportunities to improve Americans' health and well-being and assist specific groups of Americans who have serious and neglected problems. The five major programs and their percentage of funding from 1980 to 1992 are 1) improvement in health care services (47%); 2) advancement of the well-being of elderly people (28%); 3) development of the capacities of young people (13%); 4) promotion of healthier lifestyles (7%); and 5) improvement of the health of minorities (9%).

The fund sponsors projects within these areas of funding; these projects include the Americans Over 55 at Work Program, the Youth Opportunities Program, the Quality of Urban Life Program, the Career Beginnings Program, and the Fellowship Program in Academic Medicine for Minority Students. Two programs of special emphasis are the Quality of Life in New York City, a project that encourages creative solutions to urban problems in New York City, and Organizations Working with Foundations, a program of support to foundations which fund mostly health-related grant making.

Sample grants:
> Alliance for Aging Research, Washington, DC. $180,000 to promote better medical research and clinical care for older Americans. Year of award: 1993
> University of California, Los Angeles, CA. $186,598 for women's health-related behavior and use of preventive services. Year of award: 1993

Culpeper Foundation, Charles E.

Subject code(s):
> 1
Point of contact:
> Linda E. Jacobs, Vice President of Programs
> (203) 975-1240
Address:
> Financial Centre
> 695 East Main Street, Suite 404
> Stamford, CT 06901

Description. The Charles E. Culpeper Foundation provides grants to organizations concerned with health, education, science and technology, arts and letters, cultural programs, and justice administration. Established in 1940 by the will of Charles E. Culpeper, the foundation provides nearly 65% of its annual funding to the fields of health, education, and the arts. The foundation also sponsors the Scholarship in Medical Science, which aims to support the career development of academic physicians. Up to three grants of $100,000/year for up to 3 years are made within this scholarship program to U.S. medical schools on behalf of the candidates who are judged by the quality of their research proposals and their potential for successful careers in academic medicine. The deadline for this annual grant program is August 15 of each year.

Sample grants:

University of California, San Francisco, CA. $324,000 to support David M. Holtzman, M.D., as a Medical Science Scholar, to research the molecular and cellular pathogenesis of Alzheimer's disease-like neurodegeneration in a mouse model of Down syndrome. Year of award: 1993

University of Texas, Dallas, TX. $97,200 to support research on value issues in psychiatric classification. Year of award: 1993

Cummings Foundation, The Nathan

Subject code(s):

11

Point of contact:

Charles R. Halpern, President

(212) 787-7300

Andrea Kydd, Director of the Health Program

Address:

1926 Broadway, Suite 600

New York, NY 10023

Description. Established in 1949, the Nathan Cummings Foundation is a national grant making organization dedicated to the wellbeing of all people. It focuses this philosophy by supporting four major programs in the arts, health, environment, and Jewish life. The foundation's approach to its grant making carries basic themes in all its programs: concern for the underserved, poor, and disadvantaged, respect for cultural differences, education, and empowerment of the powerless. The foundation seeks to fund projects that are innovative and risk-taking.

The health program of the foundation stresses three issues: 1) promotion of health among the underserved, particularly low-income children and their families; 2) support of the field of mind/body and behavioral medicine and comprehensive patient-centered health care; and 3) cancer prevention and treatment from the perspective of the patient.

Sample grants:

Beth Israel Hospital, Boston, MA. $68,035 to determine the extent to which people nationwide use and pay for alternative medical therapies. Year of award: 1990

Mind/Body Medical Institute, Boston, MA. $151,486 for a school-based relaxation-response curriculum for troubled and healthy children. Year of award: 1990

University of Louisville School of Medicine, Louisville, KY. $60,000 for the development of a medical school curriculum on mind/body techniques and to encourage professional careers in clinical services and research related to mind/body medicine. Year of award: 1993

Harvard Community Health Plan Foundation, Cambridge, MA. $150,000 to support the study of mind/body approaches to healing and the development of new skills for building trust between the patient and physician. Year of award: 1993

National Academy of Sciences, Washington, DC. $100,000 to support a study by the Institute of Medicine on mind/body medicine. Year of award: 1993

Dana Foundation, The Charles A.

Subject code(s):
1 2 17 24
Other subject areas:
Genetic research
Point of contact:
Robert N. Kreidler, President
(212) 223-4040
Stephen Foster, Executive Vice President
Address:
745 Fifth Avenue, Suite 700
New York, NY 10151

Description. Since 1991, The Dana Foundation, which has been providing grants since 1950, has emphasized programs in health, particularly neuroscience research, and higher education. In its health-related funding, the foundation makes major grants for collaborative research on diseases and disorders of the brain in order to advance diagnosis, treatment, and prevention of such diseases. Research is generally carried out by consortia of scientists from medical centers that have research strength in neuroscience.

In 1993, the foundation established the Dana Alliance for Brain Initiatives and has committed $25 million to foster breakthroughs in brain research and mental illness. Topics of research interest include genetic links to brain disorders, drug development for specific diseases and central nervous system injuries, development of agents to block addictive substances, and study of neuronal mechanisms associated with learning and memory. The various consortia coordinate with the alliance in their research goals.

As of 1994, the foundation has been involved with the creation of consortia that address memory loss in older persons, genetic basis of manic-depressive illness, language-based learning disorders, therapy for HIV dementia, and neuroimaging leadership training. The foundation also supports a program of research grants to test experimental and innovative ideas that may advance clinical applications of neuroscience research.

The Dana Foundation also sponsors the Charles A. Dana Awards for Pioneering Achievements in Health and Education, which provide $50,000 annually to senior individuals to honor innovative ideas that have had demonstrated potential with the hope of furthering their impact by encouraging further development and dissemination; up to five awards may be given each year.

Sample grants:

The Dana Consortium on the Genetic Basis of Manic-Depressive Illness. $2.5 million over 3 years to be shared by Cold Spring Harbor Laboratory, Cold Spring Harbor, NY; Johns Hopkins Medical Institutions, Baltimore, MD; and Stanford University School of Medicine, Stanford, CA. Year of award: 1993

The Dana Consortium on Language-Based Learning Disabilities. $2.3 million over 3 years to be shared by the State University of New Jersey, Rutgers, Newark, NJ; University of California, San Francisco, CA; Harvard Medical School, Boston, MA; New York University Medical Center, New York, NY; and Washington University School of Medicine, St. Louis, MO. Year of award: 1993

The Dana Consortium on Therapy for HIV Dementia and Related Cognitive Disorders. $1.9 million over 3 years to be shared by Columbia University College of Physicians and Surgeons, New York, NY; Johns Hopkins School of Medicine, Baltimore, MD; and University of Rochester School of Medicine and Dentistry, Rochester, NY. Year of award: 1993

Stanford University, Stanford, CA. $124,000 for research train-

ing of physicians in neuroscience. Year of award: 1993
Neuroscience Research Foundation, Inc., New York, NY. $25,000
for general support. Year of award: 1993
Washington University School of Medicine, St. Louis, MO.
$1,222,000 for the training of scientists to incorporate PET
into neurobiological research. Year of award: 1993
University of California, Los Angeles, CA. $1,154,100 for the
training of scientists to incorporate PET into neurobiological
research. Year of award: 1993

Diamond Foundation, The Aaron

Subject code(s):
1 16 18 20 24
Other subject areas:
Local giving in New York, NY
Point of contact:
Isabel Dane, President
(212) 757-7680
Address:
1270 Avenue of the Americas, Suite 2624
New York, NY 10020

Description. The Aaron Diamond Foundation is dedicated to improving the quality of life in New York City by supporting biomedical and social science research on AIDS and drug abuse, minority education, and cultural activities. Administered by the New York State Health Research Council, the Aaron Diamond Foundation Postdoctoral Research Fellowships in the Biomedical and Social Sciences support research in understanding AIDS and drug abuse by linking new investigators with mentors in New York research institutions. The foundation will distribute all of its capital by 1997.
Sample grants:
Aaron Diamond AIDS Research Center, New York, NY.
$1,750,000 to support AIDS research. Year of award: 1992
Capital District Center for Drug Abuse Research and Development, Albany, NY. $100,000 to create a center to develop new
treatments for drug addiction. Year of award: 1992
Children's Blood Foundation, New York, NY. $60,000 to study
HIV-positive infants and the risk of developing *Pneumocystis*

carinii pneumonia. Year of award: 1992

Mount Sinai Medical Center, New York, NY. $75,000 to study severely disruptive behavior in preschool children. Year of award: 1992

Ford Foundation, The

Subject code(s):
1 4 10 16 20 24
Other subject areas:
Poverty and urban issues
Point of contact:
Barron M. Tenny, Vice President
(212) 573-5000
Address:
320 East 42nd Street
New York, NY 10017

Description.   The Ford Foundation, founded in 1936 by automotive industrialist Henry Ford, is a private philanthropic institution dedicated to international peace and to advancing the well-being of people throughout the world. Primary emphasis is to fund projects designed to produce significant advances on problems of worldwide importance. In recent years, the Ford Foundation has turned to the formation of partnerships with other private and public organizations on both the national and local level to create programs of greater impact.

The major program areas supported by the foundation are 1) urban poverty, 2) rural poverty and resources, 3) human rights and social justice, 4) governance and public policy, 5) education and culture, 6) international affairs, 7) other program allocations, including populations activities and special program actions, and 8) unanticipated needs within the major programs. Nearly 35% of program monies are spent abroad on programs in developing nations. Programs that may be of particular interest to psychiatric research include the urban poverty program, the rural poverty and resources program, and the fellowship programs for minorities.

The urban poverty program focuses on multiple approaches to addressing the needs of people living in poverty. This program, since the late 1960s, has supported community development corporations to revitalize distressed neighborhoods three ways. It creates community partnerships, funds assistance organizations, and evaluates this impact. Areas of concern in this program include housing, economic and business development, and the improvement and study of services to children, youth, and families with the aim of developing successful models that can be reproduced on a widespread scale.

The foundation sponsors two minority fellowship programs: 1) The Predoctoral and Dissertation Fellowships for Minorities (PDFM) and 2) Postdoctoral Fellowships for Minorities (PFM). The PDFM are awarded to minorities for research-based programs in the social/behavioral sciences, physical sciences, biological sciences, engineering, humanities, and interdisciplinary. Annual stipend is $11,500/year for 3 years, $6,000 for institution. The PFM follows the same criteria with stipends of $25,000/year, $3,000 for travel costs, and $2,000 for host institutions for training in research and teaching.

The rural poverty and resources program emphasizes programs that strengthen the economic and social development and increase employment opportunities in rural areas, especially for women and minorities. The foundation supports efforts to analyze rural problems and advise public/private organizations on rural poverty policies. Special emphasis is placed on analyses of income, poverty, and employment generation, strengthening research capacities of local private/public organizations, and promoting discussion of issues affecting rural populations.

Foundation for Child Development

Subject code(s):
    10 16
Point of contact:
    Barbara Blum, President
    (212) 697-3150
    Sheila Smith, Director of Research
    Claudia Conner, Grants Manager
Address:
    Room 700
    345 East 46th Street
    New York, NY 10017

Description. The Foundation for Child Development, founded in 1900 as a voluntary agency in New York, has focused its funding interests on policies and programs directly affecting children and families at risk. Grants given by the foundation are designed to improve the lives of at-risk and poverty-level children and families in the fields of research, policy, and direct service.

The research component of the foundation stresses the integration of action and research. Researchers should make explicit the potential connections between children and families at risk, implying the public policy or direct action that may result from their findings. All services initiatives are for projects in New York City. All proposals are reviewed three times a year (March, June, and December); proposals should be submitted 2 months before these review meetings.
Sample grants:

  Albert Einstein College of Medicine, Bronx, NY. $6,391 for research on mentally retarded adults. Year of award: 1990

  Bank Street College of Education, New York, NY. $50,000 for an analysis of data in a study of homeless and low-income housed families. Year of award: 1990

French Foundation for Alzheimer Research, The

Subject code(s):
  1 17
Point of contact:
  Thomas Ennis, President
  (310) 445-4650
  Gwen Waggoner, Research Administrator
Address:
  11620 Wilshire Boulevard
  Los Angeles, CA 90025

Description. The French Foundation for Alzheimer Research, founded in 1983, funds research into the cause, cure, and prevention of Alzheimer's disease and creates model care facilities in conjunction with hospitals, universities, and other institutions. The foundation research support sponsors neuroscientists and brain researchers in studies on genetic, environmental, neurochemical, and infectious factors. The program in model facilities attempts to create treatment centers specially assisting the needs of Alzheimer's disease patients.

The foundation also provides funding for fellowships in Alzheimer's research.

Fulbright Scholar Program

Subject code(s):
   1 24
Other subject areas:
   International education
Point of contact:
   Council for International Exchange Scholars (CIES)
   (202) 686-7877
Address:
   3007 Tilden Street, NW, Suite 5M
   Washington, DC 20008

Description. The Fulbright Program is authorized by Public Law 87-256 with the purpose of "enabling the government of the United States to increase mutual understanding between the people of the United States and the people of other countries and to assist in the development of friendly, sympathetic, and peaceful relations between the United States and other countries of the world." Grants are made to U.S. citizens and nationals of other countries for a variety of educational activities, primarily university teaching, advanced research, graduate study, and elementary/secondary school teaching. The Scholar Program enables Americans to learn firsthand about other countries and cultures and allows those from other cultures to learn about America, and to promote academic and professional development. It has funded about 27,000 Americans to lecture or conduct research abroad and brought 30,200 visiting scholars to the United States.

The grant categories are 1) research, 300 awards in most disciplines; 2) lecturing, 700 awards for university lectureships and possible research; 3) lecturing/research, with equal distribution between both activities; 4) distinguished lecturing, for scholars outstanding in their discipline; 5) junior lecturing and junior research, designed for younger scholars who are recent Ph.D.s or advanced Ph.D. candidates; and 6) travel awards for transportation to the country of choice. Candidates must have a doctorate or comparable qualifications, and decisions are made on professional and personal qualifications, research project, project statement for lecturing, previous experience, invitation, qualifications, and geographic distribution. Deadlines vary according to host location from June 15 to August 1 to November 1 to January 1.

Glenn Foundation for Medical Research

Subject code(s):
   2 17
Point of contact:
   Paul Glenn, President
   (805) 565-3363
Address:
   1250 Coast Village Road, Suite K
   Santa Barbara, CA 93108

Description.   The Glenn Foundation, founded by venture capitalist Paul Glenn, supports research in the biology of aging. The foundation supports junior investigators, students, and start-up projects that may lay the groundwork for significant research.

   The Glenn Foundation invites proposals and accepts recommendations for funding from the American Federation for Aging Research (AFAR) and the aging research community. A Glenn Foundation committee of scientists recommends investigators for fellowship awards.

Grant Foundation, William T.

Subject code(s):
   1 4 7 9 10 11 16 19 20 23
Point of contact:
   Beatrix Hamburg, M.D., President
   (212) 752-0071
   Lonnie R. Sherrod, Ph.D., Vice President
Address:
   515 Madison Avenue
   New York, NY 10022

Description.   The William T. Grant Foundation's primary mission is to support research and evaluation studies relevant to the health and psychological and social development of children and youth. Foundation support is provided through five mechanisms, all of which are investigator-initiated: 1) research on the development of children, adolescents, and youth; these research grants are given to investigate developmental issues, origins, and outcomes of problem behaviors; 2) research to evaluate broadly based social interventions and innovative community-based interventions aimed at reducing problem behaviors in youth; 3) the faculty scholars program, which supports young investigators in various disciplines whose research is relevant to the mental health of youth; up to 5 years for five investigators per year with funding up to $175,000/year is given in order to protect the research time of scholars early in their careers; these scholars are nominated by their institutions and must devote at least 50% of their time to research; 4) consortia—support is given for individuals from various disciplines/institutions to meet and coordinate research; and 5) small grants programs, which provide for support of research, education and training, or community service projects within the interests of the foundation. These awards are usually for 1-year terms and meet special needs.

Grass Foundation, The

Subject code(s):
    1 2
Point of contact:
    Mary G. Grass
    (617) 773-0002
Address:
    77 Reservoir Road
    Quincy, MA 02170

Description. The Grass Foundation is a fund devoted to the support of research and education in neurophysiology through supporting fellowship grants. Other projects include support of courses in neurobiology and several lectureships in neuroscience.

Guggenheim Foundation, The Harry Frank

Subject code(s):
    15 19 20 23

Point of contact:
James M. Hester, President
(212) 644-4907
Karen Colvard, Program Officer
Address:
527 Madison Avenue
New York, NY 10022

Description. The Harry Frank Guggenheim Foundation sponsors an international program of scientific research and scholarly study into the causes and consequences of dominance, aggression, and violence. The foundation was endowed in 1929 for general philanthropic purposes; in 1959, the focus shifted to its current objective of investigating man's relationship to man. The initial focus was on dominance and was enlarged in the early 1970s to include aggression and violence.

Areas of research support include anthropology, psychology, neurobiology, pharmacology, animal behavior, primatology, and sociology. Areas of particular funding interest since 1985 include juvenile violence, family violence, war, and drug-related violence. Grants are awarded to individuals, projects, and career development. Applications are considered twice a year, with due dates February 1 and August 1. Most grants range from $15,000 to $35,000 a year for periods of 1–2 years.

Sample grants:
Medical College of Pennsylvania, Philadelphia, PA. Serotonin in impulsive aggression: neuropsychopharmacologic studies in personality disordered patients. Year of award: 1993

State University of New York, Buffalo, NY. Understanding family sub-abusive violence against children. Year of award: 1993

University of California, Los Angeles, CA. A model of aggressive, violent, and alternative behavior among individuals. Year of award: 1993

University of Illinois, Chicago, IL. Interparental conflict and child aggression. Year of award: 1993

Rutgers University, New Brunswick, NJ. Male aggressive behavior and t-complex genotype. Year of award: 1993

University of Medicine of New Jersey, Trenton, NJ. The development and socialization of anger in human infants. Year of award: 1993

Mount Sinai School of Medicine, New York, NY. Neural basis of anabolic-androgenic steroid action. Year of award: 1993

University of Southern California, Los Angeles, CA. Criminal violence and mental illness in a birth cohort. Year of award: 1993

Harris Foundation, The

Subject code(s):
    4 16
Point of contact:
    Ruth K. Belzer, Executive Director
    (312) 621-0566
Address:
    2 North LaSalle Street, Suite 605
    Chicago, IL 60602

Description. Incorporated in 1945, the Harris Foundation supports research and demonstration projects that advance the knowledge, understanding, and prevention of family dysfunction, particularly in young families. Further support is also provided for prevention of teenage pregnancy and infant mortality/morbidity, infant mental health, and early childhood development. Funding can be for research, projects, equipment, publications, and conferences and seminars, operating budgets, among other categories.

Hartford Foundation, The John A.

Subject code(s):
    10 17
Point of contact:
    Stephen C. Eyre, Executive Director
    (212) 832-7788
    Richard S. Sharpe, Program Director
Address:
    55 East 59th Street
    New York, NY 10022

Description. The John A. Hartford Foundation, established in 1929, seeks to improve health care in America. It pursues this goal by supporting two major programs with its funding activity: 1) The health care cost and quality program emphasizes the need to balance quality and cost containment in U.S. health care. Specifically, the program supports the development, evaluation, and dissemination of prototype systems and other projects that offer potential national impact in assistance to health. 2) The aging and health program supports research into the long-term needs of the elderly, particularly in the area of reducing functional deterioration of hospitalized elders.

Hood Foundation, The Charles H.

Subject code(s):
 2 16
Point of contact:
 Raymond Considine, Executive Director
 (617) 695-9439
Address:
 95 Berkeley Street, Suite 201
 Boston, MA 02116

Description.   Charles H. Hood founded this fund in 1931 to carry out charitable activities, stressing his long-standing interest in the health of children. Since 1942, the foundation has continuously maintained an active program devoted to research grants, especially those that benefit child health in New England. Emphasis is on the initiation or furtherance of medical research and related projects contributing to a reduction of health problems and needs of large numbers of children. Traditionally the foundation has focused on start-up projects and promising young investigators and also emphasizes research that leads to practical clinical applications. Deadline for applications is October 14.

Howard Hughes Medical Institute (HHMI)

Subject code(s):
 1 2 3 24
Other subject areas:
 International
Point of contact:
 Purnell W. Choppin, M.D., President
 (301) 215-8500
 Joseph Perpich, M.D., J.D., Vice President for Grants

Address:
   Office of Grants and Special Programs
   4000 Jones Bridge Road
   Chevy Chase, MD 20815

Description. The Howard Hughes Medical Institute (HHMI) is the largest active foundation in the United States, combining elements of a traditional foundation and a medical research organization. Unusual among private philanthropies, the HHMI was established in 1985 by the late Howard Hughes; he gave sole title to Hughes Aircraft Company. Unlike foundations, however, HHMI is designated as a "medical research organization," an entity that must be actively engaged in medical research in conjunction with a hospital. Facilities that receive funding become HHMI facilities; individual scholars supported by the HHMI become employees. In exchange, the HHMI is able to avoid many of the burdens the tax law places on private foundations.

HHMI Medical Program: The core program of the HHMI, the medical program, is directed toward the conduct of intramural biomedical research in five broad scientific areas of the basic sciences: cell biology and regulation, genetics, immunology, neuroscience, and structural biology. The research is dictated by the individual, not the project, and it focuses on fundamental research and is not oriented toward any particular disease category. The HHMI maintains programs both for senior and younger researchers. Currently, over 175 senior HHMI researchers are working in 30 HHMI units affiliated with medical schools and universities across the country. Recommended by medical school deans, other senior scientists, or HHMI advisory panel members, and selected through a very rigorous process by peer review boards in each of the five areas of interest, these scientists are given infrastructure support, staff, and salary in the form of an annual budget for 3, 5, or 7 years. While encouraged to maintain alternative sources of funding, HHMI researchers enjoy substantial support.

There are also HHMI "select units," where hospitals or universities with special research programs are funded and allow one or two highly qualified and directed researchers to be chosen to work as HHMI employees at these sites. The selection process is rigorous, with the expectation of growth in the "select" research program. Postdoctoral fellows work in these HHMI laboratories on a case-by-case basis. As of 1992, postdoctoral research fellowships for physicians numbered 75 for 3 years of training at 45 academic and research institutions, totaling $5 million annually.

HHMI Research Scholars: While the conduct of research by HHMI investigators remains central, HHMI has broadened its program to support science education. The Cloister project, also known as the HHMI/NIH Research Scholars Program, is a joint teaching effort with the NIH to encourage medical students to pursue research careers. This program allows medical students to take a year off and spend it in an NIH laboratory. As of 1992, research training fellowships for medical students numbered nearly 60 fellows per year, with an additional 40 in continuing activities, totaling $2.3 million annually.

HHMI Education Program: The grants program, begun in 1987, focuses on science education across a range of educational levels. HHMI supports graduate education through its predoctoral fellowships in the biological sciences, funding about 300 graduate students at 51 academic institutions at a cost of $7.5 million annually. These HHMI doctoral fellows receive a stipend for at least 3 and up to 5 years and their institutions also receive a stipend. The fellowships, made to those who have demonstrated superior scholarship and promise for future achievement in biomedical research and education, are intended for students at or near the beginning of their graduate study in the biological sciences.

Of particular interest to those in medical education are the postdoctoral research fellowships for physicians and research training fellowships for medical students. Postdoctoral research fellowships provide 3 years of postdoctoral training in studying basic biological processes and disease mechanisms at an academic or not-for-profit research institution. The fellowships for medical students allow 1 year of full-time research in a laboratory at their medical school or another academic institution studying basic biological processes. Dates for beginning this fellowship are arranged for each fellow with the institution.

Reaching back in the educational process, HHMI awards 5-year awards to research and doctorate-granting universities to improve undergraduate biological education programs. These awards are usually between $400,000 and $2 million, with total funding in 1992 reaching $52.5 million. Aiming toward the education of even younger students, the grants program also supports a study by the National Research Council/National Academy of Sciences (NAS) of high school biology education. The NAS study will focus on curricula and the teaching process. This will assist in the development of the third area of the grant program's interest—public and precollege science education. In 1992, $6.4 million was distributed in 5-year awards to 29 science museums nationwide to assist in the public education effort.

Huntington's Disease Society of America

Subject code(s):
    22
Point of contact:
    Claudia Archimede, Executive Director
    (212) 242-1968
Address:
    140 West 22nd Street, 6th Floor
    New York, NY 10011

Description. The mission of the Huntington's Disease Society of America is to cure Huntington's disease (HD) and to improve the lives of those affected by HD. This organization supports basic and applied research and research training in scientific areas of interest to HD, such as neuroscience and molecular genetics.
Sample grants:
    Rosalinda Roberts, Ph.D., Maryland Psychiatric Research Center, Baltimore, MD. Study of synaptic reorganization in striata of lesioned rats and Huntington's patients. Year of award: 1992
    Bruce Jenkins, Ph.D., Massachusetts General Hospital, Boston, MA. In vivo neurochemical studies of Huntington's disease using magnetic resonance spectroscopic imaging. Year of award: 1992

Ittleson Foundation, Inc.

Subject code(s):
    1 3 4 9 10 11 16 17 18 23 24
Other subject areas:
    Underserved populations
Point of contact:
    Anthony C. Wood, Executive Director
    (212) 838-5010

Address:
645 Madison Avenue, 16th Floor
New York, NY 10022

Description.   The Ittleson Foundation's primary focuses are mental health projects that address the underserved populations such as the elderly, poor, and minorities; the environment; AIDS; and, added in 1992, crime, violence, and justice. The foundation is interested especially in projects that fuse formal professional expertise to informal networks of support to make services available to excluded populations. The foundation also supports projects that address the effects of AIDS on people's mental health. Grants generally range from $10,000 to $50,000. Deadlines for applications are April 1 and September 1.
Sample grants:
Winthrop-University Hospital, Mineola, NY. $20,000 to train geriatric fellows and medical residents in neuropsychology. Year of award: 1992
Harvard School of Public Health, Boston, MA. $35,00 to study and develop a community-based violence prevention program and subsequently a national demonstration project. Year of award: 1992
National Alliance for the Mentally Ill, Arlington, VA. $25,500 for research and education regarding the incarceration of mentally ill in jails. Year of award: 1992
New York Interface Development Project, Inc., New York, NY. $30,000 to study school violence intervention. Transferred to the Welfare Research Institute in mid-1992. Year of award: 1992

Jacobs Foundation, Johann

Subject code(s):
1 16 24
Other subject areas:
International funding
Point of contact:
Dr. Laszlo Nagy, President
Address:
Seelfeldquai 17
PO Box 101
CH 8034 Zurich
Switzerland

Description.   The Johann Jacobs Foundation undertakes and/or finances programs aimed at research on adolescence and youth-related research, action, and social policy. It focuses its programs on four areas: 1) analysis of adolescent development in context of a rapidly changing world and as part of the whole course of life; 2) analysis of the nature of social forces in developing both positive and negative adolescent reactions and behavior; 3) development of new programs designed to improve the opportunities of adolescents throughout life; and 4) promoting respect for the environment and conservation. The foundation operates internationally and promotes research, education, communications, and interdisciplinary cooperation.

Funding support is given through 1) research grants, addressing adolescent concerns; 2) dissertation grants of $5,000; 3) young investigator grants of $10,000 in the field of adolescence/youth; 4) scholarships and travel stipends for travel and short-term work between scholars or mentor and students, particularly from socialist and the third world countries; 5) visiting professorship in Switzerland given to a scholar who will lecture and perform research in the area of human development and youth; and 6) young scientist sabbatical program.

JM Foundation, The

Subject code(s):
    10 11 19 20 24
Other subject areas:
    Rehabilitation
Point of contact:
    Chris K. Olander, Executive Director
    (212) 687-7735
Address:
    60 42nd Street, Suite 1651
    New York, NY 10165

Description.   The JM Foundation was founded in 1924 by Jeremiah Milbank to support organizations in the areas of medical research, rehabilitation of people with disabilities through comprehensive rehab centers, and projects supporting the strengthening of values essential for a free society. Recent years have seen a strong interest in combining education and social policy issues. Two programs, sponsored and emphasized by the foundation, are 1) the JM Foundation Medical Student Program in Alcohol and Other Drug Dependencies, which has introduced 1,300 medical students to drug and alcohol issues since 1984, and 2) the JM Foundation National Search for Excellence Awards in Chemical Dependency, which recognizes public and private programs that provide services to people with drug or alcohol abuse problems.

Sample grants:

Memorial Sloan-Kettering Cancer Center, New York, NY. $200,000 to support interdisciplinary training program in the biomedical sciences for postdoctoral fellows (5-year, $1,000,000, 4:1 challenge grant). Year of award: 1990

Center for Alcohol Studies, Rutgers University, New Brunswick, NJ. $12,000 for medical student program in alcohol and other drug dependencies. Year of award: 1990

Center for Policy Studies, Minneapolis, MN. $25,000 to design a community-based system that provides access to health insurance for the uninsured. Year of award: 1990

Rehabilitation Institute, Chicago, IL. $50,000 to develop, evaluate, and disseminate a model substance abuse program for people with disabilities. Year of award: 1990

Johnson Foundation, The

Subject code(s):
24
Other subject areas:
Conferences
Point of contact:
Gail Kirby, Program Secretary
(414) 639-3211
Address:
PO Box 547
Racine, WI 53401

Description. The Johnson Foundation, Inc., was established in 1959 and devotes its resources primarily to supporting conferences at its headquarters in Racine, WI. These sponsored conferences offer full support in planning and logistics, meals, and other amenities such as local transportation. The foundation's funding priorities

for the period of 1990-1994 include international affairs, education
and child development, family, science and the humanities, and various proposals for southeastern Wisconsin. The foundation also
supports the Keland Endowment Fund, which supports conferences that are designed to promote the arts; assist persons with physical, developmental, or mental disabilities; or preserve or enhance the
environment.

Johnson Foundation, The Robert Wood (RWJ)

Subject code(s):
    1 10 19 20
Point of contact:
    Edward H. Robbins, Proposal Manager
    (609) 452-8701
Address:
    PO Box 2316
    College Road East & US Hwy No 1
    Princeton, NJ 08543

Description. The Robert Wood Johnson Foundation, one of the
largest private philanthropies in the nation, disburses nearly $100
million each year toward finding and implementing solutions to
America's health care problems. In past years, most grants went to
large, multisite, national programs overseen by experts from leading
institutions; current activity now includes community organizations and institutions so there is an equal balance between the two
recipients. In August 1991, RWJ redirected its giving programs to
focus on specific health care problems. These specific areas of interest
include assuring basic health care for all Americans; identifying and
correcting problems in the health service area for those with chronic
health problems; research on risking health care costs; and reducing
substance abuse through education, intervention, and treatment,
with particular emphasis on integrating services with specialty services such as AIDS and mental health services. Funding percentages
of RWJ 1992 grants in these areas are: 1) health care access programs
(28%); 2) substance abuse programs (23%); 2) chronic health care
services (19%); 3) medical cost containment research (4%); and
5) other local programs in New Jersey (26%).

This general focus is concentrated on 10 specific areas: infants, children, and adolescents (including dysfunctional families/home-lessness); chronic illness and disability (including elderly); AIDS; destructive behavior (including substance/drug abuse); mental illness (including deinstitutionalization/health care services); organization/financing of health care; quality of care; ethical issues; health manpower; and impact of medical advances. Specific fellowship programs focusing on health care and its national impact are also available.

Sample grants:
>   American Academy of Pediatrics, Inc., Elk Grove Village, IL. $113,362 for the classification of mental health of children in primary care settings. Year of award: 1992
>
>   Consumers Union of the United States, Yonkers, NY. $100,000 for 15 months supporting research enabling revision of a substance abuse source book. Year of award: 1992
>
>   Harvard University, Cambridge, MA. $998,254 for a 2.5-year study of college drinking patterns and practices. $32,968 for a study of substance abuse linkage to a criminal behavior study. Year of award: 1992
>
>   Pacific Institute of Medical Research, Los Angeles, CA. $42,140 for a 2-year study of the mental health of homeless children. Year of award: 1992
>
>   Institute for Health, Health Care Policy, and Aging Research, Rutgers University, New Brunswick, NJ. $199,868 for a 2-year study of informal caregivers for the seriously mentally ill. Year of award: 1992
>
>   University of Colorado Health Sciences Center, Denver, CO. $199,821 for the analysis of data on the long-term course of severe mental illness. Year of award: 1992

Kaiser Foundation, The Henry J.

Subject code(s):
>   1 10 16 19 20 24

Other subject areas:
>   Minority and women's issues

Point of contact:
>   Barbara Kehrer, Vice President
>   (415) 854-9400
>   Karen P. Sparks, Grants Manager

Address:
    Quadras
    2400 Sand Hill Road
    Menlo Park, CA 94025

Description. From its inception in 1948 until the early 1970s, the Henry J. Kaiser Foundation devoted the largest share of its funding to establishing the HMO health care system. Since the early 1970s, the emphasis has focused on broader priorities: medical education and curricula development, primary health care, research training, health promotion, humanism in medical care, and minority support. Programs of support include 1) the Kaiser Faculty Scholar Awards, which enable academic general internists at the junior faculty level to pursue research interests; 2) Project on the General Professional Education of the Physician and College Preparation for Medicine, which has influenced regular program support in the area of curricula development/educational reform within medical schools. Support is given for research, fellowships, professorships, special projects, and publications, among other areas. Recent funding with the foundation's poverty and health program aims to combat health problems of low-income and minority Americans involving health care access and cost, lack of insurance, and lifestyle. Projects focusing on teen pregnancy, substance abuse, and poor nutrition are of particular interest.

Keck Foundation, W. M.

Subject code(s):
    2
Point of contact:
    Joan F. DuBois, Program Vice President
    (213) 614-0934
Address:
    555 South Flower Street, Suite 3230
    Los Angeles, CA 90071

Description. The W. M. Keck Foundation, established in 1954 by William Myron Keck, stresses three primary areas for support: higher education, medical research, and science. Projects for medical research support include molecular genetics, neuropsychiatry, immunochemistry, mapping the human genome, and the upgrading of medical equip-

ment and laboratories. Giving is mostly focused in Southern California.
Sample grants:

University of Richmond, Richmond, VA. To purchase equipment for faculty-student research in biology and neuroscience. Year of award: 1993

Brandeis University, Waltham, MA. To support construction of a Center for Complex Systems for research on higher brain function. Year of award: 1993

University of Alabama, Birmingham, AL. To develop a molecular/neuronal imaging facility within the Neurobiology Research Center. Year of award: 1993

University of Wisconsin, Madison, WI. To support a laboratory for neural imaging. Year of award: 1993

Kenworthy–Sarah H. Swift Foundation, Inc., Marion E.

Subject code(s):
16
Point of contact:
Maurice V. Russell, Ed.D., ACSW, President
(212) 685-4918
Address:
300 East 34th Street, Suite 19-C
New York, NY 10016

Description. The Kenworthy–Swift Foundation, established in 1963, awards grants for mental health programs, social services, education programs for minorities, family services, drug abuse, welfare and legal services, and the advancement of psychiatry. Current grants are awarded primarily to requests involving children and/or families. Awards range from $1,000 to $40,000/year to organizations with nonprofit status. Deadlines for review of grant applications are April 1 and November 1.

Klingenstein Fund, Inc., The Esther A. and Joseph

Subject code(s):
1 2 3

Point of contact:
  President
  (212) 492-6181
Address:
  787 Seventh Avenue, 6th Floor
  New York, NY 10019

Description. The Klingenstein Fund, established in 1946 as a vehicle for expressing the personal philanthropic interests of Esther and Joseph Klingenstein, has broadened its funding interest into three major programs: 1) epilepsy, with a primary emphasis on basic research in neuroscience; 2) independent secondary education and faculty development through the Klingenstein Center at Columbia University, NY; and 3) Klingenstein Fellowship Awards in the Neurosciences that support young investigators in the early stages of their careers who are engaged in clinical or basic research that may lead to a better understanding of the etiology, treatment, and prevention of epilepsy. Awards are $100,000 for 3 years beginning in July, and up to nine fellows may be appointed annually; deadline is October 15. Besides these main programs, other funding is provided on issues of public policy, health care, and social welfare.

Life and Health Insurance Medical Research Fund

Subject code(s):
  2 3
Point of contact:
  Eve Katz, Ph.D., Executive Director
  (202) 624-2312
Address:
  1001 Pennsylvania Avenue, NW
  Washington, DC 20004

Description. The Life and Health Insurance Medical Research Fund is a nonprofit corporation supported by member companies of the American Council of Life Insurance and the Health Insurance Association of America and by the National Association of Life Companies, the Million Dollar Round Table Fund, and other individuals and groups. Its mission is to support basic medical research and scholarship primarily but not exclusively in the areas of cancer, heart disease, immunology, and metabolic disease with an emphasis on studying underlying molecular biology. Areas of particular interest to psychiatric researchers include studies in neuroscience, behavior, and neurological disease treatments. Awards are generally solicited from medical schools each January, with awards being given in June of each year.

Lilly Endowment Inc.

Subject code(s):
   1 4 11 16 23
Point of contact:
   John M. Mutz, President
   (317) 924–5471
   Joan Lipsitz, Ph.D., Research Grants
Address:
   PO Box 88068
   2801 North Meridian Street
   Indianapolis, IN 46208

Description. Lilly Endowment Inc., an Indianapolis-based private philanthropy created in 1937, funds grants in the areas of religion, education, and community development, emphasizing particularly projects that benefit young people and promote leadership education. Although it funds some national and international projects, its main emphasis is funding within the state of Indiana.

A program of special interest to psychiatric researchers involves the youth and caring grant program. The endowment funds research that addresses youth and families. Topics include antecedents of caring behavior; linkage between children's caring attitudes and caring behavior; consequences of caring behavior; gender, age, and ethnic differences in development and definition of caring; and societal structures nurturing caring behavior.

Sample grants:
   Brandeis University, Waltham, MA. $304,255 to study national policy concerning early adolescence. Year of award: 1992
   Harvard University, Indiana University Foundation, Trenton State College, University of Medicine of New Jersey, University of Pittsburgh. $192,033 for five grants in the research program on youth and caring. Year of award: 1992

MacArthur Foundation, The John D. and Catherine T.

Subject code(s):
  6 10 11 13 16 17 23
Point of contact:
  Adele Simmons, President
  (312) 726-8000
  Victor Rabinowitch, Senior Vice President
  Denis J. Prager, Director of the Health Programs
Address:
  140 South Dearborn Street
  Chicago, IL 60603

Description.   The John D. and Catherine T. MacArthur Foundation was created in 1978 for charitable and public service purposes and currently funds eight programs: 1) the health program, devoted to research on mental health and on the biology of parasitic disease; 2) the MacArthur Fellows program, which awards fellowships to exceptionally creative individuals regardless of field; 3) the program on peace and international cooperation; 4) the world environment and resources program; 5) the special grants program, which supports cultural/community activities in Chicago, IL, and Palm Beach, FL; 6) the general program, focusing on mass communications and special initiatives; 7) the education program; and 8) the world population program.

The health program has supported research on the fundamental processes underlying mental health and illness. This program emphasizes human development research, focusing on research topics affecting individuals across the entire life span (early childhood, adolescence, midlife, and aging) and exploring these life stages as important factors in normal and pathological mental functioning. Additional topics of research interest are pathologic development research that stresses adaptive rather than maladaptive behavior and the "Mind in Context," which explores the relationship between mental and physical health. The health program also funds a smaller, eclectic set of programs designed to generally enhance the field (e.g., DSM-IV data reanalysis project, support for several publications).

The foundation is committed to a collaborative research strategy that allows networks of scientists of varying disciplines to share research interests. These special, foundation–sponsored networks are

the Network on the Psychobiology of Depression and Other Affective
Disorders, the Network on Early Childhood Transitions, the Network
on Health and Behavior, the Network on Development and Criminal
Behavior, and the Network on Mental Health Law and Policy. The
general field enhancement grants totaled $1,076,700 in 1992, and in-
ternational health grants totaling $500,000 were also awarded. Total
grant support in the health program in 1992 was $30.39 million.
Sample grants:

> Mental Health Law Project, Washington, DC. $250,000 to sup-
> port the transition of the project to the David L. Bazelon Cen-
> ter for Mental Health Law. Year of award: 1992
>
> Western Psychiatric Institute and Clinic, Pittsburgh, PA.
> $600,000 for work on the Network on the Psychobiology of
> Depression. Year of award: 1992
>
> Institute of Behavioral Science, University of Colorado, Boulder,
> CO. $5,121,297 for interdisciplinary research on youth grow-
> ing up in adverse conditions and examining factors that con-
> tribute to success in such environments. Year of award: 1992
>
> Life Trends, Inc., Vero Beach, FL. $198,472 for activities of the Net-
> work on Successful Midlife Development. Year of award: 1992
>
> Program on Conscious and Unconscious Mental Processes, Uni-
> versity of California, San Francisco, CA. $1,600,000 to sup-
> port program studying the effect of unconscious processes
> on mental functions, emotions, and behavior. Year of award:
> 1992
>
> Harvard University, Boston, MA. $10,000,000 for a 5-year
> study of the factors contributing to the development of
> criminal behavior in urban youth. Year of award: 1992
>
> Rush-Presbyterian-St. Luke's Medical Center, Chicago, IL.
> $35,000 to support collaborative research on the impact of
> stress on health status. Year of award: 1992

Mailman Family Foundation, Inc., A. L.

Subject code(s):
> 16 23

Point of contact:
> Luba H. Lynch, Executive Director
> (914) 681-4448
> Victoria S. Frelow, Program Officer

Address:
    707 Westchester Avenue, Suite 401
    White Plains, NY 10604

Description.   The A. L. Mailman Family Foundation is committed
to strengthening the family and enhancing the ability of families to
support the development and well-being of their children. Special
interest is in disadvantaged and minorities issues, and emphasis in
the 1990s will be placed on child care, early intervention, and value-
oriented education for children. The types of support that this foundation provides include start-up/seed money and special projects.
The foundation is interested in projects that propose innovative approaches to long-standing problems, develop a model for replication,
and include a long-term financial plan. Applied research that is consonant with program objectives is also encouraged. Deadlines for
board review of proposals are March 15 and October 15.

Sample grants:
    Purdue University, West Lafayette, IN. $16,949 to review parent
        education programs serving young children (birth to
        8 years), describing the current status of parent education
        activities, identifying strengths and limitations, and offering
        direction on research and policy. Year of award: 1991
    Fordham University, Tarrytown, NY. $5,000 to study violence
        prevention. Year of award: 1991
    Georgia State University, Atlanta, GA. $9,982 for a process
        evaluation of the Parent Services Project model of family sup-
        port in Atlanta in family child care settings, particularly the
        impact of the program on family day care providers and par-
        ents. Year of award: 1991

McDonnell Foundation, James S.

Subject code(s):
    1 2
Point of contact:
    John T. Bruer, President
    (314) 721-1532
    For McDonnell-Pew Cognitive Neuroscience program:
    Michele Symcak at Princeton University
    (609) 258-5014

Address:
   1034 South Brentwood Boulevard, Suite 1610
   St. Louis, MO 63117

Description. Established in 1950 by aerospace industry magnate James McDonnell, the James S. McDonnell Foundation has focused its funding on biomedical research, innovation in education, and research related to global understanding. Most of the foundation's support is provided to foundation-initiated programs within these three fields of interest. Proposals are reviewed that are outside these foundation programs, and support may be provided if funding is available.

Specific areas of McDonnell funding are 1) research that improves the quality of life, particularly research in the biological and behavioral sciences, especially if they integrate behavioral and biological approaches to the study of higher brain function or improvement in diagnostic, therapeutic, and preventive interventions; 2) research and innovation in education, particularly research in the cognitive, behavioral, and social sciences that improves curricula, learning, and teacher training; implementation of cognitive, behavioral, and social research in the classroom; and innovative/experimental programs in improving educational excellence in St. Louis, MO; and 3) efforts to improve global understanding.

The foundation initiative in biomedical research, supported in conjunction with the Pew Charitable Trusts, is the McDonnell-Pew Program in Cognitive Neuroscience, which allocates funding to establish research centers and training programs to study the brain and all basic cognitive processes. (Refer to the entry for the Pew Charitable Trusts.)

McKnight Endowment Fund for Neuroscience, The

Subject code(s):
   1 2 3
Point of contact:
   Kathy Rysted, Administrator
   (612) 333-4220
Address:
   600 TCF Tower
   121 South Eight Street
   Minneapolis, MN 55402

Description. The McKnight Awards, initiated by the McKnight Foundation in 1977, support neuroscience research in three categories: research projects, development, and scholar grants. In 1986, the foundation decided to make a permanent commitment to the support of fundamental research in neuroscience, especially as it pertains to memory and its biological substrates, by establishing the McKnight Endowment Fund for Neuroscience. Awards for research and development are given every 3 years and are by invitation only. Scholar awards are given annually by competitive selection.

Merck Fund, The John

Subject code(s):
    1 16 24
Other subject areas:
    International issues
Point of contact:
    Francis W. Hatch, Chairman
    (617) 723-2932
    Ruth Hennig, Secretary & Administrator
Address:
    11 Beacon Street, Suite 600
    Boston, MA 02108

Description. The John Merck Fund primarily focuses its support on research on children's developmental disabilities at teaching hospitals; in 1986, it expanded its programs to include environmental issues, international human rights, and population control.
Sample grants:
    Rose-Mary Boustany, M.D., Duke University, Durham, NC. $240,000 for a 3-year grant for research on mutations leading to metabolic neurogenetic diseases. Year of award: 1990
    Linda Restifo, M.D., Ph.D., University of Arizona, Scottsdale, AZ. $240,000 for a 4-year grant to study hormonally regulated genes involved in the development of the central nervous system. Year of award: 1991
    American Association for the Advancement of Science, Washington, DC. $25,000 for training and research of Guatemalan medical students in forensic sciences for human rights investigations. Year of award: 1992

University of Sao Paulo, Sao Paulo, Brazil. $20,000 to support the Center for the Study of Violence, which conducts research and policy analysis on the social factors underlying human rights violations in Brazil. Year of award: 1992

Milbank Memorial Fund

Subject code(s):
   4 7 10 24
Other subject areas:
   Conferences
Point of contact:
   Daniel M. Fox, President
   (212) 570-4800
   Kathleen S. Andersen, Senior Program Officer
Address:
   One East 75th Street
   New York, NY 10021

Description.   The Milbank Memorial Fund was chartered in 1905 with the mission "to improve the physical, mental, and moral condition of humanity and generally to advance charitable and benevolent objects." The fund has focused this philosophy in supporting grants for conferences, publications, fellowship support, and research. Areas of interest within the field of health policy include demography, mental health, epidemiology, public health, and the influence of clinical and social sciences in contributing to improved health policy and services. Projects interested in funding should initially write the fund, since most projects are solicited.
Sample grants:
   Allan V. Horwitz, Ph.D., Rutgers University, New Brunswick, NJ. $28,160 to study the role of siblings in the provision of care to the seriously mentally ill. Year of award: 1990
   Eileen M. Crimmins, Ph.D., University of Southern California, Los Angeles, CA. $13,577 to study meeting the functional needs of older Americans. Year of award: 1990

Mott Fund, Ruth

Subject code(s):
4 9 10 11 19 20
Point of contact:
Deborah Tuck, Executive Director
(810) 232-3180
Robert Stix, Program Officer
Address:
1726 Genessee Towers
Flint, MI 48502

Description. The Ruth Mott Fund supports grants fostering prevention issues and promoting sensible health practices, especially focusing on problems of low-income populations in improving nutrition, stress control, exercise, smoking cessation, reduced drug and alcohol use, and health care access.
Sample grants:
American Friends Service Committee, Philadelphia, PA. $20,000 for support of the Maquiladora Project, which researches and addresses health and safety problems arising from industrial expansion along the U.S.-Mexican border. Year of award: 1992

Center for Budget and Policy Priorities, Washington, DC. $20,000 for support to improve maternal and child health. Year of award: 1992

National Alliance for Research on Schizophrenia and Depression (NARSAD)

Subject code(s):
1 2 5 6 8 12 13
Point of contact:
Connie Lieber, Executive Director
(516) 829-0091
Brenda Berman, Grants Administrator
(312) 641-3483
Address:
60 Cutter Mill Road, Suite 200
Great Neck, NY 11021

Description. NARSAD is an alliance founded by the National Alliance for the Mentally Ill (NAMI), the National Mental Health Association (NMHA), the Schizophrenia Foundation, and the National Depressive and Manic Depressive Association (NDMDA), to provide support for research into severe and persistent mental illnesses. Its research program was developed by distinguished scientists in neuroscience and psychiatry with the purpose of awarding grants to young and established investigators throughout the United States and Canada. This alliance is composed of citizens, foundations, organizations, and corporations that donate funds to initiate and accelerate mental illness research. Since its inception, NARSAD has grown to be the largest private sector, philanthropically supported funder of mental illness research. As of 1993, it has provided 503 grants to 315 investigators at 78 universities, medical schools, and research institutions.

Funds are distributed through its two grant programs, the Young Investigator Awards and Established Investigator Awards. These research awards are given for 1 year and range from $25,000 to $100,000 and are available to scientists who are associate professors or above and/or principal investigators on a federal grant. Second year renewal is possible. Research may focus on basic or clinical research or combination thereof. In 1993, the Young Investigator Program supported 30 scientists in basic science, 28 in clinical research, and 10 who combined clinical and basic research; the Established Investigator Program funded nine scientists.

Sample grants:

Established Investigator—David Shaffer, M.D., Columbia University, New York, NY, for pilot studies on the effect of thyrotropin-releasing hormone on human brain function. Year of award: 1992

Established Investigator—Alfred L. Lewy, M.D., Ph.D., Oregon Sciences University for research on hormone melatonin for medication for chronobiologic or mood disorders. Year of award: 1992

Established Investigator—Paul Greengard, Ph.D., Rockefeller University, New York, NY, for study of the mechanisms of interactions between dopamine and glutamate neurotransmitter systems and their significance in psychosis. Year of award: 1992

Established Investigator—Alan S. Bellack, Ph.D., Medical College of Pennsylvania, Philadelphia, PA, for the development of updated social skills training protocol based on contemporary understanding of the neurology and phenomenology of schizophrenia. Year of award: 1992

Young Investigator—Steven E. Arnold, M.D., University of Pennsylvania, Philadelphia, PA, to study microtubule-associated proteins missing from some hippocampal neurons in schizophrenia patients. Year of award: 1992

Young Investigator—Peter F. Buckley, M.D., Case Western Reserve University, Cleveland, OH, for the study of a posited neurodevelopmental basis for schizophrenia. Year of award: 1992

Young Investigator—Michael R. Johnson, M.D., Medical University of South Carolina, Charleston, SC, to study patients with major depressive illness and panic disorder responding to imipramine and MAO inhibitor phenelzine. Year of award: 1992

Young Investigator—Robert C. Malenka, M.D., Ph.D., University of California, San Francisco, CA, to study the cellular mechanisms responsible for short-term and long-term modulation of synaptic transmission. Year of award: 1992

Young Investigator—Adelaide S. Robb, M.D., National Institute of Mental Health, Rockville, MD, to study improvements in identifying genes responsible for predisposition to psychiatric disease. Year of award: 1992

Young Investigator—Madhukar H. Trivedi, M.D., University of Texas, Dallas, TX, for the study of amphetamine, a pharmacological probe in identifying circuits in the brain associated with mood changes. Year of award: 1992

Young Investigator—Ralf Zimmerman, M.D., Mayo Clinic, Rochester, MN, for the development of a test involving tryptophan depletion that will predict ability of an individual with depression to respond to medication inhibiting serotonin reuptake. Year of award: 1992

National Alliance for the Mentally Ill (NAMI)

Subject code(s):
1 2 5 8 12 13
Point of contact:
E. Fuller Torrey, M.D., Chairperson
(703) 524-7600
Kitty Clark

Address:
2101 Wilson Boulevard, Suite 302
Arlington, VA 22201

Description. NAMI was founded in 1979 by parents who were dissatisfied with the treatment their children with mental illness had been receiving. A membership organization with 140,000 members and 1,000 chapters, NAMI focuses on all severe, biologically linked mental illnesses; its main goal has been "to improve the conditions of the mentally ill and to eradicate the stigma attached to mental illnesses." NAMI supports advocacy, research, and public education programs on mental illness. It monitors the media, commercial products, and organizations to uncover inaccurate information on mental illness, and it produces public service announcements for public education.

NAMI also awards more than $1 million annually in mental health research funds and administers the Theodore and Vada Stanley Foundation Research Awards. These awards support established scientists in research directly related to causes of serious mental illnesses, such as schizophrenia, bipolar disorder, and major depression. These grants are also intended to attract established scientists from other areas of biology and medicine, such as biochemistry and neurology, into research on severe mental illnesses and to provide support for innovative research. Awards are from 1 to 2 years and may be up to $50,000 each year. Scientists from other areas of biology and medicine and those with innovative research proposals are strongly encouraged to apply. Deadline for applications is April 1.
Sample grants:
> Fritz Henn, Ph.D., M.D., State University of New York, Stony Brook, NY. PET scan studies of pedigree families with major affective disorders using Mu receptor ligand. Year of award: 1992
>
> Robert Kerwin, M.D., Institute of Psychiatry, London, and Oxford, England. Testing with postmortem brains from patients with schizophrenia neurodevelopmental hypothesis by studying isoforms glutamate receptors. Year of award: 1992
>
> Ezra Susser, M.D., New York State Psychiatric Institute, New York, NY. Identification of individuals who have developed serious mental illness from cohorts of birth. Year of award: 1992
>
> Shon Lewis, M.D., Ann Stewart, M.D., and Robin Murray, Institute of Psychiatry, London, England. Follow-up of low-birth-

weight babies to ascertain incidence of schizophrenia and major affective disorders. Year of award: 1992

Lori Altshuler, M.D., University of California, Los Angeles, CA. Conducting MRI studies on the temporal lobe structures in patients with schizophrenia and bipolar disorder. Year of award: 1992

B. M. Cohen, M.D., McLean Hospital, Belmont, MA. Studying schizophrenia as a developmental disorder by making lesions in the temporal cortex of rats. Year of award: 1992

S. C. Schulz, M.D., Case Western Reserve University, Cleveland, OH. Conducting studies on adolescents with first episode schizophrenia or bipolar disorder using MRI, neuropsychology, and eye tracking, and retesting 1 year later. Year of award: 1992

T. Young, M.D., Clarke Institute, Toronto, Canada. Conducting studies to follow up the findings of high incidence of protein G in postmortem brain tissue from individuals with bipolar disorder. Year of award: 1992

National Parkinson Foundation

Subject code(s):
   22
Point of contact:
   Paula Conley, Research Grants
   (305) 547-6666
Address:
   1501 NW 9th Avenue
   Miami, FL 33136

Description.   The National Parkinson Foundation supports basic research on Parkinson's disease by funding studies using experimental physiological, biochemical, or molecular biologic procedures that focus on the basic mechanisms involved in the disease process. Research must have the potential of finding the causes and/or means of preventing Parkinson's disease. Up to $40,000 per year is available for direct expenses. The aim of this research program is to attract scientists in this field of research and provide them with seed money for initial studies with the hope of competing successfully for major federal grants. The annual deadline is February 1.

New-Land Foundation, Inc., The

Subject code(s):
  2 10 16 22
Point of contact:
  Robert Wolf, President
  (212) 479-6162
Address:
  1114 Avenue of the Americas, 46th Floor
  New York, NY 10036

Description. The New-Land Foundation provides funding for mental health, population control, peace and arms control, civil rights, child development, the environment, leadership development, and minority education. Grant support is provided for general purposes, research, conferences, and internships. Deadlines for all considerations for support are February 1 and August 1.

Packard Foundation, The David & Lucile

Subject code(s):
  1 10 16
Point of contact:
  Colburn S. Wilbur, Executive Director
  (415) 948-7658
  Richard E. Behrman, M.D., Director of Center for the Future of Children
Address:
  300 Second Street, Suite 200
  Los Altos, CA 94022

Description. The David and Lucile Packard Foundation was founded in 1964 to support and encourage organizations dependent on private funding and volunteer leadership. This is reflected in its support for the following areas of commitment: 1) science and education, especially ocean science, fellowship support in engineering and science, historically black colleges and universities; 2) population and conservation; 3) local giving in southern California; and 4) children, especially support from the foundation's Center for the Future of Children, a multidisciplinary applied research, policy, and grant-making program on behalf of children and their families. Research on pregnancy and birth outcomes, child care and early intervention, and medical outcomes and prevention/treatment research are significant areas of current funding.

Proposals are due quarterly—January 2, April 1, July 1, and October 1. For those interested in applying for support from the Center for the Future of Children, proposal deadlines are December 15, March 15, June 15, and September 15.

Sample grants:

Families and Work Institute, New York, NY. $31,681 to study the quality and nature of family child care. Year of award: 1992

Miramonte Mental Health Services, Palo Alto, CA. $35,000 to assist the Association of Mental Health Contract Agencies of Santa Clara County in conducting a study of the cost effectiveness of mental health care delivery and possible alternatives. Year of award: 1992

Northwestern University, Chicago, IL. $14,697 to study the ethnic differences in lifestyles, psychological factors, and medical care in pregnancy. Year of award: 1992

Pew Charitable Trusts, The

Subject code(s):
1 3 10 16 24

Other subject areas:
Poverty issues; local funding around Philadelphia, PA

Point of contact:
Thomas W. Langfitt, M.D., President
(215) 575-9050
Carolyn H. Asbury, Health Program Director
(215) 575-4939

Address:
One Commerce Square, Suite 1700
2005 Market Street
Philadelphia, PA 19103

Description.   The Pew Charitable Trusts is a national and international philanthropy composed of seven trusts with a special commitment to Philadelphia. It provides support in the areas of conservation and the environment, culture, education, health and human services, public policy, and religion. It encourages grants that promote individual development and personal achievement, cross-disciplinary approaches, and innovative solutions to current social needs.

Psychiatric research funding is supported through the health and human services program, which aims to improve the opportunities of disadvantaged Americans to join the economic and social mainstream and to assist the health care system to respond more effectively to the health needs of Americans. The program's "Children at Risk" initiative seeks to address the problems and needs of poverty-stricken children and their families and increase economic and social opportunities. Also of interest are the health care services grants, which seek to improve accountability, quality, organization, and distribution of health care and public health services, and the Biomedical Sciences Initiative, which promotes linkages among biomedical research specialties and institutional collaboration. Outcomes research on medical practice organization, education, and training is supported.

One foundation program in biomedical research, supported in conjunction with the James S. McDonnell Foundation, is the McDonnell-Pew Program in Cognitive Neuroscience, which allocates funding to establish research centers and training programs to study the brain and all basic cognitive processes. (Refer to the entry for the James S. McDonnell Foundation.)

Sample grants:

McDonnell-Pew Program in Neuroscience 1992-1994 Awards (all for 2 years): The Johns Hopkins University, $135,000; Massachusetts Institute of Technology, $829,255; Princeton University, $293,938; University of Arizona Foundation, $528,000; University of California, Davis, $87,500; and University of Oregon, $480,000. Year of award: 1992

Brown University, Providence, RI. $150,000 for the Center for Gerontology and Health Care Research in analyzing data on the settings of long-term care used by elderly people. Year of award: 1993

National Academy of Social Insurance, Washington, DC. $350,000 to support an analysis of disability policy as it relates to people with serious mental illness. Year of award: 1993

Dartmouth College, Hanover, NH. $50,000 to develop a cognitive neuroscience training video. Year of award: 1992

Wistar Institute of Anatomy and Biology, Philadelphia, PA.

$1,000,000 for a 2-year grant to strengthen three of the institute's research programs. Year of award: 1992

Foundation for Health Services Research, Washington, DC. $370,000 over 2 years to develop and implement an information system on ongoing health services research projects. Year of award: 1991

New York University, New York, NY. $1,000,000 over 3 years to develop a research and demonstration project on substance abuse prevention among high-risk adolescents. Year of award: 1991

The Johns Hopkins University, Baltimore, MD. $155,000 for a 2-year grant to support a survey of Medicaid-eligible women and their access to prenatal care services. Year of award: 1991

American Psychiatric Association, Washington, DC. Support for state-university collaboration project in psychiatry. Year of award: 1991

Retirement Research Foundation, The

Subject code(s):
    4 9 10 17
Other subject areas:
    Chicago, IL grants are given precedence
Point of contact:
    Marilyn Hennessy, Executive Director
    (312) 714-8080
Address:
    8765 West Higgins Road, Suite 401
    Chicago, IL 60631

Description. The Retirement Research Foundation, established by John D. MacArthur in 1950, is a private philanthropy dedicated to improving the quality of life of older persons in the United States. This mission is focused on four main objectives: 1) to increase the availability and effectiveness of community programs for older persons to maintain independence; 2) to improve the quality of nursing home care; 3) to provide new and expanded opportunities for older persons to engage in employment and volunteer work; and 4) to support basic, applied, and policy research on problems of the aged.

Research grants are to be project grants, and grants from the Chicago metropolitan area are given priority over those grants nationwide that are of equal significance. Applications are reviewed three times each year, with deadlines of February 1, May 1, and August 1.

Sample grants:

University of Illinois, Urbana-Champaign, IL. $23,622 for a national survey of suicide prevention centers to examine how potential cases of elderly suicide are managed. Year of award: 1993

University of California, Los Angeles, CA. $214,500 for a 3-year grant to launch a competitive pilot grant program in geriatrics and gerontology. Year of award: 1993

Coalition of Advocates for the Rights of Infirm Elderly, Philadelphia, PA. $125,000 for a 2-year grant to examine and research neglect and abuse issues in personal care homes and develop a training curriculum for personal care facilities. Year of award: 1993

Population Resource Center, Princeton, NJ. $20,000 to develop a research agenda to assess the impact of changing status of women on future health and well-being in retirement. Year of award: 1993

Alliance for Aging Research, Washington, DC. $75,000 for a 3-year grant to support advocacy for increased funding for aging research. Year of award: 1993

University of Notre Dame, South Bend, IN. $1,000 to provide second-year support for a survey on the current availability and level of support for gerontological and geriatric specialization within core health and mental health professions. Year of award: 1992

Center for Elderly Suicide Prevention and Grief-Related Services, San Francisco, CA. $271,550 over 3 years for the evaluation of the effectiveness and efficiency of three intervention techniques in the prevention of suicide in older adults. Year of award: 1992

Medicate Advocacy Project, Los Angeles, CA. $35,500 to study hospital admission patterns for the senior population of Los Angeles, CA. Year of award: 1992

Loyola University Medical Center, Maywood, IL. $49,975 to continue research evaluating Z-HUP-A, a chemical variant of HUP-A, as a potential agent for treatment of Alzheimer's disease. Year of award: 1992

RGK Foundation, The

Subject code(s):
    2 22 24
Other subject areas:
    Mental health conferences
Point of contact:
    Ronya Kozmetsky, President
    (512) 474-9298
Address:
    2815 San Gabriel
    Austin, TX 78705

Description. Founded in 1966, the RGK Foundation provides support for medical and educational research. It sponsors studies in areas of national and international concern, including health, corporate governance, energy, and economic analysis. Major emphasis has been on connective tissue diseases, particularly scleroderma, and spinal cord injury. Areas of mental health research focus include neuroscience and neurological research.

Sample grants:

The University of Texas Health Science Center, San Antonio, TX. Conference entitled, "Health Policy and the Hispanic: The Economic and Social Impact of Public and Private Sector Strategies." Year of award: 1989

Harvard Medical School, Division on Aging. Support for conference, "Geriatric Care—Clinical Dilemmas and Ethical Solutions." Year of award: 1991

National Ataxia Foundation. Research on hereditary ataxias and other neurological disorders. Year of award: 1989

Texas Foundation for Mental Health and Mental Retardation. Support for second annual Helen Farabee Conference on Mental Health and Mental Retardation. Year of award: 1991

National Spinal Cord Injury Association. Prevention campaigns, services, and research programs on spinal cord injuries. Year of award: 1989

Texas Foundation for Mental Health. Support for the third annual conference on mental health and mental retardation. Year of award: 1992

The Johns Hopkins University School of Medicine, Kennedy Institute, Baltimore, MD. Research on the fragile X syndrome and social disability in female children. Year of award: 1991

Sandoz Foundation for Gerontological Research

Subject code(s):
   17
Point of contact:
   Robert N. Butler, M.D., President
   (201) 503-8544
   Bill Connelly, Secretary
Address:
   59 Route 10
   East Hanover, NJ 07936

Description.   The Sandoz Foundation was created in 1986 to promote scientific research concerned with aging and the problems faced by the aging individual. This support encourages scientists to undertake innovative research projects in the biological sciences, pharmacology, geriatric internal medicine, and geriatric psychiatry. The foundation funds direct costs, equipment expenses, travel, publications, and administrative costs. Maximum grant support for 1 year is $35,000; renewals are infrequent. Annual deadlines for funding consideration are May 1 and November 1.

Supreme Masonic Council, 33, Scottish Rite

Subject code(s):
   2 5 8 12
Point of contact:
   Steven Matthysse, Ph.D., Research Director
   (617) 862-4410
   Nancy L. Maxwell, Administrator
Address:
   PO Box 519
   33 Marrett Road
   Lexington, MA 02173

Description.   The Supreme Council, 33, Scottish Rite of Freemasonry inaugurated the Benevolent Foundation Schizophrenia Research Program in 1934 to support research into the nature and causes of schizophrenia. There has been a steady increase in the level of support directed to this research by the program: more than $9 million has been allocated to the program since creation, and it currently awards grants and fellowships in excess of $600,000 each year.

Two research funding mechanisms constitute the schizophrenia research program: Research Grant Awards and Dissertation Research Fellowship Awards. The Research Grant Awards support funding for clearly defined projects that advance understanding of the nature/causes of schizophrenia, preferably pilot projects. It is the expectation that 1–2 years of support will provide the foundation for other long-term funding. Deadline for a letter of intent is December 15, with proposals due March 15. The Dissertation Research Fellowship Awards supports exceptionally promising students during the preparation of their doctoral dissertations in fields relevant to schizophrenia research. Fields include biochemistry, epidemiology, genetics, neuroscience, pharmacology, and psychiatry. Criteria for this award include creativity, schizophrenia research advancement, and project relevance. Deadline for fellowship sponsor letters of intent is February 1, with final applications due March 15.

Sample grants:

George Bartzokis, M.D., and Stephen R. Marder, M.D., University of California, Los Angeles, CA. Neuroleptic effects of T2 relaxation times of the basal ganglia nuclei. Year of award: 1990

Lisa Dixon, M.D., and Robert Conley, M.D., Maryland Psychiatric Research Center, Baltimore, MD. Psychoactive substance use assessment in schizophrenia. Year of award: 1990

Kenneth S. Kendler, M.D., Medical College of Virginia, Richmond, VA. A multitrait twin study of schizotypy. Year of award: 1990

Stanley J. Watson, Ph.D., M.D., Huda Akil, Ph.D., and James Meador-Woodruff, M.D., University of Michigan, Ann Arbor, MI. Acquisition and neuropathological characterization of postmortem schizophrenic CNS material for molecular biological analysis. Year of award: 1990

Steven E. Hyman, M.D., and Robert J. Birnbaum, Ph.D., M.D., Massachusetts General Hospital, Boston, MA. Developmental regulation of tyrosine hydroxylase gene expression. Year of award: 1990

Robert R. Conley, M.D., and Carol Taminga, M.D., Maryland Psychiatric Research Center, Baltimore, MD. Evaluation of clozapine effects on dopamine and serotonin receptors. Year of award: 1990

Adityanjee, M.D., Medical College of Virginia, Richmond, VA. M-CPP challenge response as the predictor of response to clozapine in neuroleptic-resistant schizophrenia patients. Year of award: 1992

Jonathan A. Javitch, M.D., Ph.D., and Arthur Karlin, Ph.D., Columbia University, New York, NY. Molecular mapping of antipsychotic drug binding sites in the dopamine D2-like receptor family. Year of award: 1992

James L. Kennedy, M.Sc., M.D., and Arturas Petronis, M.D., Ph.D., University of Toronto, Ontario, Canada. Molecular genetic investigation of unstable DNA sites in schizophrenia. Year of award: 1992

Jean-Piere Lindenmayer, M.D., Albert Einstein College of Medicine, Bronx, NY. Methylphenidate challenge response as predictor of clozapine response in neuroleptic refractory schizophrenics. Year of award: 1992

Alfred Pope, M.D., McLean Hospital, Belmont, MA. Biology of human prefrontal cortex. Year of award: 1992

USX Foundation, Inc.

Subject code(s):
   10 17 24
Other subject areas:
   Equipment
Point of contact:
   Peter B. Mulloney, President
   (412) 433-5237
Address:
   600 Grant Street
   Pittsburgh, PA 15219

Description. The USX Foundation, Inc., provides financial support related to charitable, medical-health, educational, civic, cultural, and scientific endeavors. Medical research funding has been provided for research and research training, construction, and Alzheimer's dis-

ease. In 1992, the foundation supported 12 grants totaling $109,500 to medical and health-related organizations.
Sample grant:
> Alzheimer's Disease Alliance of Western Pennsylvania. Construction of a model care and research center. Year of award: 1991

---

van Ameringen Foundation, Inc.

Subject code(s):
> 16 24

Other subject areas:
> Broad support in mental health and psychiatric research issues

Point of contact:
> Henry van Ameringen, President
> (212) 758-6221
> Eleanor Sypher, Ph.D., Executive Director

Address:
> 509 Madison Avenue, Suite 2010
> New York, NY 10022

Description.   The van Ameringen Foundation is a private grant-making foundation located in New York City and active principally in the urban Northeast. The foundation was established by Arnold Louis van Ameringen in 1950. From its beginning the foundation has sought to stimulate prevention, education, and direct care in the mental health field with an emphasis on those individuals and populations having a disadvantaged background and deprived opportunities. Support is also given for child development, medical education, and other related health fields. Under support from the van Ameringen Foundation, the American Psychiatric Association has developed the Psychiatric Research Resource Center, a project advancing the recruitment, retention, and training of scientists in psychiatric research (which includes the development of this manual).

Sample grants:
> The General Hospital Corporation, Boston, MA. A 2-year grant of $129,600 for community outreach and ongoing research in identifying and treating psychiatrically ill pregnant women and women suffering from postpartum depression. Year of award: 1992
> The Mount Sinai Hospital, New York, NY. $100,000 for a 2-year

grant to improve and expand a clinical data base of risk factors for patients with Alzheimer's and other dementias. Year of award: 1992

The General Hospital Corporation, Boston, MA. $129,600 to fund community outreach and ongoing research in identifying and treating psychiatrically ill pregnant women and women suffering from postpartum depression. Year of award: 1992

Institute for Experimental Psychiatry Research Foundation, Merion Station, PA. $152,200 for a 3-year grant supporting personnel costs for the completion of a clinical study of the effects of hypnosis on children in pain with sickle cell disease. Year of award: 1990

Memorial Sloan Kettering Cancer Center, New York, NY. $70,000 for a 1-year grant for the support of an additional clinician for the study entitled, "Parent Guidance Prevention Program for Bereaved Children." Year of award: 1990

Episcopal Mission Society, New York, NY. $67,960 to design a model program and policy recommendations for abused children and their battered mothers. Year of award: 1992

Harvard University, Cambridge, MA. $36,000 for a 1-year grant for developing an interdisciplinary and collaborative support and research center for guidance counselors in Massachusetts. Year of award: 1992

NARSAD, Great Neck, NY. $200,000 for a 4-year grant supporting research efforts concerned with schizophrenia and depression. Year of award: 1990

Emory University—The Carter Center, Atlanta, GA. $40,000 for a 1-year grant in support of the Sixth Annual Rosalyn Carter Symposium on Mental Health Policy, sponsored by the Carter Presidential Center at Emory University. Year of award: 1992

Whitehall Foundation, Inc.

Subject code(s):
    1 2
Point of contact:
    Laurel T. Baker, Secretary
    (407) 655-4474
    George M. Moffett II, President

Address:
    251 Royal Palm Way, Suite 211
    Palm Beach, FL 33480

Description. The Whitehall Foundation, through its program of grants and grants-in-aid, assists scholarly research in the life sciences. The foundation's policy is to assist those areas of basic biological research that are not heavily supported by the federal government or other foundations. In order to respond to the changing environment, the Whitehall Foundation periodically reassesses the need for financial support by the various fields of biological research. Currently, the foundation is interested only in the area of neurobiology, specifically invertebrate and vertebrate neurobiology, exclusive of human beings, investigating neural mechanisms as they relate to behavior. Support is provided through 1) Research Grants, which are available to established scientists of all ages working at accredited institutions; applications are judged on the scientific merit of the proposal and competence of the applicant, and grants, normally between $10,000 and $40,000 for up to 3 years, will be provided; a single 2-year grant is also possible; and 2) Grants-in-Aid, for researchers at the assistant professor level who experience difficulty in competing for research funds; these awards are for 1-year periods and do not exceed $15,000. Deadlines are open, with three grant review sessions each year.

Wills Foundation, The

Subject code(s):
    22
Point of contact:
    Alice E. Pratt, President
    (713) 965-9043
Address:
    PO Box 27534
    Houston, TX 77227

Description. The Wills Foundation provides research funding relevant to Huntington's disease for U.S. institutions. Grants and post-doctoral fellowships are available, ranging up to $20,000, depending on the nature of the research. Investigators interested in applying must send a letter of intent by either September 1 or March 1, the two preapplication deadlines, in order to receive funding by January or July, respectively.

◆ Section 3: Foundation Profile Subject Index

This subject index lists foundations that indicate an interest or have funded grants in mental health and psychiatric-related research and are profiled in Section 2. These organizations are listed alphabetically within each subject area. Please note the limitations of this subject listing. Many of these foundations are not necessarily a perfect fit to all the tracked categories, and foundations may change the emphasis of their funding interests. Use the listing as a guideline to obtain more detailed information about the foundation.

Research Training Funding/Career Development

Allied-Signal Foundation
Alzheimer's Disease and Related Disorders Association
American Medical Association Education and Research Foundation
Burroughs Wellcome Fund, The
Commonwealth Fund, The
Culpeper Foundation, Charles E.
Dana Foundation, The Charles A.
Diamond Foundation, The Aaron
Ford Foundation, The
French Foundation for Alzheimer Research, The
Fulbright Scholar Program
Grant Foundation, William T.
Grass Foundation, The
Howard Hughes Medical Institute
Ittleson Foundation, Inc.
Jacobs Foundation, Johann
Johnson Foundation, The Robert Wood
Kaiser Foundation, The Henry J.
Klingenstein Fund, Inc., The Esther A. and Joseph
Lilly Endowment Inc.
McDonnell Foundation, James S.

McKnight Endowment Fund for Neuroscience, The
Merck Fund, The John
National Alliance for the Mentally Ill
National Alliance for Research on Schizophrenia and Depression
Packard Foundation, The David and Lucile
Pew Charitable Trusts, The
Whitehall Foundation, Inc.

Basic Biological Sciences/Neuroscience

American Paralysis Association
Bristol-Myers Squibb Foundation, Inc.
Burroughs Wellcome Fund, The
Dana Foundation, The Charles A.
Glenn Foundation for Medical Research
Grant Foundation, William T.
Grass Foundation, The
Hood Foundation, The Charles H.
Howard Hughes Medical Institute
Keck Foundation, W. M.
Klingenstein Fund, Inc., The Esther A. and Joseph
Life and Health Insurance Medical Research Fund
McDonnell Foundation, James S.
McKnight Endowment Fund for Neuroscience, The
National Alliance for the Mentally Ill
National Alliance for Research on Schizophrenia and Depression
RGK Foundation, The
Supreme Masonic Council, 33, Scottish Rite
Whitehall Foundation, Inc.

Behavioral/Cognitive Sciences

Klingenstein Fund, Inc., The Esther A. and Joseph
Life and Health Insurance Medical Research Fund
McKnight Endowment Fund for Neuroscience, The
Pew Charitable Trusts, The
Sandoz Foundation for Gerontological Research
Spinal Cord Research Foundation, The

Social Sciences, including cross-cultural issues

AARP Andrus Foundation
Carnegie Corporation of New York
Ford Foundation, The
Grant Foundation, William T.
Harris Foundation, The
Ittleson Foundation, Inc.
Lilly Endowment Inc.
Milbank Memorial Fund
Mott Fund, Ruth
Retirement Research Foundation, The

Clinical Psychobiology

National Alliance for the Mentally Ill
National Alliance for Research on Schizophrenia and Depression
Supreme Masonic Council, 33, Scottish Rite

Diagnosis/Nosology

MacArthur Foundation, The John D. and Catherine T.
National Alliance for the Mentally Ill
National Alliance for Research on Schizophrenia and Depression
Supreme Masonic Council, 33, Scottish Rite

Epidemiology

Grant Foundation, William T.
MacArthur Foundation, The John D. and Catherine T.
Milbank Memorial Fund

Psychopharmacology

Burroughs Wellcome Fund, The
National Alliance for the Mentally Ill

National Alliance for Research on Schizophrenia and Depression
Supreme Masonic Council, 33, Scottish Rite

Psychosocial Treatments

Grant Foundation, William T.
Ittleson Foundation, Inc.
Mott Fund, Ruth
Retirement Research Foundation, The

Health/Mental Health Services Research

AARP Andrus Foundation
American Health Assistance Foundation
Burden Foundation, Florence V.
Commonwealth Fund, The
Ford Foundation, The
Foundation for Child Development
Grant Foundation, William T.
Hartford Foundation, The John A.
Ittleson Foundation, Inc.
JM Foundation, The
Johnson Foundation, The Robert Wood
Kaiser Foundation, The Henry J.
MacArthur Foundation, The John D. and Catherine T.
Milbank Memorial Fund
Mott Fund, Ruth
Packard Foundation, The David and Lucile
Pew Charitable Trusts, The
Retirement Research Foundation, The
USX Foundation, Inc.

Consultation-Liaison Psychiatry/Behavioral Medicine

Cummings Foundation, The Nathan
Grant Foundation, William T.
Ittleson Foundation, Inc.
JM Foundation, The

Lilly Endowment Inc.
MacArthur Foundation, The John D. and Catherine T.
Mott Fund, Ruth
Retirement Research Foundation, The

See also Section 2 (e.g., American Cancer Society, American Heart Association, American Diabetes Association).

Psychotic Disorders/Schizophrenia

National Alliance for the Mentally Ill
National Alliance for Research on Schizophrenia and Depression
Supreme Masonic Council, 33, Scottish Rite

Affective/Mood Disorders

MacArthur Foundation, The John D. and Catherine T.
National Alliance for the Mentally Ill
National Alliance for Research on Schizophrenia and Depression

Anxiety/Stress-Related Disorders

Howard Hughes Medical Institute
National Alliance for Research on Schizophrenia and Depression

Personality Disorders

Guggenheim Foundation, The Harry Frank

Child/Adolescent Mental Disorders

Alcoholic Beverage Medical Research Foundation
Burden Foundation, Florence V.
Carnegie Corporation of New York
Clark Foundation, The Edna McConnell
Commonwealth Fund, The

Diamond Foundation, The Aaron
Ford Foundation, The
Foundation for Child Development
Grant Foundation, William T.
Guggenheim Foundation, The Harry Frank
Harris Foundation, The
Hood Foundation, The Charles H.
Ittleson Foundation, Inc.
Jacobs Foundation, Johann
Kaiser Foundation, The Henry J.
Kenworthy—Sarah H. Swift Foundation, Inc., Marion E.
Lilly Endowment Inc.
MacArthur Foundation, The John D. and Catherine T.
Mailman Family Foundation, Inc., A. L.
Merck Fund, The John
New-Land Foundation, Inc., The
Packard Foundation, The David and Lucile
Pew Charitable Trusts, The
van Ameringen Foundation, Inc.

Geriatric Psychiatry/Dementia, Delirium, and Other Cognitive Disorders

AARP Andrus Foundation
Allied-Signal Foundation
Alzheimer's Disease and Related Disorders Association, Inc.
American Health Assistance Foundation
Burden Foundation, Florence V.
Clark Foundation, The Edna McConnell
Commonwealth Fund, The
Dana Foundation, The Charles A.
Diamond Foundation, The Aaron
French Foundation for Alzheimer Research, The
Glenn Foundation for Medical Research
Hartford Foundation, The John A.
Ittleson Foundation, Inc.
MacArthur Foundation, The John D. and Catherine T.
Retirement Research Foundation, The
Sandoz Foundation for Gerontological Research
USX Foundation, Inc.

AIDS

Diamond Foundation, The Aaron
Howard Hughes Medical Institute
Ittleson Foundation, Inc.

Alcohol Abuse

AARP Andrus Foundation
Alcoholic Beverage Medical Research Foundation
Grant Foundation, William T.
Guggenheim Foundation, The Harry Frank
JM Foundation, The
Johnson Foundation, The Robert Wood
Kaiser Foundation, The Henry J.
Mott Fund, Ruth

Other Drug Abuse

AARP Andrus Foundation
Clark Foundation, The Edna McConnell
Diamond Foundation, The Aaron
Ford Foundation, The
Grant Foundation, William T.
Guggenheim Foundation, The Harry Frank
JM Foundation, The
Johnson Foundation, The Robert Wood
Kaiser Foundation, The Henry J.
Mott Fund, Ruth

Movement Disorders and Other Neurologic Conditions

American Paralysis Association
Huntington's Disease Society of America
National Parkinson Foundation
RGK Foundation, The
Wills Foundation, The

See also Section 2 (e.g., spinal cord injury).

Forensic/Legal/Violence Issues

Burden Foundation, Florence V.
Clark Foundation, The Edna McConnell
Grant Foundation, William T.
Guggenheim Foundation, The Harry Frank
Ittleson Foundation, Inc.
Lilly Endowment Inc.
MacArthur Foundation, The John D. and Catherine T.
Mailman Family Foundation, Inc., A. L.

Other Subject Areas
(listing of organization and interest)

AARP Andrus Foundation: Older women's issues; geriatric public
    policy
American Suicide Foundation: Suicide and related research issues
Arca Foundation, The: International issues; human rights abuse
Commonwealth Fund, The: Urban issues, particularly in New York
    City
Dana Foundation, The Charles A.: Genetic research
Diamond Foundation, The Aaron: Local giving in New York City
Ford Foundation, The: Poverty and urban issues
Fulbright Scholar Program: International education
Ittleson Foundation, Inc.: Underserved populations
Jacobs Foundation, Johann: International issues
JM Foundation, The: Rehabilitation
Johnson Foundation, The: Conferences
Kaiser Foundation, The Henry J.: Minority and women's issues
Merck Fund, The John: International issues
Milbank Memorial Fund: Conferences
Pew Charitable Trusts, The: Poverty issues; local funding in
    Philadelphia, PA
RGK Foundation, The: Mental health conferences
USX Foundation, Inc.: Equipment
van Ameringen Foundation, Inc.: Broad support in mental health
    research

◆ Section 4: Foundations Supporting General Biomedical Research; Supporting Research on Particular General Medical Conditions With Potential Support of Related Psychiatric Research, or Having Limited Support of Mental Health Research

American Academy of Family Physicians Foundation
8880 Ward Parkway
Kansas City, MO 64114
Rachelle Rediwine
1 (800) 274-2237
(Family medicine)

American Cancer Society, Inc.
1599 Clifton Road NE
Atlanta, GA 30329
Research Department
(404) 320-3333
(Cancer)

American Diabetes Association
1660 Duke Street
Alexandria, VA 22314
Lauren Smith, Director of Research Programs
(703) 549-1500
(Diabetes)

American Foundation for AIDS Research
5900 Wilshire Boulevard, 23rd Floor
Los Angeles, CA 90036
Bernie Dempsey, Grants Department
(213) 857-5900
(AIDS)

American Heart Association
7272 Greenville Avenue
Dallas, TX 75231
Division of Research Administration
(214) 706-1453
(Coronary heart disease)

American Philosophical Society
104 South Fifth Street
Philadelphia, PA 19106
Ellie Roach, Director of the Grants Office
(Research training in clinical medicine; scholarly research)

Association for Health Services Research
1350 Connecticut Avenue, NW, Suite 1100
Washington, DC 20036
Alice Hersh, Director
(202) 223-2477
(Health services research)

Bader Foundation, Inc., Helen
777 East Wisconsin Avenue, Suite 3275
Milwaukee, WI 53202
Daniel J. Bader, President
Robert Pietrykowski, Program Office for Families and Children
(414) 224-6464
(Child and family issues research; Alzheimer's disease)

Baker Trust, The George F.
767 Fifth Avenue, Suite 2850
New York, NY 10153
Rocio Suarez, Executive Director
(212) 755-1890
(Research on child issues)

Baxter Foundation, The
One Baxter Parkway
Deerfield, IL 60015
Patricia Morgan, Executive Director
(708) 948-4605
(Primary care; autoimmune and genetic disorders)

Cancer Research Foundation of America
700 Princess Street, Suite 5
Alexandria, VA 22314
Carolyn R. Aldige, President
(703) 836-4412
(Cancer)

Diabetes Research and Education Foundation
PO Box 6168
Bridgewater, NJ 08807
Herbert Rosenkilde, M.D., Executive Director
(908) 658-9322
(Diabetes)

Doheny Foundation, The Carrie E.
911 Wilshire Boulevard, Suite 1750
Los Angeles, CA 90017
Robert A. Smith III, President
Shirley Bernard, Grants Coordinator
(213) 488-1122
(Broad biomedical research)

Emerson Electric Co. Charitable Trust
MR8000 West Florissant
St. Louis, MO 63136
Jo Ann Harmon, Vice President
(314) 553-2000
(Child)

Epilepsy Foundation of America
4351 Garden City Drive
Landover, MD 20785
Ruby Gerald or Joe Giffles, Research Administration
(301) 459-3700
(Epilepsy)

FHP Foundation
401 East Ocean Boulevard, Suite 206
Long Beach, CA 90802
Sandra Lund Gavin, Executive Director
(310) 590-8655
(Health care delivery)

Hearst Foundation/The Hearst Foundation, Inc., William Randolph
888 7th Avenue, 27th Floor
New York, NY 10106
Robert M. Frehse Jr., Executive Director
Ilene Mack, Senior Program Officer
(212) 586-5404
(Health care delivery, broad biomedical research)

Juvenile Diabetes Foundation International
432 Park Avenue South, Suite 206
New York, NY 10016
Barbara Lermand, Grants Administrator
(212) 889-7575
(Diabetes)

Kellogg Foundation, W. K.
One Michigan Avenue East
Battle Creek, MI 49017
Norman A. Brown, President
Nancy A. Sims, Grants Management
(616) 968-1611
(Health services for children and aging)

Kettering Family Foundation, The
1440 Kettering Tower
Dayton, OH 45423
Charles T. Kettering III, President
Jack L. Fischer, Secretary
(513) 228-1021
(Broad biomedical research)

Kleberg Foundation, The Robert and Helen
700 North St. Mary's Street, Suite 1200
San Antonio, TX 78205
Robert Washington, Grants Coordinator
(512) 271-3691
(Broad biomedical research)

Kresge Foundation, The
PO Box 3151
3215 W. Big Beaver Road
Troy, MI 48007
Elizabeth C. Sullivan, Program Officer
(810) 643-9630
(Medical equipment purchases)

March of Dimes Birth Defects Foundation
1275 Mamaroneck Avenue
White Plains, NY 10605
Dr. Michael Katz, Vice President for Research
Tanya Pezzullo, Social and Behavior Research
(914) 997-4511
(Birth defects)

Metropolitan Life Foundation
One Madison Avenue
New York, NY 10010
Sibyl Jacobson, President
(212) 578-6272
(Basic research; health care delivery; child)

National Easter Seal Society
70 East Lake Street
Chicago, IL 60601
Norman D. Grunewald, Vice President
(312) 726-6200
(Services delivery issues; cerebral palsy)

National Multiple Sclerosis Society
733 Third Avenue
New York, NY 10017
Michael Dugan, President
Robert Enteen, Director, Health Research and Policy Programs
(212) 986-3240
(Multiple sclerosis)

Pediatric AIDS Foundation
1311 Colorado Avenue
Santa Monica, CA 90403
Trish DeVine, Program Coordinator
(310) 395-9051
(Pediatric AIDS)

Pharmaceutical Manufacturers Association Foundation
1100 Fifteenth Street, NW
Washington, DC 20005
Maurice Q. Bectel, President
Donna Moore, Director of Programs
(202) 835-3470
(Pharmacology and therapeutics)

Prudential Foundation, The
751 Broad Street, 15th Floor
Newark, NJ 07102
Peter Bushyeager, Program Office for Health and Human Services
(201) 802-7354
(Health care delivery; child)

Ronald McDonald Children's Charities
One McDonald's Plaza
Oak Brook, IL 60521
Programs Director
(708) 575-7048
(Research on child issues)

Rubenstein Foundation, Helena
405 Lexington Avenue
New York, NY 10174
Diane Moss, President
(212) 986-0806
(Women and children)

Scholl Foundation, Dr.
11 South LaSalle Street, Suite 2100
Chicago, IL 60603
Mr. Jack E. Scholl, Executive Director
(312) 782-5210
(Training; research on child issues, developmentally disabled, and aging)

Simon Foundation, Jennifer Jones
411 West Colorado Boulevard
Pasadena, CA 91105
Janet H. Ellis, Administrative Assistant
(213) 681-2484
(Has supported mental health research, but its funds are committed and awards are given by invitation only)

Smokeless Tobacco Research Council, Inc.
420 Lexington Avenue
New York, NY 10170
Kathy Traystman, Executive Vice President
(212) 697-3485
(Smoking; tobacco)

Spinal Cord Research Foundation, The
Paralyzed Veterans of America
801 18th Street, NW
Washington, DC 20006
C.M. Chaunaud, Associate Director of Research
(202) 416-7659
(Spinal cord)

The Eppley Foundation for Research
575 Lexington Avenue
New York, NY 10022
Rivington R. Winant, President
Huyler C. Held, Secretary
(Basic research)

Thrasher Research Fund
50 East North Temple Street
Salt Lake City, UT 84150
Robert M. Briem, Ed.D., Associate Director
(801) 240-4753
(Research on child issues)

Tobacco Research-USA, Inc., The Council for
900 Third Avenue
New York, NY 10022
Harmon McAllister, Ph.D., Research Director
Arthur D. Eisenberg, Ph.D, Associate Research Director
(212) 421-8885
(Smoking; tobacco)

Tourette Syndrome Association
42-40 Bell Boulevard
Bayside, NY 11361
Sue Levy-Pearl, Scientific Liaison
(718) 224-2999
(Tourette syndrome)

Weight Watchers Foundation, Inc.
Jericho Atrium
500 North Broadway
Jericho, NY 11753
Xavier Pi-Sunyer, M.D., Executive Director
Susan A. Witze, Foundation Administrator
(516) 949-0462
(Eating disorders; weight-related research)

Whitaker Foundation, The
4718 Old Gettysburg Road, Suite 405
Mechanicsburg, PA 17055
Miles J. Gibbons Jr., Executive Director
(717) 763-1391
(Biomedical engineering)

Whitney Foundation, The Helen Hay
450 East 63rd Street
New York, NY 10021
Barbara M. Hugonnet, Administrative Director
(212) 751-8228
(Training; basic biomedical research)

◆ Section 5: Local Foundations That Have Supported Psychiatric or Related Research

Alden Trust, John W.
c/o State Street Bank and Trust Co.
PO Box 351
Boston, MA 02101
Deborah A. Robbins, Vice President
(617) 654-3343
Funding region: Eastern Massachusetts

Buhl Foundation, The
Room 1522
Four Gateway Center
Pittsburgh, PA 15222
Doreen E. Boyce, Director
(412) 566-2711
Funding region: Western Pennsylvania

Cargill Foundation, The
Box 9300
Minneapolis, MN 55440
Audrey Tulberg, Program Director
(612) 475-6122
Funding region: Minnesota

Casey Foundation, The Annie E.
One Lafayette Place
Greenwich, CT 06830
Peggy McCormick
(203) 661-2773
Funding region: Connecticut

Chicago Community Trust, The
222 North LaSalle Street, Suite 1400
Chicago, IL 60601
Sandy Cheers, Grants Manager
(312) 372-3356
Funding region: Chicago, Illnois, and environs

Columbus Foundation, The
1234 East Broad Street
Columbus, OH 43205
James I. Luck, President
(614) 251-4000
Funding region: Ohio

Cummings Foundation, Inc., James H.
Room 112
1807 Elmwood Avenue
Buffalo, NY 14207
William J. McFarland, Executive Director
(716) 874-0040
Funding region: Buffalo, New York, and Toronto, Canada

Dean Foundation for Health, Research and Education
8000 Excelsior Drive, Suite 203
Madison, WI 53717
William J. Brink, President
(608) 836-7000
Funding region: Wisconsin

Farish Fund, The William Stamps
10000 Memorial, Suite 920
Houston, TX 77002
Caroline Rotan
(713) 686-7373
Funding region: Texas

Fyssen Foundation
194, Rue de Rivoli
75001 Paris, France
Colette Kouchner, Redacteur en chef
33 (1) 42.97.53.16
Funding region: International

Gerstacker Foundation, The Rollin M.
PO Box 1945
Midland, MI 48641
E. N. Brand, President
(517) 631-6097
Funding region: Michigan

Jewett Foundation, George Frederick
The Russ Building
235 Montgomery Street, Suite 612
San Francisco, CA 94104
Theresa A. Mullen, Executive Director
(415) 421-1351
Funding region: Pacific Northwest

Kansas City Community Foundation and Affiliated Trusts,
  The Greater
1055 Broadway, Suite 130
Kansas City, MO 64105
Janice C. Kreamer, President
(816) 842-0944
Funding region: Kansas City, Missouri

Lowe Foundation
2 East 14th Avenue
Denver, CO 80203
Justice Luis D. Rovira
(303) 837-3750
Funding region: Colorado

Lowenstein Foundation, Inc., Leon
126 East 56th Street
New York, NY 10022
John F. Van Gorder, Executive Director
(212) 319-0670
Funding region: New York

McGraw Foundation
3436 North Kennicott Drive
Arlington Heights, IL 60004
James F. Quilter, Vice President
(708) 870-8014
Funding region: Illinois

McInerny Foundation
PO Box 3170
(c/o Bishop Trust Co., Ltd., 130 Merchant Street)
Honolulu, HI 96802
Lois C. Loomis, Vice President
(808) 523-2111
Funding region: Hawaii

Meadows Foundation, The
Wilson Historic Block
3883 Swiss Avenue
Dallas, TX 75204
Dr. Sally R. Lancaster, Grants Administrator
(214) 826-9431
Funding region: Texas

Monika Foundation, Anna (Anna–Monika–Stiftung)
Am Kaiserhein 19
D–4600 Dortmund 1 FRG
Benno Hess
(0231) 13905-11
Funding region: International

New York Community Trust
Two Park Avenue
New York, NY 10016
Joyce M. Bove, Vice President of Programs
(212) 686-0010
Funding region: New York, New York

North Dakota Community Foundation
1025 N. 3rd Street
Bismarck, ND 58502
Dr. Richard H. Timmins, President
(701) 222-8349
Funding region: North Dakota

Ontario Mental Health Foundation
365 Bloor Street East, Suite 1708
Toronto, Ontario, CN
M4W 3L4
Dugal Campbell, Ph.D., Executive Director
(416) 920-7721
Funding region: Ontario, Canada

Richardson Foundation, Sid W.
309 Main Street
Fort Worth, TX 76102
Valleau Wilkie Jr., Executive Vice President
(817) 336-0494
Funding region: Texas

Richardson Fund, Anne S.
c/o Chemical Bank
270 Park Avenue
New York, NY 10017
Patricia Kelly
Funding region: New York, New York

Scaife Family Foundation
Three Mellon Bank Center
525 William Penn Place, Suite 3900
Pittsburgh, PA 15219
Joanne B. Beyer, Vice President
(412) 392-2900
Funding region: Western Pennsylvania
(Please write.)

Scranton Area Foundation
204 Wyoming Avenue, Suite 207
Scranton, PA 18503
Jeanne A. Bovard, Executive Director
(717) 347-6203
Funding region: Scranton, Pennsylvania

Staunton Farm Foundation
Center City Tower
650 Smithfield Street, Suite 240
Pittsburgh, PA 15222
Marilyn H. Ingalls, Grant Administrator
(412) 281-8020
Funding region: Western Pennsylvania

Towsley Foundation, The Harry A. & Margaret D.
670 City Center Building
220 East Huron Street
Ann Arbor, MI 48104
Margaret Ann Riecker, President
(313) 662-6777
Funding region: Michigan

CHAPTER

5

Research Capacities and Activities of State Mental Health Agencies

Theodore Lutterman, Vera Hollen, and
Noel Mazade, Ph.D.

State mental health agencies (SMHAs) are the primary entities that fund and provide mental health services in the nation. A recent study reports that SMHA-controlled expenditures for mental health in fiscal year 1990 totaled over $12 billion (NASMHPD Research Institute 1993). Research to determine the effectiveness of services is at the heart of improving the quality of the services that states deliver. To better serve individuals with serious mental illnesses, the state agencies are involved in many research projects. Several recent studies by the Research Institute of the National

Inquiries should be made to Mr. Lutterman at the NASMHPD Research Institute, 66 Canal Center Plaza, Suite 302, Alexandria, VA 22314. The authors would like to acknowledge the assistance of Kirby Smith, Department of Psychiatry, University of Pennsylvania School of Medicine, for his assistance in conducting an inventory of SMHA research projects, and Dee Roth, M.A., Director, Office of Research, Ohio Department of Mental Health, for her review of the manuscript.

Association of State Mental Health Program Directors (NASMHPD) have begun to reveal the types and quantities of services research in which states are involved.

This chapter provides an overview of mental health research efforts conducted or funded by SMHAs. Although the states conduct and fund clinical research projects that may include efforts to assess the results of medications, examine the characteristics of persons with various psychiatric diagnoses, and other patient-focused studies, this chapter will focus on SMHA services research projects. Brief attention will also be paid to models of state funding for mental health research and factors that influence state funding for such research.

In fiscal year 1993, the 52 reporting SMHAs expended approximately $80.7 million on research and evaluation activities. Half (52%) of these funds came from state government sources, 40% from federal government sources, and the rest from other sources such as foundations. State expenditures for research and evaluation ranged from a high of $57 million in New York to a low of $5,000 in South Dakota. The median SMHA expenditure was approximately $143,000 (NASMHPD Research Institute 1993).

A separate 1990 study of 26 SMHAs identified more than 218 mental health services research projects. Of these, over 130 reported details on the project's funding. More than 70% of these projects were supported with some SMHA funds; overall, 40% of the total research funds were provided by the SMHA (NASMHPD Research Institute 1991). These projects did not include any clinical research activities. Figure 5–1 gives the source of funding of the research projects done by these 26 SMHAs.

◆ Mental Health Services Research Defined

Mental health services research encompasses a broad arena of investigation about the planning, organization, implementation, and evaluation of various types of mental health services offered under SMHA auspices. These services can include any combination of inpatient, outpatient, residential, emergency, case management, social support, and other types of services. In general, the portfolio of mental health services research projects includes the following.

◆ Service system and treatment outcome studies as related to the design, management, and evaluation of service systems; effectiveness of various treatment programs; approaches in relation to cost per episode of care; and efforts to study inpatient utilization.

◆ Financing of mental health services, including prospective payment systems, alternative funding mechanisms, cost-finding and rate-setting studies, alternative insurance models, direct and unintended effects of policy changes, and cost-effectiveness issues.

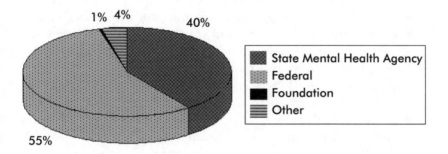

Total Dollar Amount From Various Funding Sources

Total Funding: $37,338,816
Number of Projects Reporting Total Funding: 131

Total State Mental Health Agency Funds: $14,865,797
Number of Projects Reporting SMHA Funds: 92

Total Federal Funds: $20,643,244
Number of Projects Reporting Federal Funds: 56

Total Foundation Funds: $280,224
Number of Projects Reporting Foundation Funds: 9

Total "Other" Funds: $41,395,551
Number of Projects Reporting "Other" Funds: 17

Figure 5–1. Sources of research funding for projects of 26 state mental health agencies.

◆ Organization of services issues, including public and private operation, service system models, developing state typologies, centralized versus decentralized structures, and resource allocation
   models.
◆ Performance measures research, including development of
   norms for hospital-based and freestanding services; benefits
   among dimensions of performance (efficiency-effectiveness);
   cost benefits of public care models; and issues of data reliability,
   validity, manipulation, safeguards, and risks.
◆ Work force issues, including shifting loci of care; staffing levels
   and mix; work force retention; performance and productivity
   standard impacts; supply, demand, and cost; projecting human
   resource needs; and conditions of employment such as licensing,
   standards, professional organizations, unions, personnel practices, and classification systems.
◆ Special populations, including persons with serious mental illness, children, elderly persons with mental illness, forensics, and
   dual-diagnosed persons; topics include service needs of these
   groups, incidence and prevalence, appropriate services mix, and
   determining unique service needs and service delivery systems.
◆ Legal issues and their impact on protection and advocacy, right
   to refuse treatment, state insurance laws, insanity statutes, zon-
   ing and placement of services, commitment statutes and policies,
   and impact of state and local consent decrees (Lutterman 1992;
   NASMHPD 1989; NASMHPD Research Institute 1991).

◆ SMHA Research
Capacity and Interests

In the late 1980s, the National Association of State Mental Health
Program Directors (NASMHPD), as the membership organization of
the 55 state and territorial mental health commissioners, conducted
several studies to determine SMHA involvement in mental health services research and areas that states felt needed additional research.
These studies demonstrated that SMHAs were becoming actively involved in efforts to analyze the services they provide. In 1988, 64%
of SMHAs (33 of 52 SMHAs responding; includes Washington, DC,
Guam; Puerto Rico; and the Virgin Islands) reported that they were
conducting or directly funding mental health services research.
   SMHAs have developed a number of approaches to conducting

services research and evaluation regarding their services and clients. Some SMHAs conduct intramural research carried out by SMHA-based researchers. Others fund universities and other research entities to conduct research on state mental health programs, and still others have state-owned research institutes. Some states utilize all three approaches.

◆   30 SMHAs reported they had SMHA employees conducting research;
◆   25 reported collaboration with institutions of higher education;
◆   20 reported collaborating or contracting with agencies or groups other than higher education;
◆   19 awarded contracts or grants to higher education to complete research;
◆   16 provided student research placements; and
◆   7 conducted services research under other arrangements (NASMHPD 1988).

In late 1988, NASMHPD formally developed a research agenda to guide the states and itself in the development and utilization of research. The agenda was developed from a recognition that the numerous changes in the public mental health service delivery system were creating a greater need for improved services research. In addition to the general trend of reduced finances for services, some of the recognized changes included the shift in government responsibility among federal, state, and local auspices; the continuing trend from institutional toward community-based care; the increasing influence on SMHA programs of judicial and legislative entities; the development of a large proprietary mental health sector; and the needs of new populations with serious mental illness.

NASMHPD's research agenda was based on several principles.

◆   SMHAs require services research that is generalizable, has scientific credibility, and is relevant to policy formulation and program development;
◆   Research should relate to the SMHA's management responsibility and capacity for information systems, planning, monitoring, and regulation;
◆   Research should be expanded to NASMHPD and its member state units, and research results should be shared with other national organizations, proprietary mental health providers, foundations, and federal agencies;

◆ There should be a substantial increase in federal, state, and private sector financial resources to conduct services research;

◆ Whenever possible, NASMHPD policy development should be predicated on relevant research findings and should specify knowledge gaps and needed research resources and identify further priority questions and issues;

◆ NASMHPD's internal capacity and that of the independent NASMHPD Research Institute, Inc., should focus on national policy-relevant projects that are highly linked to the research agenda;

◆ The research agenda should help define NASMHPD's priorities for research sponsored by the federal government; and

◆ The agenda should be periodically updated.

The NASMHPD research agenda provides details on a number of research priorities. These priority arenas include ascertaining the needs and preferences of persons with a serious and persistent mental illness; increasing the understanding of service delivery processes and outcomes; analyzing the organization and delivery of mental health services; examining fiscal coverage and financing; exploring human resource-related issues; increasing research on legal issues; improving the availability and use of data for policy definition, decision making, and research; and increasing the methodological sophistication of services research.

The agenda influenced development of the NASMHPD Research Institute, Inc. (a separate not-for-profit corporation), in early 1990 and served as a reference for NASMHPD in defining its own needs for data and in identifying research priorities that were communicated to the federal government, particularly the National Institute of Mental Health and the Center for Mental Health Services, which fund state-related services research.

◆ SMHA Profiling

The NASMHPD Research Institute is currently updating the information on the SMHAs' involvement in services research and evaluation through the SMHA profiling system, which is funded by the federal Center for Mental Health Services. Results (52 SMHAs reporting) show that 65% of the SMHAs are involved in mental health research and 52% are involved in program evaluation. Twenty-two of the 52 reported that research and evaluation functions are combined into one special office. In addition, 14 SMHAs reported that they either operate a Mental Health Research Institute (8 SMHAs) or fund such an institute (6 SMHAs) (NASMHPD Research Institute 1993).

In addition to directly conducting research, 16 SMHAs operate a research grant or contract program to support research outside of the SMHA and 16 use grants for research within the SMHA. Nine SMHAs use grants or contracts to support evaluations outside of the SMHA.

In the 1993 SMHA profiling system, states were asked about the locus of their mental health services research and evaluation. Thirteen states reported that the research function is located outside of the SMHA, in such organizations as local programs or universities; 30 reported the research function is within the SMHA; 8 reported having no research function; and 4 have no evaluation function. Of the latter, only North Carolina reported operating research grants or contract programs to support internal research.

Five states reported that the organizational location of the evaluation function is outside the SMHA (such as in private institutes or universities), 38 reported that it was located within the SMHA, and four (Indiana, Nevada, South Carolina, and Wyoming) reported having no evaluation function. South Carolina reported supporting a SMHA-operated research center/institute.

Although some states reported having neither a research nor an evaluation function within the SMHA, the reports cited above are evidence that many of these states have dedicated funds for research independent of the SMHA, either to a research center/institute or through research grants or contracts to support internal or external research and/or evaluation.

Eight states support a SMHA-operated research center/institute: Arkansas, Illinois, Michigan, New York, Rhode Island, South Carolina, Utah, and Virginia. Six states support a SMHA-funded (but not operated) research center/institute: Maryland, Massachusetts, Missouri, New Hampshire, South Dakota, and Washington. SMHA researchers in 40 states have collaborative relationships with researchers in universities, and in 16 states SMHA researchers collaborate with other organizations such as other human service agencies or local providers of mental health services. These figures are an indication that many states are expanding their services research capacities by involving researchers outside of the boundaries of the SMHA.

◆ Research Directory

In 1990, the NASMHPD Research Institute initiated a directory of SMHA services research projects. SMHAs were asked to submit a brief report on each, along with information on its professional staff. For this directory, 26 states submitted a total of 218 research projects. The number in any one state varied from 59 in New York to one in 4 states (Alabama, Florida, Minnesota, and Nebraska); the median number was 5.

The research projects can be grouped according to the types of projects or keywords. The six most commonly cited keywords are listed in Table 5–1.

Of the 218 projects entered in the research directory, slightly more than one-half identified the primary entity that initiated each of the projects: 54% indicated SMHA personnel, 25% indicated university/college personnel, 19% indicated a joint initiation between personnel at the SMHA and a university or college, and 2% indicated another group (for example, the Alliance for the Mentally Ill or a consumer group).

Of those respondents identifying who was primarily responsible for completing the project, 46% stated SMHA personnel, 33% stated university or college personnel, and 21% stated that both the SMHA and the university or college had responsibility.

In the initial survey used to compile the directory, respondents were asked to indicate all organizations that were involved in the project. A total of 394 responses were made. A university or college was cited the most (85 times), followed closely by a SMHA research office (79 times), and a state mental hospital (70 times). Other or-

Table 5–1. Six most commonly cited keywords

Keyword	Number of projects	Number of states
Serious and persistent mental illness	50	16
Case management	34	17
Outcome measures	31	10
Therapy outcomes	21	10
Family systems	15	10
Institutional systems	13	11

ganizations indicated several times included a SMHA operations office (35 times), a local community mental health program (31 times), and other mental health service provider (35 times).

Data on staffing indicate that approximately 15% of the researchers were psychiatrists. Psychologists comprised 30%; the rest were nurses, social workers, sociologists, and other nonmental health professionals including mathematicians, administrators, political scientists, and economists (see Figure 5–2).

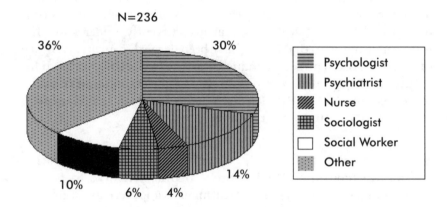

"Other" includes:

Administration	3	Other MH Professional	5
Anthropology	2	Other Physician	1
Biometrics	1	Pharmacology	1
Child Development	1	Pharmacy	2
Criminal Justice	2	Political Science	4
Economist	3	Public Health	1
Education	1	Public Policy	1
Epidemiology	3	Research	4
Geography	1	Social Ecology	1
Math	5	Social Policy	1
Occupational Therapy	1	Religious Studies	1

Figure 5–2. Disciplines of researchers listed in state mental health agencies services research projects directory.

◆ Issues in Mental Health Services Research Facing SMHAs

One primary goal of mental health services research studies in recent years has been the utilization of research findings in policy development and management decision making. As a senior staff person on the frontline of service delivery, the director of research in the SMHA must strive to rapidly translate findings into implications for policy and practice.

The linkage of research findings to policy and practice is best illustrated by examining the specific types of research projects conducted and funded by SMHAs that are currently under way. The topics and subtopics that follow have been derived from an inventory of SMHA research projects conducted by the NASMHPD Research Institute and from a review of proposals and presentations in response to the last three NASMHPD Research Institute annual conferences on state mental health agency research.

◆ New research technology, computer application, and mathematical modeling: Application of neural networks to patient triaging, computer-assisted treatment, computerizing state hospital databases, determining appropriate sizing of inpatient facilities, and mathematical modeling of services.

◆ Client characteristics, population group description, and analysis of client types: Examining assaultive behavior, day treatment interventions, results of clustering persons with a severe mental illness, age shifts in state hospital resident populations, and determining why patients remain hospitalized.

◆ Case management and assertive community treatment programs: Determining cost effectiveness, comparison group studies of case management models, determining the impact of differing reimbursement mechanisms on provider agency behavior, case management service client outcome studies, impact of substance abusers on the mental health system, and the role of psychotropic medication and compliance in case management and assertive community treatment programs.

◆ Psychopharmacology and impact of medications on the mental health system: Cohort studies of patients taking clozapine and utilization of medications in community support programs.

◆ Mental health service types and assessment of outcomes: Ecology of inpatient services, control group studies on peer support services, forensic program evaluations, predictive models of service utilization, cross-state comparative studies of capitated services, studies of organizational and system change, and person- versus program-centered research studies to assess program outcome.

◆ Infrastructure for conducting mental health services research: Consortium arrangements between SMHAs and academic institutions, postdoctoral research fellowship training program models, predoctoral training needs in mental health services research, and the impact of various organizational structures for managing SMHA research.

◆ Housing, housing support, and evaluation of housing initiatives: Housing and support service preferences of persons with a serious mental illness, methodologies for evaluating diverse housing service delivery models, and urban and rural differences in approaches to supported housing.

◆ Family supports, preferences, and involvement in services system: Long-term needs of families and significant others who provide care for persons with severe mental illness, roles of family members and mental health professionals, and adequacy of resources to family members.

◆ Policy formulation and analysis: Impact of interventions and approaches to assist SMHA managers with complexities of choosing alternative courses of action under conditions of fiscal and other resource scarcity and uncertainty.

◆ Mental health services consumer/survivor studies: Impact of consumers as direct service providers in the SMHA network of services; relationships among consumers, their families, and case managers; consumer preference surveys and analysis; impact of consumers on SMHA policy and decision making; and alternative methods for facilitating consumer empowerment.

◆ Financing of mental health services: Level and types of disability as a factor in the cost of providing services; impact of SMHA funding incentives of local programs; analysis of SMHA-controlled revenues and expenditures; studies of Medicaid paid claims files and identification of heavy user populations; other state agency expenditures on mental health-related services; and analysis of SSI, SSDI, Medicare, and other federal expenditures for mental health services.

◆ Outcome research: Explorations of methodologies, research protocols, subject characteristics, instrumentation, and informed consent.

◆ Research on state hospitals and other SMHA psychiatric inpatient services: Measuring services system outcomes using life table analysis; determining actual and expected length of stay; trends in admissions and discharges; roles of the state hospital; and analysis of hospital and/or unit closures, consolidations, reconfiguring, and downsizing.

◆ Rural mental health services research: Characteristics of agency and professional providers; effects of poverty, stigma, isolation, and availability of supports; degree of congruity between SMHA policies and rural conditions; epidemiology of disorders among rural populations, including migrant workers, Native Americans, elderly persons, and children; economic issues; access to services; and research training programs for rural researchers.

◆ Research on methodological issues: Improved definition of instruments and measurement used in field settings; identifying research methods that are not now widely used but have promise for mental health services research (e.g., use of large data sets, qualitative methods, single subject designs, etc.); improved communication of research needs, projects, findings, and applied results among the states; and improved models for assessing research needs.

◆ Models of State Research Funding

As already noted, the main emphasis of this chapter has been on mental health services research, which has become the major focus of SMHA-funded research in most states. There has also been a tradition in some states of more broad-based support for mental health research incorporating basic biological, behavioral, and clinical research as well as health services research. Across all these categories of research, a 1988 American Psychiatric Association study (Ridge et al. 1989) described four general mechanisms under which SMHAs support mental health research: the joint state-university research unit, research grants, state in-house research, and contracts. These models reflect a broad range of costs, resource needs, degree of SMHA direction in the selection of research topics, and capacity to produce an intellectual core from which further externally funded research might emanate. The models are not mutually exclusive; states with larger research programs may employ several mechanisms of support.

◆ Factors Influencing State Funding

The APA study also sought to identify the factors underlying support of mental health and substance abuse research. The findings indicated that neither a large population base nor a large state mental health authority budget was a prerequisite to a state's willingness to invest in mental health research. Other factors were likely to be far more important, including the advocacy efforts of academic and citizens groups and their influence on the state political environment and the nature of the leadership of the state mental health system.

A political environment conducive to research programs is generally characterized by budget stability, strong leadership within the state government itself, with officials who are sympathetic to mental health issues, and active external advocacy by citizens groups and the research community. It has been noted that a state's political environment is extremely fragile and on occasion volatile, subject to the electoral process in both the legislature and the governor's office and subject also to changing economics.

Individual leadership both inside and outside the government structure is of great value in establishing or preserving state commitment to mental health research. In the APA survey cited above, several states with strong state-supported efforts in mental health research traced their beginnings to individuals who worked against the odds to establish these programs. The individuals were characterized as having a deep commitment to mental health, an ability to understand the political environment, and the tenacity to see a program through to completion.

◆ Conclusions

◆ States are expanding their capacity for research, especially mental health services research.
◆ There is a broad range of topics of relevance to mental health services research.
◆ Research funding overall is supported under four broad mechanisms.
◆ Leadership and activism within the SMHAs, citizen groups, and academia are the most important factors in expanding state support of mental health research.

◆ References

Lutterman T (ed): Special Issue on Assertive Community Treatment. Alexandria, VA, NRI Outlook 2(2), 1992

National Association of State Mental Health Program Directors: Survey of State Level Research Interests and Capacity (Study No 87–597). Alexandria, VA, National Association of State Mental Health Program Directors, 1988

National Association of State Mental Health Program Directors: NASMHPD Research Agenda. Alexandria, VA, National Association of State Mental Health Program Directors, adopted by the NASMHPD membership July 12, 1989

National Association of State Mental Health Program Directors Research Institute: Directory of State Mental Health Agency Services Research Projects. Alexandria, VA, National Association of State Mental Health Program Directors Research Institute, 1991

National Association of State Mental Health Program Directors Research Institute: The State Mental Health Agency Profiling System (data file). Alexandria, VA, National Association of State Mental Health Program Directors Research Institute, 1993

Ridge R, Pincus HA, Blalock R, et al: Factors that influence state funding for mental health research. Hosp Community Psychiatry 40:377–382, 1989

Resources 5–1
State Mental Health Agency Research Contacts

Alabama
Brian H. McManus
Director, Bureau of Mental Illness
200 Interstate Park Drive
PO Box 3710
Montgomery, AL 36109-0710
(205) 271-9253 Fax: (205) 240-3195

Alaska
Leonard Abel
Community Mental Health Administrator
PO Box 110620
Juneau, AK 99811
(907) 465-3370 Fax: (907) 465-2668

Arizona
Rhonda Baldwin
Department of Health Services
Division of Behavioral Health Services
2122 Highland Street, Suite 100
Phoenix, AZ
(602) 381-8999 Fax: (602) 553-9140

Arkansas
Bob Gale, M.D., J.D.
Assistant Director for Clinical Services
Director of Research & Training Institute
4313 West Markham Street
Little Rock, AR 72205-4096
(501) 686-9045 Fax: (501) 686-9182

California
William DeRisi, Ph.D.
Chief, Program Development & Evaluation Branch
Department of Mental Health
1600 Ninth Street, Room 120
Sacramento, CA 95814
(916) 654-2635 Fax: (916) 654-2804

Colorado
Christine Engleby
Director, Decision Support
3520 W. Oxford Avenue
Denver, CO 80236
(303) 762-4081 Fax: (303) 762-4373

Connecticut
Susan Essock, Ph.D.
Department of Mental Health
90 Washington Street
Hartford, CT 06106
(203) 566-4726 Fax: (203) 566-6195

Delaware
Maurice L. Tippett
Manager of Computer & Application Support
Division of Alcoholism, Drug Abuse, & Mental Health
Administration Building, 1st Floor
1901 North Dupont Highway
New Castle, DE 19720
(302) 577-4478 Fax: (302) 577-4486

District of Columbia
Jean H. Thrasher, Ph.D.
Grants Management Officer
2700 Martin Luther King Jr. Avenue, SE
Washington, DC 20032
(202) 373-7521 Fax: (202) 373-5427

Florida
Linda Buckhalt
Senior Human Services Program Specialist
Alcohol, Drug Abuse & Mental Health Program Office
1317 Winewood Boulevard
Tallahassee, FL 32399-0700
(904) 487-1301 Fax: (904) 487-2239

Georgia
Margaret Taylor
Mental Health Section
Department of Mental Health, Mental Retardation, & Substance Abuse
878 Peachtree Street, NE, Room 315
Atlanta, GA 30309
(404) 894-6333 Fax: (404) 894-6561

Guam
Pramilla Sullivan, M.A.
MIS Specialist
790 Gov. Carlos G. Camacho Road
Tamuning, GU 96911
(671) 647-5400 Fax: (671) 649-6948

Hawaii
Howard Gudeman, Ph.D.
Box 3378
Honolulu, HI 96801
(808) 586-4677 Fax: (808) 586-4745

Idaho
Roy Sargeant, A.C.S.W.
Bureau Chief, Bureau of Mental Health
450 West State Street, 7th Floor
Boise, ID 83720
(208) 334-6500 Fax: (208) 334-6664

Illinois
Randy Pletcher
Department of Mental Health & Mental Retardation
401 South Spring Street
Springfield, IL 62765
(217) 785-7226 Fax: (217) 782-9535

Indiana
John Giandelone
Deputy Director of Contract Management
Division of Mental Health
402 West Washington Street, W353
Indianapolis, IN 46204
(317) 232-7872 Fax: (317) 233-3472

Iowa
Harold Templeman
Acting Administrator
Department of Human Services, 5th Floor
Hoover State Office Building
Des Moines, IA 50319
(515) 281-5126 Fax: (515) 281-4597

Kansas
Randy Proctor
Administrator of Decision Support
Mental Health & Mental Retardation
Docking State Office Building, 5th Floor North
Topeka, KS 66612
(913) 296-4222 Fax: (913) 296-6142

Kentucky
Richard T. Heine, Ph.D.
Research Psychologist
Department of Mental Health & Mental Retardation Services
275 East Main Street
Frankfort, KY 40517
(502) 564-4448 Fax: (502) 564-3844

Louisiana
Randall Lemoine, Ph.D.
Director, Program Evaluation & Research
Office of Mental Health
PO Box 4049, Bin #12
Baton Rouge, LA 70821
(504) 342-5835 Fax: (504) 342-5066

Maine
Stanley Fabisak
Bureau of Mental Health
State House Station #40
Augusta, ME 04333
(207) 287-4203 Fax: (207) 287-4268

Maryland
Tim Santoni
Room 416
201 West Preston Street
Baltimore, MD 21201
(410) 225-6540 Fax: (410) 333-5402

Massachusetts
Fred Altaffer, Ph.D.
Director of Research
Department of Mental Health
25 Staniford Street
Boston, MA 02114
(617) 727-5500 Fax: (617) 727-5500

Michigan
Marilyn Hill
Department of Mental Health
Lewis Cass Building, 6th Floor
Lansing, MI 48913
(517) 373-6440 Fax: (517) 335-6775

Minnesota
Jeff Tenney
Research Analyst, Senior
Department of Human Services
444 Lafayette Road
St. Paul, MN 55155-3828
(612) 296-4467 Fax: (612) 296-6244

Mississippi
Mardi Carter, Ph.D.
Director, Division of Human Resources
Department of Mental Health
1101 Robert E. Lee Building
239 North Lamar Street
Jackson, MS 39201
(601) 359-1288 Fax: (601) 359-6295

Missouri
Dorn Schuffman
Deputy Director
Department of Mental Health
PO Box 687
Jefferson City, MO 65102
(314) 751-9484 Fax: (314) 751-7815

Montana
Sandra Harris
Research & Analysis Manager
Mental Health Division
1539 11th Avenue
Helena, MT 59620
(406) 444-4922 Fax: (406) 444-4920

Nebraska
Peter Beeson, Ph.D.
PO Box 94728
Lincoln, NE 68509
(402) 471-2851 Fax: (402) 479-5145

Nevada
Peter Steinmann
Chief of Planning, Evaluation
Room 403
Kinkead Building
505 E. King Street
Carson City, NV 89507
(702) 688-2157 Fax: (702) 687-4773

New Hampshire
Bret Longgood
Program Coordinator
Division of Mental Health & Developmental Services
State Office Park South
105 Pleasant Street
Concord, NH 03301
(603) 271-5053 Fax: (603) 271-5058

New Jersey
Gayle Reisser, Ph.D.
Planning Coordinator
2-98 East State Street
Trenton, NJ 08655-0727
(609) 777-0822 Fax: (609) 777-0835

New Mexico
Rosemary M. Moya
Chief, Community Programs Bureau
Division of Mental Health
PO Box 26110
Santa Fe, NM 87502
(505) 827-2666 Fax: (505) 827-2695

New York
David Shern, Ph.D.
Director of Research
44 Holland Avenue
Albany, NY 12229
(518) 473-7358 Fax: (518) 474-6995

North Carolina
Gustavo Fernandez
Head, Program Evaluation Branch
325 North Salisbury Street, Suite 1124
Raleigh, NC 27603
(919) 733-7013 Fax: (919) 733-9455

North Dakota
Sam Ismir
Director
Division of Mental Health Services
600 East Building Avenue, Judicial Wing
Bismarck, ND 58505-0271
(701) 224-2766 Fax: (701) 224-2359

Ohio
Dee Roth
Chief of Program Evaluation & Research
30 East Broad Street, Suite 1340
Columbus, OH 43266-0414
(614) 466-8651 Fax: (614) 466-9928

Oklahoma
Steve Davis, Ph.D.
Director, Evaluation & Data Analysis
PO Box 53277
Oklahoma City, OK 73152-3277
(405) 271-8752 Fax: (405) 271-7413

Oregon
Marilyn Wachal
Manager, Program Analysis
2575 Bittern Street, NE
Salem, OR 97310
(503) 378-2248 Fax: (503) 373-7327

Pennsylvania
Donn S. Flores
Division Chief for Planning, Evaluation & Management Information
Systems
Room 631, Health Welfare Building
PO Box 2675
Harrisburg, PA 17105
(717) 783-5132 Fax: (717) 787-5394

Rhode Island
Richard L. Wagner, M.D.
Director of Research
Rhode Island Medical Center
600 New London Avenue, LP-4
Cranston, RI 02920
(401) 464-3220

South Carolina
Jack Balling
Director, Budget Planning
PO Box 485
Columbia, SC 29202
(803) 734-7772 Fax: (803) 734-7879

South Dakota
Kelly A. Wheeler
Director of Mental Health
East Highway 34
500 East Capitol
Pierre, SD 57501
(605) 773-5991 Fax: (605) 773-5483

Tennessee
Julie Hinton
Director
Office of Planning & Evaluation
Department of Mental Health & Mental Retardation
706 Church Street, Suite 300
Nashville, TN 37243-0675
(615) 532-6767 Fax: (615) 532-6737

Texas
William Rago
PO Box 12668
Austin, TX 78711-2668
(512) 465-4817 Fax: (512) 465-4851

Utah
Ray Preston, Ph.D.
Center for Program Evaluation & Research
1300 East Center Street
Provo, UT 84606
(801) 344-4634 Fax: (801) 375-7526

Vermont
John A. Pandiani, Ph.D.
Chief of Research & Statistics
Department of Mental Health
103 South Main Street
Waterbury, VT 05671-1601
(802) 241-2639 Fax: (802) 241-3052

Virginia
J. Randy Koch, Ph.D.
Director, Research & Evaluation
PO Box 1797
Richmond, VA 23214
(804) 478-6608 Fax: (804) 478-6924

Washington
Paul Peterson, Ph.D.
Chief, Human Resource Development & System Research
The Washington Institute
PO Box 94500
Fort Steilacoom, WA 98494-0500
(206) 756-2851 Fax: (206) 756-3987

West Virginia
Robert E. Hess, Ph.D.
Director, Office of Behavioral Health Services
1900 Kanawha Boulevard
East Building 6, Room B717
Charleston, WV 23505
(304) 558-0627 Fax: (304) 558-1008

Wisconsin
Martha Mallon
Department of Health & Social Services
PO Box 7851
Madison, WI 53707
(608) 266-6661 Fax: (608) 266-0036

Wyoming
James R. Lewis, Ph.D.
Substance Abuse Consultant
Division of Behavioral Health
452 Hathaway Building
Cheyenne, WY 82002
(307) 777-6493 Fax: (307) 777-5580

CHAPTER

6

Industry and Academia Collaboration in Psychiatric Research

Joyce West, M.P.P., Deborah A. Zarin, M.D.,
Tricia Hill, and Harold Alan Pincus, M.D.

Over the past several decades, as the growth in federal and philanthropic support for basic and clinical research has leveled off and the process of obtaining research awards has become increasingly competitive, investigators have sought research funding support from alternative sources. During this time, large corporations and businesses have taken a greater interest in funding and investing in basic as well as applied research, resulting in a growing number of commercial collaborations and ventures between industry and academia. In the early 1980s in particular, a number of biomedical research institutions formed collaborations with biotechnology, pharmaceutical, and for-profit health care industries.

The federal government has played an active role in fostering these relationships and encouraging industry-funded research to promote technology transfer and to increase the market competitiveness of the United States. The 1980 Bayh-Dole Act enabled institutions and investigators receiving federal research funding to retain patent ownership rights or to license patents to companies interested in developing marketable products (Witt et al. 1994). The 1986 Federal Technology Transfer Act also fostered collaboration between federal scientists and industry through Cooperative Research and Development Agreements (CRADAs), which created a mechanism for federal laboratories to work collaboratively with industry in order to accelerate the number of commercial products derived from the government's research investment.

The most recent estimates indicate that nearly one-half of all biotechnology firms support research in universities and that 90% of the top 100 universities conducting biotechnology research receive financial support from industrial sources (Blumenthal et al. 1986a). Industry-sponsored support for psychiatric research, however, has lagged behind industry-sponsored support associated with overall biomedical research both with regard to the overall level of funding as well as the pace at which newer models of collaboration, such as CRADAs and venture capital start-ups, have developed.

Although the National Institutes of Health (NIH) estimates that private industry currently supports approximately 50% of all health-related research and development efforts (NIH 1993), the proportion of research and development costs supported by industry in mental and addictive disorders is estimated at only about 17% (Pincus and Fine 1992). Reasons for the disparities between industry support of psychiatric and biomedical research include a number of specific barriers, including regulatory impediments related to the abuse potential of psychoactive drugs; the lengthy and expensive drug approval process; the perception of limited marketing potential for psychotropic drugs due to the stigma of mental illnesses and limited reimbursement for the treatment of psychiatric disorders; the enormous expense of psychopharmacology research, which requires the cooperation of clinical populations that are difficult to recruit and maintain compliance with clinical trial protocols; and the clinical costs of conducting research on severely disabled patients, who may require inpatient drug washout periods or placebo control conditions (Pincus and Fine 1992).

This chapter describes the goals and benefits of collaborative research, the structure and characteristics of common models of collaboration, and the potential problems and conflicts of interest resulting from collaborative research; suggestions are offered for investigators to avoid potential problems and conflicts of interest in participating in industry-sponsored research.

◆ Goals and Benefits of Collaborative Research

The primary purpose of academic and industry collaboration in research is to facilitate the conduct of research and the transfer of the products of research to appropriate parties. These relationships also result in a number of important secondary benefits to academic investigators, their institutions, and to the sponsoring corporations. Collaborative research also can result in significant benefits to society.

Benefits to Investigators

In addition to benefiting from having funding to support the direct costs of their research, investigators participating in industry-supported research may benefit from having access to funds that often involve less red tape than similar support from the government. Industry sponsors may cover ancillary expenses such as travel as well as provide funds for additional technical support. Academic investigators benefit by obtaining access to scientists working in industry with whom they can consult. Participation in industry-sponsored research also enables researchers to accelerate their publication and patent development rates and advance their careers (Blumenthal et al. 1986b). In fact, researchers participating in industry-sponsored research tend to participate in more administrative and professional activities and earn more than colleagues without such support (Blumenthal et al. 1986b). Researchers participating in industry-sponsored research also may tend to produce research that generates more immediate, practical applications (AMA Council on Scientific Affairs and Council on Ethical and Judicial Affairs 1990).

Benefits to Investigators' Institutions

Academic research institutions benefit from having their researchers collaborate with industry by receiving external funding to offset the direct and indirect costs of research and the opportunity to obtain patents with subsequent financial rewards. Other benefits include the potential for expansion of the institutions' physical plant and staff (AMA Council on Scientific Affairs and AMA Council on Ethical and Judicial Affairs 1990).

Benefits to Corporations

Corporations sponsoring academic research enhance their ability to focus research on areas of potential profit and the opportunity for immediate product development based on experimental results. In fact, corporate investments in academic research appear to be significantly more successful than other forms of corporate research in yielding patent applications (Blumenthal et al. 1986a). Collaboration may also offer financial advantages in reducing corporations' taxable holdings (AMA Council on Scientific Affairs and AMA Council on Ethical and Judicial Affairs 1990).

Industry sponsors collaborating with researchers in academia also obtain direct access to university researchers and facilities without the need to duplicate or "tool up" their research laboratories for new projects. In addition, they garner a positive public relations image and enhance their opportunities to achieve corporate goals while making valuable contributions to society (AMA Council on Scientific Affairs and AMA Council on Ethical and Judicial Affairs 1990).

Benefits to Society

There are two primary benefits to society resulting from academia and industry collaboration in research. First, with industry increasingly assuming responsibility for conducting research, these funds augment the public investment in research. Second, research and research breakthroughs themselves constitute a "public good" in that society ultimately benefits from research findings and the new products and technologies that may result.

Given that the private sector has long profited from the products and technologies developed as a result of federally funded research, a case can also be made that corporations have a moral responsibility to assume at least some of the costs of conducting basic and clinical research.

◆ Common Models of Collaboration

A myriad of collaborative relationships between academia and industry have emerged. Although these arrangements have been characterized as heterogeneous and complex, these relationships can be conceptualized or broadly categorized into five general types of models of collaboration: joint venture, consultantship, award program, venture capital start-up, and contracted research. In the summary descriptions of each model that follow, a brief description of the model is provided that characterizes the model with regard to the following features: 1) the focus of research; 2) the role of the scientist in relationship to both academia and industry; and 3) the degree of openness in the collaboration. Other distinguishing features and the major advantages and disadvantages of each model are also outlined. Table 6–1 provides a summary of each model, highlighting the features listed above.

The **focus** of the collaborative research can be categorized as being general, targeted, or specific. A general area of research provides the scientist the freedom to choose a subject within a broad field that he or she wishes to investigate. Research that is targeted takes place within a fairly narrow branch of a particular field. Finally, research with a specific focus refers to research conducted in a highly specified area or a particular type of study, such as a clinical trial of a specific drug.

The **relationship between the researcher and industry** can take several different forms, such as consultant, full-time employee, or part-time employee. Each relationship varies in terms of contractual commitments, financial arrangements, and potential conflicts of interest. The **degree of openness** refers to the extent to which researchers are allowed to publish, communicate, or share their knowledge freely with other researchers.

Joint Venture

A joint venture model of collaboration generally consists of a formal agreement between academia and industry to establish a long-term joint research venture. It is based on the exchange of capital from industry to fund research projects in academia in return for access to scientific knowledge and, in many cases, exclusive licenses to patents.

Under this type of arrangement, the corporation may set up a fully equipped research laboratory within the university and provide funds to support a full-time staff. Although the corporation funds the staff salaries, the staff is employed by the university or research institution. The corporation may, however, reserve the right to place some of its scientists in the laboratory to keep apprised of the project's progress and to learn from the academic researchers.

Table 6–1. Models of industry/academia research collaboration: summary of distinguishing characteristics

	Joint venture	Consultantship	Award program	Venture capital start-up	Contracted studies
Focus of research	Broad	Narrow	Broad or narrow	Broad	Narrow
Relationship of scientist to industry	Employed by the academic institution, but industry may fund salary	Usually employed by the academic institution; in some cases employed by industry	Employed by the academic institution	Investigator typically employed/affiliated with both parties	Employed by academic institution
Patent policy and control of the use of research	University has patent rights, but industry may acquire licenses to research products	Industry has patent rights	Some companies request right of first refusal or exclusive rights to patents	The research corporation has patent rights	Industry has patent rights
Compensation for results of research	Investigators may receive royalties from resulting products	Only in rare instances, in exclusive consulting arrangements, are royalties received	Varies; royalties may be awarded to investigators	Investigators may receive royalties, but patents & products owned by the start-up company	No royalties, investigators compensated only for the conduct of research

Information dissemination/ openness of communication	May require confidentiality or approval to publish or engage in other corporate-sponsored research	Confidentiality requirements imposed	Varies; if industry has exclusive rights to patents, restrictions on confidentiality and dissemination likely	Confidentiality required on projects under way	Confidentiality and information dissemination requirements established contractually
Freedom to choose path or change direction of research	Freedom	Limited freedom	Significant freedom	Depends on investigator's role/leverage	Limited freedom

The research conducted under a joint venture arrangement is most commonly in a general basic science area—a research program under which any number of discoveries could be made. Few or no restrictions are placed on the investigators' choice of research projects. Requirements of the investigators include submitting periodic progress reports or holding annual symposia; requesting approval from the sponsor prior to engaging in other consulting activities; and mandatory review of all papers related to the research prior to submission to a journal in order to protect the proprietary interests of the corporation (Kenney 1986).

Ownership of all patents belongs solely to the research institution, but licenses are granted to the corporation to develop and market products that result from the corporate-sponsored research. In some cases, the corporation maintains exclusive patent privileges regarding any research findings. In addition, the academic institution and sometimes individual researchers are given a percentage of the royalties from products that are developed and marketed as a direct result of the research.

Under a joint venture arrangement the corporation does not require patent rights and has few reporting and confidentiality requirements. The primary benefits of this type of collaboration to investigators and their institutions are access to funding for research programs that otherwise would not be implemented, new facilities in which to conduct research, and funds to support staff. Some joint venture models also provide opportunities for career advancement and personal financial gain (Kenney 1986). Benefits received by the industry are access to the latest medical technologies, direct access to academic researchers, the inside track on promising young postdoctoral and graduate researchers, and, in many cases, potential remuneration from patentable discoveries.

Although joint ventures offer a number of attractive advantages to investigators and their institutions, they are criticized for the dampening effect they can have on the flow of information within the academic community. Efforts have been made to protect the free flow of information; these include establishing confidentiality requirements that are in effect only long enough for patents on discoveries to be filed. Despite efforts like these, some say that the free flow of information in the research community has been adversely affected (Culliton 1989).

Another criticism of the joint venture arrangement is the potential for conflicts of interest that some collaborations, particularly those with significant financial remuneration, may pose. Although the scientist is not an employee of the corporation, if he or she stands to gain financially from the development of a new product, some bias may adversely affect the scientific integrity of the research.

CRADAs are one type of joint venture arrangement in which the federal government and private industry invest roughly equal amounts in collaborative research. Through CRADAs, the federal government developed a mechanism for federal laboratories to work collaboratively with industry in order to turn federally funded research into commercial products and foster technology transfer. In return, the company receives first rights to intellectual property developed as a result of the collaboration and the researcher gains access to industrial technology, laboratories, and resources (Anderson 1993). In addition, federal researchers may receive royalties if projects are successful (Culliton 1989). Since the establishment of CRADAs by the Federal Technology Transfer Act of 1986, hundreds have developed, with the NIH at the forefront. However, in recent years their popularity, particularly at the NIH, has been thwarted by problems related to "reasonable pricing" clauses (developed in response to the controversy surrounding Burroughs Wellcome's pricing of the AIDS drug AZT) and administrative delays in the approval and processing time. Because of the fair-pricing provision, many pharmaceutical and biotechnology companies have been reluctant to invest in these agreements, since their return on investment may be restricted by the government (Anderson 1993). Smaller companies and start-up companies have, however, continued to pursue these arrangements despite these problems. The NIH is currently seeking to streamline the review process (Anderson 1994).

Although the government has encouraged research institutions to collaborate and form joint ventures with industry to turn federally funded science into commercial products, in recent years these arrangements have raised controversy. In 1993, the Switzerland-based Sandoz Pharmaceutical Corporation formed a 10-year, $300 million joint venture with the Scripps Research Institute, potentially gaining exclusive rights to what was estimated to be more than a billion dollars' worth of taxpayer-funded research, raising concerns among the public and members of Congress. In order to respond to these concerns, the NIH formed an ad hoc panel of academic and industrial scientists and research administrators to recommend guidelines for agreements covering research funded by a combination of government and industry funding (Anderson 1994).

Consultantship

A consultantship is the most common model of industry/academia collaboration, one that has endured through many changes in the relationship of academia and industry. Under consulting arrangements, pharmaceutical or other interested corporations seek out scientists as consultants and use the consultants' expertise in guiding their own research programs toward the drugs that are needed in the market, evaluating the design of research projects, and in incorporating newer, more advanced research models and animal experiments to update their research programs. Researchers who serve as consultants sometimes also carry out clinical trials for the same corporation. This allows the investigator to both design and carry out clinical trials for the corporation.

Scientists may consult for numerous companies during their careers and often consult for several companies at one time. Conversely, one company usually has a pool of consultants from different institutions working on the same project. Consulting scientists agree not to discuss information about one company's project with another company for which they consult in order to protect the proprietary interests of the companies. Some senior scientists have more exclusive relationships with one company, where they may design drug testing or other research programs. In these cases, a formal contract is signed by the scientist, who agrees not to disclose information about the projects. Ownership of products and patents is vested in the company; only in a few cases, typically an exclusive consulting relationship, are royalties received by consultants.

The consultant model enables the private sector to obtain the expert advice of a university scientist and incorporate this advice into their research and development (R&D) programs. At the same time, this relationship provides the consultant with a glimpse of what is going on in commercial laboratories.

Award Program

Some large corporations have scientific research award programs under which specific investigators who are producing exemplary work in a field that is of particular interest to the company are selected to receive funds. Usually this award is for a specified period (e.g., 3–5 years). During this time, the award is used to cover the costs of conducting basic research in a targeted area. Many award programs allow substantial flexibility with regard to the focus of research so that a shift in the direction of research, when appropriate, is possible.

By accepting the award, the researcher does not become an employee of the sponsoring corporation; depending on the intentions of the corporation, there may or may not be any constraints on the researcher's freedom to immediately publish findings. Some companies may expect to be granted the right of first refusal or an exclusive license to patents obtained on commercially exploitable findings. In such cases, it is expected that findings and other proprietary information will be kept confidential only as long as it takes for a patent to be filed.

Corporations implement award programs as part of their R&D agendas largely because they provide the corporations with a window into the cutting edge of science, facilitate closer relationships with the scientific community, and provide seed money for good basic science (Apple 1989). In some cases, award programs may result in profits to the company.

Award programs differ from other research collaboration models in that the funding periods are usually significantly shorter and the corporation chooses only a few researchers to sponsor each year. As a result, the corporation receives the benefits of having access to numerous investigators' work in a variety of fields without the difficulties, expense, and length of time it requires to establish a full-blown partnership.

Bristol-Myers Squibb Company and Procter and Gamble Company (P & G) are two examples of corporations that support research award programs. Bristol-Myers Squibb has a $20 million unrestricted research fund that has been operating since 1977. It grants 5-year, $500,000 gifts to selected principal investigators (Apple 1989). Bristol-Myers Squibb does not request exclusive licenses to patents nor does it require reporting of data prior to publication. Its medical research awards program has expanded into many different fields, the latest being neuroscience and psychiatric research.

P & G's exploratory research program has funded basic research for over a decade. The program awards a maximum of $50,000 a year for 3 years to three investigators. The award recipients are selected from among proposals solicited in the biological and physical sciences of mutual interest to the university researchers and P & G's research staff. P & G provides a company contact for the investigators, whose role is to make available to the principal investigator expertise and facilities within the company and to provide for the flow of new information into the company in the most appropriate way.

In the event that potentially patentable discoveries are made in research funded by P & G, the company expects an option for an exclusive license under any patent granted, with royalty arrangements to be negotiated according to the policy of the university. P & G's only procedural requirement is that the investigators submit a progress report to keep the company apprised of the status of projects.

The American Psychiatric Association (APA) has sponsored industry-supported fellowship/award programs. For example, the APA Lilly Psychiatric Research Fellowship provides a 1-year fellowship for a postgraduate psychiatry trainee specifically to further develop a research career in a mentored program.

Venture Capital Start-Up

A venture capital start-up typically consists of a research corporation or contractual arrangement established by venture capitalists in the business sector and academicians. The typical capital investment ranges from $6 million to $10 million, with the research staff remaining relatively small, usually consisting of about 10 to 15 people. This type of model creates a unique opportunity for the investigator in that he or she may be formally part of both the academic community and the private sector, i.e., an investigator may be on the faculty of a university and at the same time be on the board of directors of a start-up corporation. It also provides a quicker avenue for transferring technology from the laboratory to the market.

The venture capital start-up corporation generally conducts research in a broad, usually applied technology field such as pharmaceutical development. Patents obtained on any commercially exploitable material are vested in the corporation, with royalties going to the individual and/or institutions involved. The start-up corporation may be composed of scientists who have left academia or have only loose ties with it. Thus, the entity is independent of academia. All products are owned by the start-up company, with royalties divided among investors, usually according to the size of their investments.

Investigators generally hold equity interests in and are on the research faculty of the corporation at the same time. Some corporations participating in venture capital start-ups do not have conflict of interest policies. Venture capital start-up arrangements generally include confidentiality policies, which are in effect while projects are being undertaken. At other times, investigators are free to publish as they wish and share information freely.

The venture capital start-up offers some of the same disadvantages as the joint venture model of research collaboration in that the appearance of conflict of interest is likely to bring into question the integrity of the research conducted by the company. In addition, the pace of industry is significantly faster than academia, since investors may be anxious for products and tangible results to develop from research efforts in order to receive a return on their investment.

Contracted Research

Under the contracted research model of collaboration, the traditional, commonly used mechanism for funding industry-supported clinical research studies, a corporation seeks out a particular scientist or group of scientists to conduct research with a specific goal in mind. Studies can take many forms; the most common are clinical trials and multicenter trials. A corporation funds contracted research by paying the researcher a predetermined sum, generally a fixed amount per patient, to cover the cost of the research. As an employee of the university, the researcher does not profit directly from the research. He or she may at the same time serve as a consultant to the company and assist in developing the design of the trial. Contracted research arrangements vary, depending on the contractual agreement, in the degree to which the research institution can use the research findings.

A common problem with contracted research has been characterized as "the enormous cost and demoralization involved in assembling, disassembling, and reassembling clinical research teams based on the unpredictable cycles of support" (Kane 1991, p. 353). This problem highlights the general need for a more stable, ongoing research infrastructure to more rationally sustain and support clinical research.

◆ Potential Problems and Conflicts of Interest

Problems Related to Industry-Sponsored Research

Although collaboration between academic researchers and industry offers a number of significant advantages, researchers, academic institutions, and society at large are concerned about a number of potential adverse consequences. One concern is that industry sponsorship will result in a shift in the focus of research toward more applied product- or technology-oriented research that is likely to be profitable in the private sector and away from important public health or scientific needs with less profit potential. Another potential adverse consequence is the diminished willingness of researchers to collaborate and openly share and disseminate information. In fact, in some agreements investigators have confidentiality requirements and contractual restrictions placed on them with regard to the publication, dissemination or sharing, and use of research findings.

Another area of significant concern, which is addressed in more detail below, is the potential threat posed by conflicts of interest resulting from industry-sponsored research. Some critics, including administrators of academic research institutions, also argue that in addition to conflicts of interest, participation in industry-sponsored research may also create "conflicts of commitment" among faculty members in which commercially supported consulting and research activities compete or interfere with faculty members' teaching and administrative responsibilities. Other potential problems and risks that researchers participating in industry-sponsored research may face include lack of control over the direction of research and the forfeiture of rights to patents.

Industry-Sponsored Research and Conflicts of Interest

A conflict of interest has been defined as a set of conditions in which professional judgement concerning a primary interest (such as a patient's welfare or the validity of research) tends to be unduly influenced by a secondary interest (such as financial gain) (Thompson

1993). In this sense, a conflict of interest, as distinguished from scientific misconduct, is a condition and not a behavior in that researchers who might benefit financially by distorting their work face a conflict of interest regardless of whether they actually distort their work (Kassirer and Angell 1993). It follows that the general norm of scientific behavior (including intellectual honesty, objectivity, and reasonable doubt) is not necessarily compromised when a potential conflict of interest arises (Thompson 1993).

Conflicts of interest can result in four types of potential problems for researchers. Conflicts of interest can 1) introduce bias in the actual conduct of research, adversely affecting the validity of data; 2) introduce bias in the analysis and reporting of data, resulting in false or misleading reports; 3) result in diminished acceptance or eroded confidence in the research due to perceptions of bias in the conduct or analysis of data; or 4) result in unethical or illegal financial transactions such as purchasing or selling stock in a company on the basis of preliminary research results (i.e., "insider trading").

Although conflicts of interest (both real and perceived) resulting from industry/academia collaboration pose significant threats to investigators, it should be noted that many other types of conflicts of interest (such as the pressure to produce research findings that are positive in order to attain a tenured faculty position) are also inherent in the research process and may bias the outcome of all clinical investigations (AMA Council on Scientific Affairs and AMA Council on Ethical and Judicial Affairs 1990).

◆ Suggestions for Investigators to Avoid Potential Problems and Conflicts of Interest

To avoid some of the potential problems associated with industry-sponsored research, there are a number of steps investigators can take to protect themselves. Before entering a relationship, investigators should first become familiar with the potential problems and conflicts of interest they may encounter, as outlined above. Researchers must examine their institution's formal conflict of interest guidelines. The NIH has developed proposed federal guidelines that are to apply to research funded by a combination of government and industry support. These guidelines are intended to foster the development of more uniform, national conflict of interest standards.

Perhaps most important, it is recommended that investigators interested in participating in industry-sponsored research negotiate and formally lay out the terms of their collaborative relationship. This should be done in an explicit, formal written agreement in order to assure that the terms are mutually agreeable and the investigator's research objectives can be met.

Once an investigator becomes involved in an industry-sponsored research project, in addition to complying with his or her research institution's conflict of interest guidelines, compliance with the American Medical Association (AMA) Council on Ethical and Judicial Affairs and the AMA Council on Scientific Affairs conflict of interest recommendations is also suggested. Specifically, the AMA recommends that researchers participating in industry-sponsored research:

- ◆ Only receive remuneration commensurate with the effort made on behalf of the company.
- ◆ Disclose any material ties to companies whose products they are investigating, including disclosing financial ties when participating in educational activities, research projects, consulting arrangements, or other industry-sponsored activities. Disclosure should be made to the medical center where the research is being conducted, organizations funding the research, and journals publishing research results (Lundberg and Flanagin 1989).
- ◆ Cannot ethically buy or sell the company's stock until the involvement ends and the results of the research are published or otherwise disseminated to the public.

The AMA also recommends that all medical centers develop specific conflict of interest guidelines for their staff and establish review committees to examine disclosures made by clinical staff regarding their financial relationships with commercial corporations (AMA Council on Scientific Affairs and AMA Council on Ethical and Judicial Affairs 1990). The Association of Academic Health Centers Task Force on Science Policy recently developed a publication entitled *Conflict of Interest in Institutional Decisionmaking*, which may be referenced for a more detailed account of conflict of interest issues affecting university officials in particular and academic institutions more generally.

◆ Conclusion

In recent years a variety of collaborative research relationships between industry and academia have emerged to support the conduct of basic, applied, and clinical research. These arrangements may offer an attractive source of research funding for investigators. However, before entering into such agreements, the investigator should explicitly lay out the terms of the agreement in writing to ensure that the arrangement will meet his or her research objectives and professional or personal needs. Critical issues that should be taken into consideration include whether the arrangement will affect the investigator's ability to:

◆ Choose the path or direction of research as work progresses.
◆ Publish and disseminate research findings.
◆ Communicate openly with colleagues and share information regarding the research being undertaken.
◆ Be remunerated for the results of the research, including obtaining rights to patents or royalties from the commercialization of resulting technologies.
◆ Conduct research in a scientific manner without affecting his or her objectivity.

◆ References

American Medical Association (AMA) Council on Scientific Affairs, AMA Council on Ethical and Judicial Affairs: Conflicts of interest in medical center/industry research relationships. JAMA 263(20):2790–2793, 1990

Anderson C: Rocky road for Federal Research Inc. Science 262:496–498, 1993

Anderson C: Panel proposes guidelines for industry. Science 263:603, 1994

Apple MA: The U.S. is not making a big enough investment in its own future. The Scientist, 1989

Blumenthal D, Gluck M, Louis KS, et al: Industrial support of university research in biotechnology. Science 231:242–246, 1986a

Blumenthal D, Gluck M, Louis KS, et al: University-industry research relationships in biotechnology: implications for the university. Science 232:1361–1366, 1986b

Culliton BJ: NIH, Inc.: The CRADA boom. Science 245:1034–1036, 1989

Kane JM: Obstacles to clinical research and new drug development in schizophrenia. Schizophr Bull 17(2):353–356, 1991

Kassirer JP, Angell M: Financial conflicts of interest in biomedical research. N Engl J Med 329(8):570–571, 1993

Kenney M: Biotechnology—The University-Industrial Complex. Hartford, CT, Yale University Press, 1986

Lundberg GD, Flanagin A: New requirements for authors: signed statements of authorship responsibility and financial disclosure (editorial). JAMA 262:2003–2004, 1989

National Institutes of Health: NIH Data Book 1993. Bethesda, MD, National Institutes of Health, 1993

Pincus HA, Fine T: The "anatomy" of research funding of mental illness and addictive disorders. Arch Gen Psychiatry 49(7):573–579, 1992

Thompson DF: Understanding financial conflicts of interest. N Engl J Med 329(8):573–576, 1993

Witt MD, Phar D, Gostin LO: Conflict of interest dilemmas in biomedical research. JAMA 271:547–551, 1994

Resources 6–1

Selected Resources on Industry and Academia Collaboration

Agnew B: NIH panel gives advice on tech-transfer deals. The Journal of NIH Research 6:42, 1994

Clemmitt M: U.S. drug industry's research support. Nature 361(64):757–760, 1993

Cuatrecasas P: Industry-university alliances in biomedical research. J Clin Pharmacol 32:100–106, 1992

DeVeaugh-Geiss J: Academic medical center/industry collaboration. Arch Gen Psychiatry 48(8):754–756, 1991

Freedman DX: Research funds are down: take heart! Arch Gen Psychiatry 42(5):518–522, 1985

Ginzberg E, Ginzberg D, Anna B: The Financing of Biomedical Research. Baltimore, MD, Johns Hopkins University Press, 1989

Government-University-Industrial Research Roundtable: Industrial perspectives on innovation and interactions with universities: summaries of interviews with senior industrial officials. Washington, DC, National Academy Press, 1991

Lomasky LE: Who should profit from the business of science? Hastings Cent Rep 17(3):5–7, 1987

Marshall E: When commerce and academe collide. Science 248:152–156, 1990

Mervis J: Terms of Scripps-Sandoz agreement may be more common than its critics believe. Nature 362(6417):194–195, 1993

Noble RC: Physicians and the pharmaceutical industry: an alliance with unhealthy aspects. Perspect Biol Med 36(3):376–394, 1993

Pardes H: State-academic research liaisons. Psychiatr Q 61(1):69–74, 1990

Porter R, Malone TE: Biomedical Research: The Industry and the Academic Medical Center. Baltimore, MD, Johns Hopkins Press, 1992

Relman AS: The new medical-industrial complex. N Engl J Med 303(17):963–970, 1980

Rhein R: Will NIH'S fair-price clause make CRADAs crumble? The Journal of NIH Research 6:40–43, 1993

Sims C: Business-campus ventures grow. The New York Times, December 14, 1987, p 13

Stein MD, Rubenstein L, Wachtel TJ: Who pays for published research? JAMA 269(6):781–782, 1993

Sterman AB: A research edge: new teamwork between industry and academia. Pharmacological Executive 8:38–43, 1988

Yau-Young A: Want industry funding? points to remember. The Journal of NIH Research 5:24–26, 1993

Resources 6–2

Pharmaceutical Company Research Contacts

This list provides the names, addresses, and phone numbers of the relevant research contacts for psychiatric investigators at pharmaceutical companies.

Abbott Laboratories
AP-30
One Abbott Park Road
Abbott Park, IL 60064
Thomas Larson
Product Manager, Neuroscience & Psychiatry
(708) 937-7194

Astra/Merck Group
725 Chesterbrook Boulevard
Wayne, PA 19087
Warren Cooper
Director of Medical Affairs, Drug Development Operations
(215) 695-1063

Bristol-Myers Squibb Company
PO Box 4500
Princeton, NJ 08543
John Ieni
Assistant Director, Clinical Trials for Central Nervous System
(609) 897-2824

Burroughs Wellcome Company
3030 Cornwallis Road
Research Triangle Park, NC 27709
John Asher, M.D.
Associate Director, Clinical Neurosciences
(919) 315-3259

Ciba-Geigy Pharmaceuticals
556 Morris Avenue
Summit, NJ 07901
Charles Savari
Director of Research
(908) 277-5000

Dista Products Company
Division of Eli Lilly & Co.
Lilly Corporate Center
Indianapolis, IN 46285
Gary Tollefson, M.D., Ph.D.
Executive Director of CNS, GI, & Other Medical Research
(317) 276-6559

Gate Pharmaceuticals
1510 Delp Drive
Kulpsville, PA 19443
Barry Edwards
Executive Director
(215) 723-5544

Glaxo, Inc.
5 Moore Drive
Research Triangle Park, NC 27709
Joseph DeVeaugh-Geiss, M.D.
Director of Central Nervous System Clinical Research
(919) 990-5170

Hoechst-Roussel Pharmaceuticals, Inc.
PO Box 2500
Route 202-206
Somerville, NJ 08876
Norbert G. Riedel, Ph.D.
Director of Molecular Neurobiology, Neuroscience
(908) 231-3906

Jannssen Pharmaceutica
PO Box 200
1125 Trenton-Harburton Road
Titusville, NJ 08560
Richard Meibach, Ph.D.
Director of Clinical Research
(609) 730-3135
Jennifer Hardin, M.D.
Director of Medical Development
(609) 730-3184

McNeil Pharmaceuticals
PO Box 300
Raritan, NJ 08869
Thomas P. Gibson
Executive Director, Clinical Research
(908) 218-7499

Novo Nordisk Pharmaceuticals
100 Overlook Center, Suite 200
Princeton, NJ 08540
Jan Ohrstrom, M.D.
Director, Gynecology & CNS Clinical Development
(609) 987-5800

Parke-Davis & Company
201 Tabor Road
Morris Plains, NJ 07950
John Howard
Vice President of Neurology Care
(201) 540-6945
Larry Perlow
Vice President of Medical & Scientific Affairs
(201) 540-3455

Pfizer, Inc.
Roerig Division
235 East 42nd Street
New York, NY 10017
Clinical & Scientific Affairs
(212) 573-7956

Roche Laboratories
340 Kingsland Avenue
Nutley, NJ 07110
Lenore Fleming, Ed.D., M.D.
Director of Clinical Services
(201) 235-2398

Sandoz, Inc.
Building 122
59 Route #10
East Hanover, NJ 07936
Michael Krassner, M.D., Ph.D.
Senior Associate Medical Director, Medical Services Department
(201) 503-7755

Scios-Nova Pharmaceuticals
2450 Bayshore Parkway
Mount View, CA 94043
Kira Bacon, Scios-Nova Investor Group
(415) 940-6629
(Ms. Bacon reports that Scios-Nova is not directly involved in
psychopharmacological development.)

Searle Pharmaceuticals
Lorex
5200 Old Orchard Road
Skokie, IL 60077
Stefan Allard, M.D.
Director of Research
(708) 982-3057

SmithKline Beecham Pharmaceuticals
PO Box 1510
King of Prussia, PA 19406
Ivan Gergel, M.D.
Director, CNS Clinical Research & Development—Medical Affairs
(215) 832-3945

Solvay Pharmaceuticals
901 Sawyer Road
Marietta, GA 30062
Drew Finn, M.D.
Vice President, Clinical Research & Biometrics
(404) 578-5848
Vince Houser, Ph.D.
Director, CNS Research
(404) 578-5863

The Upjohn Company
7000 Portage Road
Kalamazoo, MI 49001
Jeff Jonas, M.D.
Divisional Vice President, Worldwide Pharmaceutical Regulatory
   Affairs
(616) 329-8358

Wallace Laboratories
Half Acre Road
Cranbury, NJ 08512
Jeffrey Freitag, M.D.
Director of Research
(609) 951-2020

Wyeth-Ayerst Laboratories
PO Box 8299
Philadelphia, PA 19101
Andrew Johannsen, M.D.
Director of Clinical Research
(215) 971-5763

Zeneca Pharmaceutical Company
New Murphy Road-Concord Pike
Wilmington, DE 19877
Ron Burch, Ph.D.
Director of Research
(302) 886-8059, Ext 2744

CHAPTER

7

Research Opportunities in Child and Adolescent Mental Disorders

Peter S. Jensen, M.D.

B ecause research on children and adolescent mental disorders has lagged behind comparable research on the adult disorders, the National Institute of Mental Health (NIMH) asked the Institute of Medicine (IOM) of the National Academy of Sciences to conduct a major review of the field, examine the scope of the research problems, and recommend potential solutions. This report, *Research on Children and Adolescents with Mental, Behavioral, and Developmental Disorders* (IOM 1989), indicated that almost every area of child and adolescent mental disorders research warranted significant expansion. Although children under age 18 comprise about one-quarter of our nation's population, research on children's mental health has in times past generally consumed much less of the total NIMH research

The opinions and assertions contained in this paper are the private views of the author and are not to be construed as official or as reflecting the views of the Department of Health and Human Services or the National Institute of Mental Health.

Portions of this report were abstracted from public domain documents previously prepared by staff of the National Institute of Mental Health.

budget. This situation was the result of a combination of factors, including a lack of awareness on the part of some investigators of the critical needs and opportunities in this area, as well as a relative lack of qualified investigators. As a result, progress in mental health research in children and adolescent disorders has not kept pace with related research on adults.

The IOM report estimated that 7.5 million young people (approximately 12% of the nation's youth) have some significant mental disorder. These mental disorders in children and adolescents, according to conservative estimates, cost our nation more than $1.5 billion in treatment costs each year. Yet fewer than one-fourth of these children now receive appropriate treatment, and many of those treated—even by the best clinicians—fail to recover because their disorders are not adequately understood.

Despite this gloomy picture, dramatic advances have occurred in child and adolescent mental health research during the past two decades. A scientific base is now in place that has given clinicians powerful new tools for diagnosing and treating a number of the mental disorders that afflict children and adolescents. Our growing scientific capability can now more effectively grapple with the many disorders that severely hamper the daily lives and the future prospects of many of our children and youth. But without a concerted effort to accelerate the pace of progress, it will continue to be too slow to help the millions of young people now in need and the millions more who will soon develop mental disorders we can neither prevent nor treat.

In response to this report, and to address the need to better understand, prevent, and treat child and adolescent mental disorders, the NIMH released a new initiative in 1990 entitled *National Plan for Research on Child and Adolescent Mental Disorders* (NIMH 1990). This program is designed to greatly expand its research activities on child and adolescent mental disorders. The national plan outlines areas where research information is critically needed, including 1) a broad epidemiologic survey of child and adolescent mental disorders to provide greater insight into the prevalence and etiology of these disorders, 2) systematic investigation of the causes and determinants of childhood mental illnesses, especially the joint impact of biologic and environmental factors in modulating children's behavior and risk for mental disorders, 3) determination of effective treatments for specific disorders, 4) genetics research (of which there has been practically none), 5) longitudinal studies concerning the links between childhood psychopathology and adult disorders, 6) comorbidity studies linking mental disorders with a second diagnosis (especially problematic in studies of children and adolescents), 7) services research to evaluate and improve the efficacy, organization, delivery, and accessibility of treatment services, and 8) studies of the relations between complex psychobiological variables (e.g., attentiveness, language, and cognitive processes) and the onset of childhood psychopathology.

In addition, because of the severe shortage of appropriately trained child psychopathology researchers, increasing the size of the cadre of trained investigators via research training is a major component of the National Plan for Research on Child and Adolescent Mental Disorders. As necessary first steps to implement this plan, the NIMH has established the NIMH Consortium on Child and Adolescent Mental Disorders Research, working under the direction of the director of the NIMH, to coordinate the implementation of the national plan. Through the efforts of members of this consortium, new Program Announcements (PAs) and Requests for Applications (RFAs) are developed to build new research capacity and focus researchers' attention on much-needed areas. In addition, this consortium works to develop liaisons with other government funding agencies, private foundations, journal editors, and other parties critical to the research enterprise, with the goal of sharing information, stimulating interdisciplinary exchange, developing new approaches to complex problems that have hindered child and adolescent research, and conducting technical assistance workshops to teach new or junior investigators the ropes about the NIMH structure, funding, and the grant writing/application process.

Beyond these consortium activities, other specific steps that the NIMH took in the first 3 years (1991–1993) of the national plan included significant increases in the proportion of the NIMH monies devoted to child- and adolescent-focused studies, funding of child and adolescent studies at more favorable percentile and priority scores, holding international conferences devoted to building consensus in critical yet controversial scientific areas, implementing a multicenter national collaborative treatment trial in attention-deficit hyperactivity disorder (ADHD) (planning phase begun in 1992), and completing the first phase of a multisite methodologic feasibility study of child and adolescent mental disorders (1993).

What is the theoretical perspective that guides much of the research that the NIMH has funded or currently seeks to fund? Are there particular theoretical biases that limit the kinds of questions that may be addressed through the NIMH funding mechanisms or as envisioned in the national plan? Simply said, no. Many people incorrectly believe that the NIMH is narrowly biologically focused or that interdisciplinary rivalries limit the psychiatrist's ability to contribute to and participate in these research programs. These notions are just plain wrong; in our experience, they result from the potential investigator's lack of experience or exposure to the broad scope of the NIMH programs and theoretical and disciplinary backgrounds of funded investigators. Instead, the most critical components of fundable research are the methodologic sophistication and feasibility of the research design, preliminary evidence that the proposed research may yield new findings important to the scientific knowledge base, the skill and research capabilities of the principal investigator, and the public health significance of the area of study.

Given these caveats, however, one must still acknowledge that a keen appreciation of developmental factors is key to understanding the evolution of behavior, mental health, and mental disorders in children and adolescents. Although the entire human lifespan is shaped by the interplay between change and constancy, the theme of the progressive unfolding of human potential is the leitmotif from infancy through adolescence. These age periods are characterized by rapid qualitative and quantitative shifts in neural, behavioral, and emotional organization in some areas, while at the same time other developmental domains remain relatively constant. And, as the thrust from one developmental domain recedes, another area previously quiescent presses forward and the cycle begins anew. This developmental framework is a hallmark of state-of-the-art basic, applied, and clinical research in child and adolescent populations and provides the essential context for understanding child and adolescent mental health and disorder at molecular, intrapsychic, and interpersonal levels. Thus, the ultimate goals of neuroscientists, behavioral scientists, and applied and clinical scientists are complementary; these goals culminate in the clarification of the origins of child and adolescent mental disorders, and the development of new avenues for overcoming these disorders across the developmental epochs of infancy, childhood, and adolescence. If any, these are the "biases" of the NIMH program and review staff concerning proposed research in child and adolescent mental disorders.

To address these developmental considerations adequately, a range of basic, clinical, and applied science studies is needed, including 1) normative studies of social, emotional, and personality development; 2) developmental approaches to structural and functional changes in memory, attention, and reasoning, both in normal and disordered populations; 3) studies of the behavioral organization of sensory processes, interactive behaviors, and homeostatic behaviors and determination of the effects of their organization and interplay on developmental malleability and resilience; and 4) studies of the interactions between family dynamics and genetic factors in shaping emotional, social, and cognitive development and adaptation in healthy and mentally disordered states, and developmental psychopharmacologic studies of the effects of drugs on behavior from infancy through adolescence.

◆ Research Opportunities and Needs

Epidemiology

A major NIMH initiative was begun in 1989 to conduct methodologic research on assessment instruments and survey procedures that could be used in a full-scale multisite epidemiologic survey of child and adolescent mental disorders and service utilization. This study is known by the unwieldy title *Cooperative Agreement for Methodologic Research for Multi-Site Epidemiologic Surveys of Mental Disorders in Child and Adolescent Populations* (PHS 1990), but the name has been shortened for communication purposes by its current investigators to MECA (Methodology for Epidemiology in Mental Disorders in Children and Adolescents). The goal of the MECA study is to determine the feasibility of its methodologic approaches for application to a large-scale, developmental epidemiologic survey of child and adolescent mental disorders. This large-scale study is expected to be similar in scope to the adult Epidemiologic Catchment Area (ECA) study (Burke et al. 1990). In contrast to the adult ECA study, however, this study will place greater emphasis on children's services needs and utilization, as well as longitudinal design components and the careful examination of the continuities/discontinuities between child, adolescent, and adult forms of psychopathology.

It should be noted that the anticipated child ECA study will not be exclusive of other investigator-initiated research, however, and further epidemiologic research is needed in areas such as studies of the prevalence, incidence, and risk factors for specific disorders, as well as problem behaviors below traditional diagnostic thresholds (e.g., suicidal behaviors, adjustment reactions, aggressive and violent behaviors, and other conditions). Also, a good deal of work is needed to study the mental health of children and adolescents living in abusive situations, areas of high violence, transient housing situations, or in juvenile justice correctional facilities or social service placements. Likewise, studies are needed of the types and frequencies of mental health problems in special populations, including homeless children, minorities, children of divorced or single parents, rural children and adolescents, and children from families with criminal, mentally disordered, or substance-abusing parents or siblings. Also, innovative methodologic research is needed to examine the epidemiology, risk factors, and correlates of disorders that are rare (e.g., prevalence less than 1%).

Assessment and Diagnosis

To provide more valid and accurate methods in determining the dimensions and significance of mental disorders and associated conditions, a number of questions require immediate attention by interested investigators. Specific attention must be given to the variables affecting informants' responses about the child or adolescent as well as site differences in subject recruitment and differences among existing assessment instruments. Disorders that are first evident during early childhood (under age 10) present special assessment challenges. Because children have limited cognitive and language abilities until about age 7 or 8, they may not be able to report reliably their self-perceptions, memories, feelings, and behavior.

Thus, the task of developing reliable diagnostic and assessment methods for children of all ages must be addressed. Much greater attention must be directed to the factors that influence the judgments of clinicians, parents, and teachers about emotional and behavior problems in children and adolescents. Furthermore, investigators must determine which techniques and assessment strategies will allow better discrimination between children and adolescents with time-limited, situation-specific problems from those who will show persistent, significant psychosocial impairments and mental disorders. Also, we need to determine what tools and instruments are needed to measure accurately the outcomes of mental health treatments, and to ascertain the extent to which developmental and family assessments are required in the measurement of treatment and prevention outcomes.

Causes and Determinants

The evolution of differences in behavior from the prenatal period through adolescence depends on biologic factors, environmental factors, and their interaction. Basic science research that determines the relative contributions of genetic and environmental factors to individual differences is essential to understanding the etiology of mental disorders and to guide investigations of biological and behavioral interventions appropriate for their treatment. To address these questions, genetic factors must be examined in the realm of genomic control and regulation of neural development, as well as in the realm of genetic factors that shape emotional, social, and cognitive development and adaptation. Likewise, environmental factors require intensive exploration; these include studies of the impact of the hormonal environment on the development and functional activity of neural circuitry, an examination of the effects of psychoactive drugs on behavior, a determination of the relationship between life stressors and health-related psychological states, and investigations of the role that peer and family experiences play in healthy and abnormal psychological development and adaptation.

To address these critical questions, a range of studies is needed. For example, in the area of biologic factors and brain mechanisms, research is needed to determine what brain mechanisms underlie the development, regulation, and modulation of behavior, both in normal and disordered states. Certainly, infants, children, and adolescents are the study population of choice for many questions in this area. We need a much better understanding of the structural and functional changes in neural circuitry that occur across the life span, and knowledge of which central nervous system mechanisms mediate the effects of poor prenatal care, prematurity, low birth weight, and childbirth complications on the child's likelihood of developing mental disorders.

Other questions of great scientific interest and public health significance remain largely unanswered: What are the mechanisms whereby chronic medical conditions (e.g., leukemia, diabetes mellitus, asthma, cystic fibrosis, epilepsy, and AIDS) predispose children toward mental disorders? Which effects are mediated through repeated or chronic stresses, through interference with the child's developmental tasks, and/or through influences on the child's environment? What is the role of cognitive impairments (such as those resulting from mental retardation or brain damage) and deficits in sensory perception (including deafness and blindness) in the development of emotional and behavioral disorders? What is the impact of the hormonal environment on the development and functional activity of the neural circuitry? At which points in development are these effects most pronounced?

Genetic Studies

A major research challenge for child and adolescent mental disorders is to determine whether a given cluster of symptoms or a disorder stems from a disturbed environment, a genetic predisposition, or the interaction of both. Rapid advances in genetics research in general, as well as in the genetic study of mental disorders, have opened new doors to understanding how mental disorders arise in children and adolescents. As it is becoming possible to map the human genome, it also will be possible to identify virtually any gene or group of genes that causes disorders presumed to be hereditary. Rapid expansion of research using genetically informative research designs in basic, clinical, and epidemiologic studies is greatly needed.

Needed research strategies include studies of genomic control and regulation of neural development, studies of the role of genetic factors in social, emotional, and cognitive development, studies of the interaction of genetic factors and shared versus nonshared environments, genetic linkage studies of mental disorders and behavioral problems whose age of onset is in childhood, such as autism, ADHD, and Tourette's syndrome, and studies that include children in proposed or ongoing genetic linkage studies of mental disorders in adults, such as bipolar disorder or schizophrenia (where age of onset could be in childhood or adolescence).

Child Development and
Psychosocial Risk Factors

Improved understanding of normal developmental processes, as well as factors associated with the emergence and/or maintenance of specific mental disorders in infants, children, and adolescents, is essential. For this reason, examination of a wide array of developmental domains, psychosocial risk factors, and disease correlates is needed, including studies of the developmental, psychological, and social factors that increase the propensity of some children and adolescents to engage in behaviors that threaten health and life; studies of the effects of persistent psychological adversity, such as disorganized and inadequate schooling, on the development of mental disorders and associated mental health problems; studies of interpersonal and family variables that could be associated with adaptive outcomes in children who are at risk for developing mental disorders or who have already developed a mental disorder; studies of the effects of child abuse or neglect, disturbed family relationships, and parental mental illness; and studies of the relationships between psychosocial and biologic variables, and how these relationships are mediated.

Are there certain critical periods when environmental risk factors are more likely to significantly alter biological thresholds and set points? At which time points are such alterations of greatest concern, and which developmental lines are most likely to be affected?

In addition, potentially informative areas for research include the examination of the mental health effects of cumulative risk factors, and the determination of whether certain combinations of risk factors mediate much greater effects than others. Determination of which intrapersonal and interpersonal factors can protect children and adolescents from persistent psychosocial adversity is greatly needed. Can these factors be learned or taught? In a related area, research with populations at high risk for the development of mental disorders is encouraged, since such populations may provide models of putative pathogenic environmental variables and adverse outcomes. For example, which factors affect the development of serious long- and short-term symptoms of mental disorders in abused and neglected children? What are the effects of homelessness on children's emotional, personality, and social development? What are the causes, correlates, and mental health consequences of antisocial behavior in children and adolescents, and how can adverse outcomes be prevented? Obviously, the number of questions is very large, and our scientific advances to date (or paucity of advances) have not been limited by the lack of important research questions but by the shortage of capable, dedicated investigators and the heretofore low priority accorded child and adolescent mental disorders research.

Treatment Research

Clinical trials are ultimately the standard for evaluating treatment, but such data are available for only a few of the more commonly used treatments for children and adolescents. The NIMH seeks to greatly expand studies in this area. Emphasis is currently being given to studies of treatments used in clinical practice but as yet inadequately tested. High priority will be given to clinical studies of the efficacy and safety of medications, and the effects of medications on learning, performance, and IQ. Furthermore, the NIMH seeks to obtain reliable information about the everyday clinical treatment practices of clinicians. Such information must be gathered if funds spent on treatment research are to be put to the best use. A range of questions must be addressed and are of the highest public health significance. For example, what are the effects of treatments commonly used in clinical practice (individual therapy, family therapy, group therapy, dynamic therapy, and relationship therapy)? Are there particular disorders for which either psychosocial or pharmacological treatments are specifically effective? What is the efficacy of research-based treatment approaches, when applied to clinical settings? (Several behavior therapy and cognitive therapy techniques have shown promise in carefully evaluated research settings but have yet to be extensively evaluated in clinical practice). Also, at what stage of a child's or adolescent's illness are various treatments most effective? And how do developmental, biologic, and contextual factors alter a child's or adolescent's response to specific treatments? How does the presence of multiple disorders affect response to treatments? What factors account for the high placebo response rates in children, and what clinical trial strategies will best control for such factors? Which treatment and subject variables are associated with successful long-term outcomes?

It is also important to determine whether promising single treatments can be made more effective by combining them with other therapeutic approaches. It has been suggested, for example, that a combination of pharmacotherapy and psychosocial therapy may be more effective than either treatment alone for treating childhood depressive disorders, ADHD, and some other disorders. Combined treatments warrant research attention because many children and adolescents have multiple disorders; also, many disorders adversely affect functioning in several areas. Pharmacotherapy, behavior therapy, and cognitive therapy are all relatively well specified, focus on different facets of functioning (thus are likely to be complementary in their effects), and include procedures that can be applied to diverse disorders. However, there is almost no research to guide clinicians in identifying which therapeutic combinations work best.

Many critical questions must be answered: Are psychological and pharmacological treatments interactive or additive in their effects? Can medication increase or decrease a child's response to psychological intervention? Is a particular sequence of the various types of therapy most desirable? Are certain drug and psychological treatment combinations more effective than others? Can the presence of specific symptoms indicate which children are likely to respond to drug therapy? Carefully controlled studies are needed to answer these questions and suggest ways to make current treatment methods more effective.

Follow-up studies of the long-term effects of treatment are especially important because such effects may differ from those seen immediately after treatment. Some treatments that appear to be effective in the short run do not always show sustained effects; others produce little or no immediate effect but may result in significant improvements 1 or 2 years later. Thus, recruitment, treatment, and follow-up of patients 1–2 years after treatment are essential. Funding for investigators carrying out long-term studies of treatment is emphasized.

Larger scale studies of treatments, in which several investigators at different sites undertake simultaneous evaluations, are essential in several disorder areas. This need is particularly clear where studies to date have shown promising findings but where considerations due to sample size, statistical power, and the likelihood of treatment-responsive subgroups warrant collaboration across multiple sites. Such studies are needed to provide critical information about the reliability and reproducibility of treatment effects and to clarify the definition of treatment–responsive homogeneous diagnostic subgroups.

Existing information about the effects of treatment needs to be used more efficiently. Efforts to record, organize, and integrate existing information would strengthen the link between research and ongoing clinical activity, promote the sharing of resources, and clarify the overall state of knowledge in the field. Data from clinical settings, for example, could provide information on patients, treatments, and the effects of treatment. Analysis of such data could reveal which children and families are referred for treatment, problems for which treatment is sought, the kinds of interventions typically used for various problems, and the changes produced by these treatments. Data on patients could also aid in identifying appropriate targets for preventive efforts.

Recently expanded requirements for reporting on patients and services, coupled with the ease of access to such information through computers, make development of patient databases increasingly possible. The NIMH encourages development of database systems for use in clinical services research for children and adolescents.

Prevention Research

Research on the prevention of mental health disorders and behavioral dysfunction and the promotion of mental health in children and adolescents is a high priority of the NIMH. These studies involve populations who are either asymptomatic or who exhibit early symptoms that do not meet diagnostic criteria for mental disorder. The goal of preventive intervention research is to identify interventions that reduce the incidence of disorder or the need/demand for treatment or that enhance psychological functioning.

Preventive intervention studies are expected to specify the epidemiologic basis for the study's target population and the extent to which the group is at risk for a disorder or serious dysfunction. Such studies should include an assessment of the intervention's effect on mental health status. Promotion and prevention studies are expected to include, as distal outcomes, measures of mental health or disorder, respectively. Areas of particular interest include the prevention of socioemotional and developmental problems in infants and children at risk, the development of early intervention models for parents at risk for abusing or neglecting their children, the prevention of conduct and other behavioral disorders in children and adolescents, the prevention of anxiety and depressive disorders in children and adolescents, the prevention of suicide and suicidality in preclinical youth, the promotion of mental health through the enhancement of protective factors and coping mechanisms, the prevention of mental disorders in homeless children and adolescents, and the prevention of affective and anxiety disorders in HIV-infected children and adolescents.

Attention should be given to the following research questions: Are global interventions, targeted interventions, or some combination of both most appropriate for the proposed population? Which risk factors can be altered through the intervention, and which cannot? How can the preventive intervention have maximum impact on those risk factors that account for the greatest variance in the outcomes of interest? What are appropriate short-term outcome measures? What are appropriate longer-term outcome measures? Which aspects of the environment or setting need to be addressed in the design of the preventive intervention? How are developmental processes best incorporated into prevention research? Are multiple-stage preventive interventions timed to critical life transitions more likely to provide lasting impact than brief, one-stage interventions? What is the best way to develop preventive interventions within the existing educational, occupational, or services delivery systems so that the interventions are accepted and sustained in settings of interest?

Mental Health Services Research

Research on mental health services for children and adolescents is meager, and there are great gaps in scientific knowledge concerning service needs and services, the adequacy and effectiveness of these services, and the best ways to finance them. Particular emphasis will be given to studies that address the following range of service system research and clinical services research questions: Do strategies to provide alternatives to residential treatment through comprehensive community-based systems work effectively? How effective are innovative service approaches for children and adolescents with serious mental disorders and their families (e.g., intensive home-based services, therapeutic foster care, family support, day treatment, mobile crisis services, case management, and individualized treatment using flexible funds)? How effective and culturally appropriate are various mental health services used by minority children and adolescents and their families, and what barriers deter their service use?

The area of mental health services research is among the most neglected of all the NIMH research areas, despite the fact that this area touches most closely on the day-to-day practices of most clinicians. For example, what are the effects on the quality, cost, and appropriateness of care of different reimbursement mechanisms and funding strategies within both the public and the private sectors, and how are efforts at cost containment or new financing mechanisms, such as capitation and managed care, changing the delivery of mental health services to children and adolescents? What are the state and impact of assessment, case planning, and clinical decision-making practices in child and adolescent mental health services? What is the quality of mental health service delivery in routine health care? How accurate is diagnosis, and how effective is the treatment of children with mental disorders and their families in a variety of settings and systems of care?

How do primary care providers recognize, refer, diagnose, and treat mental disorders in children and adolescents? What is the impact of consultation/liaison psychiatry, psychiatric emergency services, and the effectiveness of mental health treatment and referral from primary care providers? What are the most effective ways for mental health providers to respond to the needs of children and adolescents with mental disorders that co-occur with alcohol and/or drug abuse?

Special Populations

Minority youth. Research that focuses specifically on the problems of minority populations is needed. Of particular interest is research dealing with the validity of various behavioral tests and assessment instruments for minority groups. Research with a specific focus on prepubertal minority children will receive special attention and support. In addition, support will be given to studies of the mental health problems of particular minority group youths, such as Native Americans or Alaska Natives, Asians/Pacific Islanders, African Americans, and Hispanics.

Rural youth. Recent evidence indicates that rural youths are at higher risk for various mental health problems than youths from urban areas. Furthermore, rural children and adolescents may be more frequently exposed to child abuse, and rural adolescents may experience levels of depression twice that of the national average. Research with a special focus on children living in rural areas will receive special attention and support.

Pediatric AIDS. The NIMH AIDS research program relevant to children and adolescents covers a broad spectrum of issues directly pertaining to mental and behavioral consequences of HIV infection and AIDS. It includes studies on brain and psychological factors associated with HIV infection in young people and their families, as well as studies on the prevention of HIV infection in women of childbearing age. This research program will potentially yield crucial information about biopsychosocial factors in AIDS and in HIV-infected young people and their caregivers, while providing vital knowledge of the most effective prevention approaches for dealing with this deadly illness. The NIMH seeks to develop steady increases in overall support for this essential research area.

Homeless.   The mental health problems of homeless and/or impoverished children and adolescents warrant systematic attention by investigators. Available evidence indicates that homeless children and adolescents are at higher risk for a range of mental health problems and associated conditions. Furthermore, the actual numbers of homeless children and adolescents are increasing. The NIMH seeks to increase research support for this important public health problem.

Centers and Program Projects

Multidisciplinary research centers are needed to move research ahead rapidly. A talented group of investigators committed to a specific area can act synergistically and maintain a high level of scientific productivity. In the child and adolescent area, such centers and program projects can provide important sites for research training, offer pathways for career development, and create unique opportunities for interdisciplinary research. Priority will be given to the creation of multidisciplinary research centers devoted to key areas of child and adolescent mental disorders research.

The following are examples of research areas within the NIMH mission that might serve as a focus for centers or program projects: research on the etiology, evaluation, and treatment of particular disorders or classes of disorders, such as schizophrenia, attention-deficit hyperactivity disorder, manic-depressive illness, conduct disorder, and autism; longitudinal studies focused on the mechanisms that underlie specific risk factors and protective factors related to mental disorders, or on certain catastrophic outcomes such as suicide; research on the development of valid and reliable diagnostic instruments for use in epidemiological or clinical studies; efforts to develop safe and reproducible approaches to treatment of children and adolescents with mental disorders; and neuroscience research on the basic brain mechanisms underlying healthy and abnormal brain development relevant to mental illness.

Research centers are needed to conduct neuroscience studies related to mental disorders of children and adolescents and to support acquisition of state-of-the-art equipment for biological research in those laboratories. Such centers would facilitate interdisciplinary research on childhood disorders (and precursors of adult disorders) by bringing together basic neuroscientists and clinicians involved in biological investigation.

Brain-imaging techniques have immeasurably expanded the potential for studying brain pathology noninvasively in children and adolescents with mental disorders. The NIMH seeks opportunities to provide funds to support collaborative research between existing imaging facilities and researchers studying child and adolescent mental disorders. A major portion of such collaborative studies should be devoted to developmental problems and to brain structure and function in child and adolescent mental disorders.

Support for multidisciplinary treatment research of child and adolescent mental disorders may be requested through clinical research center or program project grants. These proposals should be designed to provide stable, long-term funding for cadres of researchers concerned with identifying, developing, and evaluating effective treatments.

Given the complexity of the center development and application process, investigators are encouraged to contact the NIMH program staff before embarking on the development of an application for a research center in child and adolescent mental disorders.

◆ Training Opportunities

Research Training and Career Development

The NIMH has a wide variety of programs designed to provide stipend or salary support during the developmental stages of a scientist's career (see Table 7–1). Thus, support mechanisms are available to assist graduate students, postdoctoral trainees, recently trained clinicians, and junior and senior scientists. More limited types of support are available for undergraduates and medical students.

Some of the career development and training opportunities re-

Table 7–1. NIMH research training and career development opportunities

Undergraduate research training
  MARC Honors Undergraduate Training Grants (T34)
  Minority Institutions Research Development Program
  Supplements for Underrepresented Minorities

Pre-Ph.D./Pre-M.D.
  NRSA Individual Fellowships (F31)
  NRSA Institutional Training Grants (T32)
  NRSA Predoctoral Individual M.D./Ph.D. Fellowships (F30)
  MARC Faculty Fellowship Awards (F34)
  Minority Fellowship Programs
  Minority Institutions Research Development Program
  Supplements for Underrepresented Minorities

Postdoctoral and residency
  NRSA Individual Fellowships (F32)
  NRSA Institutional Training Grants (T32)
  MARC Faculty Fellowship Awards (F34)
  Supplements for Underrepresented Minorities

Early career
  Child/Adolescent Mental Health Academic Awards (K07)
  Scientist Development Awards for Clinicians (K20)
  Scientist Development Awards (K21)
  MARC Faculty Fellowship Awards (F34)
  Minority Institutions Research Development Program
  Supplements for Underrepresented Minorities

Mid- and established career
  Research Scientist Development Awards, Level 2 (K02)
  Research Scientist Awards (K05)
  Minority Institutions Research Development Program

quire application to an NIMH-supported program at a college, university, or professional association. Information on these opportunities can be obtained from department chairpersons, academic advisors, or college or university offices of sponsored research. Alternatively, information on these programs can be obtained by calling or writing one of the NIMH contacts listed at the end of this chapter. This chapter provides general information about available research training and career development programs, but for more specific and detailed information (e.g., eligibility, application form, receipt and review schedule, period of support), applicants should contact one of the NIMH staff persons listed at the end of this chapter. Copies of all announcements can be obtained by contacting Anne Cooley, Division of Extramural Activities, NIMH, Rm. 9-95, 5600 Fishers Lane, Rockville, MD 20857, (301) 443-4673.

Undergraduate research training. Available grant mechanisms at this level are designed to meet mental health research training needs of minority undergraduate students and of students enrolled in academic institutions with a substantial enrollment of minority students.

Predoctoral research training. Under the National Research Service Awards (NRSA) Institutional Research Training Grants Program, including a special NRSA for Institutional Research Training Grants in HIV Infection and AIDS, the NIMH provides support to academic institutions for supervised training in mental health research at the predoctoral level. Trainees are selected by the directors of these institutional grants and must be enrolled in a doctoral degree program at time of appointment. NRSA institutional grants are normally used to support full-time research training but may also be used to support short-term research training for 3 months or less in the area of child and adolescent mental disorders.

NRSA Individual Fellowships, including a special NRSA for Research Training for Individual Fellows in HIV Infection and AIDS, are available to individuals for full-time supervised mental health research training at the predoctoral level. Predoctoral applicants must have completed 2 years of graduate work in a Ph.D. program prior to receipt of a grant award.

Medical student and resident research training. NRSA legislation requires that the nation's overall need for biomedical research personnel be taken into account by giving special consideration to physicians who agree to undertake a minimum of 2 years of biomedical research. Support is available under the NRSA Institutional Training Grants Program, NRSA Individual Fellowships, and NRSA HIV-AIDS grants for trainees who wish to interrupt their medical school studies or residency training for a year or more to engage in full-time mental health research training.

Under the NRSA Predoctoral Individual M.D./Ph.D. Fellowships

Program, NIMH support is available to students who are enrolled in a M.D./Ph.D. program at an approved medical school and are accepted in a Ph.D. program related to mental health.

Postdoctoral research training.   Under the NRSA Institutional Research Training Grants Program, NRSA Individual Fellowship Program, and NRSA HIV-AIDS grants, support is available from the NIMH for full-time and short-term postdoctoral training in research on child and adolescent mental disorders. Trainees are selected by the directors of the institutional grants. NRSA institutional grants are normally used to support full-time research training, but mechanisms are also available to support short-term research training (3 months or less) in child and adolescent mental disorders. In addition to Institutional Training Grants, NRSA Individual Fellowships are also available to individuals for full-time supervised mental health research training at the postdoctoral level.

Research career awards.   Five types of NIMH research career development awards may be used to support the development of scientists with a commitment to a career in research on child and adolescent mental disorders.

The Child and Adolescent Mental Health Academic Award (K07) provides 5 years of salary support to assist a junior faculty member, who is a child psychiatrist, clinical psychologist, social worker, or psychiatric nurse, in the development of expertise in the research aspects of child and adolescent development and mental health. This award differs from the research scientist awards listed below in that recipients are expected to assume leadership in teaching and to be a research resource for students in addition to undertaking their own scientific research.

The Scientist Development Award for Clinicians (K20) provides 5 years of supervised research experience for individuals trained primarily as clinicians, especially physicians. Candidates must have had at least 2 years of clinical training or experience at the postdoctoral level by the time the award is made.

The Scientist Development Award (K21) provides support for highly promising scientists who need further supervised research experience in order to undertake independent research. The award provides 5 years of support for individuals who have had between 1 and 4 years of previous postdoctoral research training or experience by the time the award is made.

The Research Scientist Development Award (K02) provides 5 years of salary support for scientists who have established a record of independent research and publication.

The Research Scientist Award (K05) is designed to provide support to outstanding senior investigators that will enable them to devote full-time to research.

Minority research training and career development.   Members of minority groups are encouraged to apply for support under any of the NIMH grant mechanisms previously listed. In addition, five grant programs are specifically designed to meet the training and career development needs of minority students and faculty.

The first is the Minority Access to Research Careers (MARC) Program. Honors Undergraduate Research Training Grants are intended to increase the number of well-prepared students from institutions with substantial minority enrollment who can compete successfully for entry into doctoral-level or M.D. degree programs in disciplines related to alcoholism, drug abuse, and mental health with an emphasis on the biological sciences and neurosciences. Grants are awarded to colleges, universities, and health professional schools.

The objective of MARC Faculty Fellowship Awards is to enhance research capabilities of faculty at institutions with substantial minority enrollment. Support is available from the NIMH for predoctoral and postdoctoral research training. Recipients of these fellowships are expected to return to their home institutions following such training to teach, conduct research, and serve as a role model for minority students.

The NIMH has awarded Minority Fellowship Programs to five professional societies for the support of minority predoctoral graduate students who are interested in research careers in areas of special interest to the NIMH. Trainees are selected by the directors of these programs and may receive up to 5 years of support. In some cases, dissertation expenses will be supported.

The Minority Institutions Research Development Program (MIRDP) is intended to assist colleges and universities with substantial minority enrollment in augmenting and strengthening their capabilities to design and conduct alcohol, drug abuse, and mental health research. MIRDP grants provide support for development and enhancement of research facilities, faculty acquisition of advanced research skills, and individual faculty research projects.

Additional support from the NIMH for exceptional high school minority students, minority undergraduate students, minority graduate research assistants, and minority faculty members is available through Supplements for Underrepresented Minorities in Biomedical and Behavioral Research Supported by the former Alcohol, Drug Abuse, and Mental Health Administration. Under this program, principal investigators on active NIMH grants may apply for additional funds in order to add a minority person to their grant for the purpose of enhancing this person's research experience and capabilities. Priority is given in awarding supplements to projects involving African American, Hispanic, Native American, Pacific Islander, or other ethnic or racial group members who have been found to be underrepresented in either biomedical or behavioral research nationally.

◆ References

Burke KC, Burke JD, Regier DA, et al: Age at onset of selected mental disorders in five community populations. Arch Gen Psychiatry 47:511–518, 1990

Institute of Medicine: Research on Children and Adolescents with Mental, Behavioral, and Developmental Disorders (Publ No IOM-89-07). Washington, DC, National Academy Press, 1989

National Institute of Mental Health: National Plan for Research on Child and Adolescent Mental Disorders: A Report Requested by the U.S. Congress (DHHS Publ No (ADM)90-1683). Rockville, MD, National Institute of Mental Health, 1990

Public Health Service: Cooperative Agreement for Methodologic Research for Multi-Site Epidemiologic Surveys of Mental Disorders in Child and Adolescent Populations (MH-89-22) (Catalog of Federal Domestic Assistance No 13.242). Washington, DC, Department of Health and Human Services, 1990

Resources 7–1

Agencies Supporting Research in Child Psychiatry

The following section supplies the points of contact and the program emphases within federal institutions supporting child mental health research. Prospective applicants are urged to contact program staff listed below for further information and assistance. Personnel and telephone numbers may change, but do not hesitate to contact the programs to find the appropriate personnel for technical guidance.

◆ National Institute of Mental Health (NIMH)

Division of Epidemiology and Services Research (Darrel A. Regier, M.D., M.P.H., Director)

Services Research Branch, Rm. 10C-06 (Thomas Lalley, M.A., Chief). The Services Research Branch is the focal point in the NIMH for support of investigator-initiated research on mental health services and the mental health service system for children and youth. Support is granted for research pertaining to services provided at clinical, institutional, and system levels in specialty mental health, general health, and other settings. The branch is subdivided into three substantive programs: Primary Care, Mental Health Economics, and the Mental Health Service System. Contact Ann A. Hohmann, Ph.D., M.P.H., Mental Health Service Systems Research, (301) 443-3364; Kimberly Hoagwood, Ph.D., Children's Mental Health Services, (301) 443-3364; Kathryn Magruder, Ph.D., M.P.H., Primary Care and Mental Health, (301) 443-3364; Paul Widem, M.A., Mental Health Economics, (301) 443-4233; Primary Care and Mental Health, (301) 443-1330.

Violence and Traumatic Stress Research Branch, Rm. 10C-24 (Susan Solomon, Ph.D., Chief). The scope of the Violence and Traumatic Stress Research Branch includes 1) the etiology, course, correlates, and mental health consequences of violent and antisocial behavior in children and adolescents, as well as preventive and therapeutic interventions for such behavior; 2) the mental health consequences of direct and indirect victimization of children and adolescents from violence, sexual assault and abuse, and natural and manmade disasters, as well as the prevention and treatment of such consequences; and 3) issues at the interface of law and mental health that affect children and adolescents, such as child witnesses in abuse proceedings, involuntary civil commitment of juveniles, and mental health treatment of juveniles detained in correctional and hospital settings. Contact James Breiling, Ph.D., Antisocial and Violent Behavior Research, (301) 443-3728; Malcolm Gordon, Ph.D., Child Abuse, Neglect and Victimization, (301) 443-3728; Ecford Voit, Ph.D., Mental Health and Legal Issues, (301) 443-3728; David Stott, Ph.D., Perpetrators and Violence, (301) 443-3728.

Basic Prevention and Behavioral Medicine Research Branch, Rm. 10-104. The Basic Prevention and Behavioral Medicine Research Branch supports research on basic behavioral, genetic, biological, and social factors and psychological processes that have an impact on physical health and the maintenance of emotional well-being in children and adolescents. The branch includes three program areas: Behavioral Medicine, Populations at Risk, and Prevention and Behavior Change. These programs encompass a wide range of health-related studies on the biological, psychological, and psychosocial aspects of stress, immunology, sleep, circadian rhythms, nutrition, ingestive behavior, sexual behavior, medical illnesses, exercise, and health-related attitudes and practices in children and adolescents. Contact Fred Altman, Ph.D., (301) 443-4337.

Epidemiology and Psychopathology Research Branch, Rm. 10-09 (Charles Kaelber, M.D., M.P.H., Acting Chief). The Child and Youth Epidemiology Program of the Epidemiology and Psychopathology Research Branch supports research in the prevalence and incidence of children's mental health disorders, risk factors associated with psychiatric disorders in children, the longitudinal development and variability of psychopathological symptomatology over time, and the development of assessment techniques and diagnostic instruments suitable for large-scale surveys of children's mental health. Epidemiologic research focuses on the patterns of occurrence of mental health symptomatology and disorders in the population and the associations of biologic, genetic, environmental, or sociodemographic factors with the disorders. Contact Karen Bourdon, M.A., Child and Youth Epidemiology Program, (301) 443-3774.

Prevention Research Branch, Rm. 10-85 (Eve K. Moscicki, Sc.D., M.P.H., Chief). The Prevention Research Branch is the focal point within the NIMH for research and research training in the prevention of mental health disorders and behavioral dysfunctions and the promotion of mental health. Included are studies of preventive intervention strategies that avoid or interrupt the development of dysfunctional conditions and/or improve individual adaptive capabilities. Research aimed at changing factors that place people at risk for mental disorders is also supported, as are methodological studies especially relevant to preventive intervention research. Contact Doreen Koretz, Ph.D., (301) 443-4283, 443-4337.

Division of Neuroscience and Behavioral Science Research (Stephen H. Koslow, Ph.D., Director)

Personality and Social Processes Research Branch, Rm. 11C-10 (Mary Ellen Oliveri, Ph.D., Chief). The Personality and Social Processes Research Branch supports basic research on personality, emotional, and social processes that account for normal behavioral functioning and adaptation in children and adolescents. This includes research on processes that promote vulnerability to maladaptive outcomes as well as those processes that foster protection and resilience to mental disorders. Three broad themes characterize the child and adolescent research supported across the branch's program areas: 1) the roles of both genetic and experiential factors in shaping individual differences relevant to mental health; 2) the interactions and interrelationships among social, psychological, and biological processes; and 3) developmental changes and continuities from infancy to adulthood. Contact Mary Ellen Oliveri, Ph.D., (301) 443-3566; Lynne C. Huffman, M.D., (301) 443-3566; Della Hann, Ph.D., (301) 443-3942.

Molecular and Cellular Neuroscience Research Branch, Rm. 11C-06 (Steven Zalcman, Ph.D., Chief). The Molecular and Cellular Neuroscience Research Branch supports research focusing on the molecular genetic mechanisms underlying neural function and control in children and adolescents, and conversely, the manner in which nervous system activity regulates expression of the genome using the techniques of molecular biology; developmental neuroscience research on the role(s) that patterns of neural development play in determining function of the evolving nervous system of children and adolescents; neuroimmunology/neurovirology research on the functional interconnections between the nervous and immune systems; and neurotransmitter and neuroregulation research on synaptic mechanisms and CNS signal transduction systems. Contact Steven Zalcman, Ph.D., (301) 443-3948.

Neuroimaging and Applied Neuroscience Research Branch, Rm. 11-95 (Stephen Zalcman, M.D., Chief). The Neuroimaging and Applied Neuroscience Research Branch supports research on integrated neuronal functions in order to facilitate understanding of normal brain function and behavior in children and adolescents. The Neural Systems Program supports research on systems approaches toward understanding the anatomical, physiological, and neurochemical interactions between neurons, groups of neurons, or nuclei within the brain. The Neuroimaging Program supports research on the use and development of imaging methodologies to explore the anatomy, chemistry, and function of the brain. The Neuroscience Centers Program supports multidisciplinary research of a highly integrated and focused nature to further understanding of normal brain/behavior relationships in child and adolescent populations. Contact Henry Khachaturian, Ph.D., (301) 443-5288.

Behavioral and Integrative Neuroscience Research Branch, Rm. 11-102 (Richard Nakamura, Ph.D., Chief). The Behavioral and Integrative Neuroscience Research Branch supports research on the brain mechanisms underlying behavior in children and adolescents, with a view to understanding how behaviors develop and are maintained and regulated. The branch programs include the Cognitive Neurosciences Program, the Behavioral Neurosciences Program, and the Theoretical Neuroscience Program. Contact Richard Nakamura, Ph.D., (301) 443-1576.

Behavioral, Cognitive, and Social Processes Research Branch, Rm. 11C-16 (Stephen H. Koslow, Ph.D., Acting Chief). The Behavioral, Cognitive, and Social Processes Research Branch provides support for research on child and adolescent cognitive processes using human, animal, and computational models and on fundamental individual and social behaviors that relate to survival and adaptation of the organism and species. The branch programs include the Basic Behavioral Processes Program, the Cognition, Learning and Memory

Program, and the Theoretical and Computational Psychology Program. Contact Rodney Cocking, Ph.D., (301) 443-9400.

Division of Clinical and Treatment Research
(Jane Steinberg, Ph.D., Acting Director)

Child and Adolescent Disorders Research Branch, Rm. 18C-17 (Peter S. Jensen, M.D., Chief). The Child and Adolescent Disorders Research Branch provides support of research and research training in psychopathology, assessment, classification, etiology, genetics, clinical course, and treatment of all emotional or behavioral or associated mental disorders in infants, children, and adolescents. These studies encompass developmental, biological, biochemical, neurophysiological, psychological, and social factors associated with psychopathology in the child or family within clinical populations. The branch supports a broad spectrum of clinical research that uses the complete range of research technologies, from molecular genetics and neuroimaging to clinical interviewing and treatment trials. Contact Edith Nottelmann, Ph.D., Affective Disorders and Suicide, (301) 443-5944; Rebecca Del Carmen, Ph.D., Mental Illness/Mental Retardation, PDD/Autism, Disorders of Infancy, Anxiety Disorders, (301) 443-5944; John Richters, Ph.D., Conduct and Oppositional Defiant Disorders, (301) 443-5944; L. Eugene Arnold, M.D., ADHD, OCD, and Tic Disorders, (301) 443-5944; Euthymia Hibbs, Ph.D., Psychosocial Treatments, Eating Disorders, Childhood Onset Schizophrenia, (301) 443-5944; Benedetto Vitiello, M.D., Psychopharmacologic Treatments, (301) 443-5944.

To address correspondence to any of the above persons, use the following address: Name, Room Number (noted above after each program/branch name), Branch or Office Name (noted above in each program area), NIMH, Parklawn Building, 5600 Fishers Lane, Rockville, MD 20857.

◆ National Institute on Drug Abuse (NIDA)

NIDA supports substantial research relating to child and adolescent disorders through each of its four divisions. Unlike the NIMH, however, many of the topics for research opportunities—suicide, drug use, and AIDS—crosscut divisions. The institute has declared as one of its top priorities research on the developmental effects of abused drugs, whether at the basic, clinical, or epidemiological levels.

Division of Basic Research

The Division of Basic Research, focusing on the basic level, is supporting studies of how drug use or abuse affects development, including such issues as neuroendocrine effects, genetic predictors of susceptibility to later drug use, and the vulnerability of the developing nervous system. It also supports research in the area of drugs and pregnancy. Contact James Dingell, Ph.D., (301) 443-1887.

Division of Epidemiology and Prevention Research

This division's **Prevention Research Branch** administers a national program of prevention and early intervention research in drug abuse, focusing on drug use practices and problems; psychosocial functioning; and the effect of group behaviors on drug abuse, among others. Contact William Bukoski, Ph.D., (301) 443-1514. The same division's **Epidemiology Research Branch** undertakes many in-house and extramural projects surveying children and youth regarding drug exposure and use. Contact Arthur Hughes, (301) 443-6637.

This division's **Community Research Branch** provides research support in special areas such as minority populations (including children and youth) and access to treatment. A recent program announcement has placed emphasis on ethnic and racial minority groups and underserved populations. Contact Richard H. Needle, Ph.D., (301) 443-6702.

Division of Clinical and Services Research

The Division of Clinical Research serves as the focal point for all clinical research in drug abuse treatment. It has received a large amount of both antidrug abuse funds and AIDS funding. Each of its five branches maintains an active interest in child and adolescent issues, whether focusing on prevention, suicide, treatment research, delinquency, child abuse and runaway youth, or cocaine babies. A series of program announcements have placed increased emphasis on school-based interventions, treatment enhancement and evaluation, vulnerabilities to drug abuse, and the effect of substance abuse on pregnant women and the children born to such women. Contact Harry Haverkos, M.D. (acting), (301) 443-6697.

◆ National Institute on Alcohol Abuse and Alcoholism (NIAAA)

The three extramural divisions of the NIAAA continue to place some emphasis on issues related to child and adolescent alcohol disorders.

Division of Basic Research

The Division of Basic Research supports research on biological markers of alcohol consumption, alcohol and immunology, and alcohol and the endocrine system in the adolescent. Contact William Lands, Ph.D., (301) 443-2530.

Division of Biometry and Epidemiology

The **Biometry Branch** of the Division of Biometry and Epidemiology supports research into the incidence and prevalence of alcohol-abusing behavior in adults, children, and adolescents and is particularly interested in nosological research issues in adult and youth populations. Contact Bridget F. Grant, Ph.D., (301) 443-3306. The **Epidemiology Branch** is interested in fetal alcohol syndrome, looking at longitudinal follow-up of infants into early school years. Other areas of epidemiologic research include studies of drinking/driving behavior of high school age students as affected by minority status, peer relations, and other potential vulnerabilities to alcohol abuse. The branch is also concerned about longitudinal evaluations of alcohol abuse and violent behavior, including spouse abuse. Contact Mary C. Dufour, M.D., M.P.H., (301) 443-4897.

Division of Clinical and Prevention Research

The Division of Clinical and Prevention Research has an ongoing interest in precursors of alcohol abuse, vulnerabilities and susceptibilities to alcohol abuse, and alcoholism in the young. It supports research in the development and assessment of behavior change strategies in both youth and adult populations as well as research concerning alcoholism and high-risk sexual behavior among adolescents (AIDS-related) and other risk-taking behavior and decision-making issues resulting from economic and socioeconomic factors. The division's **Prevention Research Branch** is particularly interested in studies involved with preventive or anticipatory guidance provided in primary health care settings, with a focus on both adult and child/adolescent populations. Contact Jan Howard, Ph.D., (301) 443-1677.

◆ National Institute of Neurological Disorders and Stroke

Division of Convulsive, Developmental, and Neuromuscular Disorders

This institute maintains within its Convulsive, Developmental, and Neuromuscular Disorders Program the **Developmental Neurology Branch**, which focuses on developmental disorders of children, mental retardation and learning disorders, autism and behavioral disorders, CNS birth defects and genetic disorders, and cerebral palsy and other motor disorders. Contact Dr. Joseph S. Drage, (301) 496-6701.

◆ National Institute of Child Health and Human Development

Center for Research on Mothers and Children

This institute's Center for Research on Mothers and Children maintains a number of separate branches, each dealing with aspects of human learning. The **Endocrinology, Nutrition, and Growth Branch** has funded two specialized research centers under a congressional mandate to increase activities in childhood learning disabilities. These centers, combining biomedical and behavioral sciences, are located at Yale and Johns Hopkins Universities. The former center is looking specifically at issues of attention and conduct disorders, attentional aspects of cognition, and a longitudinal study of attention in children. The latter center hopes to discover why children develop learning disabilities and includes a mutidisciplinary staff of psychiatrists, neurologists, geneticists, psychologists, and others. Contact Ephraim Levin, (301) 496-5593.

The **Human Learning and Behavior Branch** supports research on the development of human behavior from infancy through early adulthood. The program is divided into five major areas: developmental behavioral biology, cognitive development, development of communicative skills, social and affective development, and behavioral pediatrics. Contact Dr. Norman A. Krasnegor, (301) 496-6591.

The **Mental Retardation and Developmental Disabilities Branch** supports research on the biological, behavioral, and social processes that contribute to or influence the development of mental retardation and developmental disabilities. Specific interests include developmental neurobiological studies and issues in developmental neuroscience, psychophysiology, and developmental psychopharmacology. Studies on psychological processes in retardation and developmental disabilities include cognition and information processing, perception, motor development, neuropsychology, and affective, motivational, and personality factors. Contact Dr. Felix F. Delacruz, (301) 496-1383.

◆ Health Resources and Services Administration (HRSA)

HRSA maintains a maternal and child health research program within its **Bureau of Maternal and Child Health and Resources Development.** The program aims to support applied research relating to maternal and child health services that shows promise of substantial contribution to the advancement of such services. HRSA has sought research proposals in such areas as the psychosocial aspects of physical health problems, health services research aspects of infant and child development, and care of children with special health care needs, including mental disorders. Contact Gontran Lamberty, D.P.H., (301) 443-2190.

◆ Other Agencies

Several other DHHS and non-DHHS agencies support research on child and adolescent disorders bearing on mental illness. The Department of Justice's **National Institute for Juvenile Justice and Delinquency Prevention**, for example, issues an annual research plan for extramural funding in the fiscal year. Prevention priorities have included drug abuse prevention among high school youth, drug abuse among minorities and adolescents, and prevention of adolescent victimization. Contact Ellen Grigg, (202) 724-7751. The Department of Education's **National Institute on Disability and Rehabilitation Research** (contact Ramon Garcia, Ed.D., [202] 732-1158) also maintains a regular research interest in medical, neurological, and psychological conditions that affect handicapped persons, including children and adolescents. The DHHS Office of Human Development Services' **Administration on Children, Youth, and Families** (contact Betty Steward, [202] 245-0618); the **Family and Youth Services Bureau** (contact Paget Hinch, [202] 472-4426); and the **Administration on Developmental Disabilities** (contact Will Wolfstein, [202] 245-2890) support research in such areas as child abuse and neglect, homeless and runaway youth, and social and psychological needs of the developmentally disabled. Each of these programs announces grant opportunities in the *Federal Register* in a joint Office of Human Development Services Coordinated Discretionary Fund Program Announcement. For information about the overall program, contact Ann Queen, Division of Research and Demonstrations, (202) 472-3026.

Aging and Psychiatric Research

Gene D. Cohen, M.D., Ph.D.,
Barry D. Lebowitz, Ph.D., and
Theodora Fine, M.A.

The biomedical research explosion has been a phenomenon of this last quarter of the 20th century, spurred on by new technologies and techniques that have altered fundamentally how research is conducted and how the products of research can be turned to clinical application. The blossoming of the field of geriatric psychiatry research represents a microcosm of the larger image. Today, a field that barely had a name in 1970 is bursting with vitality in both the numbers who have been attracted to the field and the magnitude of advances that have been made. Both the growth and the scientific vigor of the field of geropsychiatry are becoming increasingly critical to our future as national demographics point inexorably to the aging of our population and to the need to grapple with the physical and mental pathology that arises in the aging body and brain.

◆ Epidemiology: Growth of a Population at Risk

At the turn of the century, the average life expectancy was 47.3 years; by 1985, the average man was expected to live 71.2 years and the average woman 78.2 years (National Center for Health Statistics 1986). We have gained over 30 years of life expectancy in the course of this century, more than was realized in the history of mankind to this time. At the turn of the century, the three million Americans over the age of 65 represented 4% of our population. In 1988, they numbered 30 million and represented 12.4% of the population. The number is expected to double again, to 66 million—22% of all Americans—by the year 2030 (Division of Health Promotion and Disease Prevention, Institute of Medicine 1990). The so-called old-old persons age 85 or older, are the fastest-growing segment of our population today. During the next 60 years, this population at greatest risk for illness and disability will increase sixfold (National Institute on Aging, unpublished data). The most frail population will grow to more than 17 million persons—the size of the present population of Australia. In significant part, this "demographic revolution" (Butler et al. 1992) is the product of the parallel revolution in biomedical and behavioral science.

The remarkable growth in the average life span realized during this century presents important challenges to clinicians and researchers alike. The Institute of Medicine captured one of the primary issues in the title of its 1991 report, *Extending Life, Enhancing Life*, underlining the importance of the quality of life, not just its duration. Unfortunately, with additional years the incidence and prevalence of disorders and concomitant disability rise. These disorders are predominantly chronic in nature, requiring ongoing medical attention and, over time, increasing amounts of assisted living. Mental disorders and disturbances are numbered among the problems that increase in number and severity over the life span, affecting as many as 25% of all persons 65 years and older. Those with clinically significant depressive symptoms (including those with diagnosable major depressive disorder, the most prominent of the mental disorders) represent as many as 15% of this population group (Blazer 1986; Blazer et al. 1987).

Concomitant with the rise in depression, suicide reaches a peak in white men in the eighth decade of life (National Research Council

1991). More than one-fifth of all suicides occur in persons over the age of 65 (Blazer et al. 1986; Manton et al. 1987; Division of Health Promotion and Disease Prevention, IOM 1990). Moreover, the incidence of organic mental disorders, including Alzheimer's disease and other dementias, rises significantly in old age, increasing the incidence of disability. Psychosis increases after 65 and even more beyond age 75 (Anthony and Aboraya 1992).

The human and economic costs of these disorders are staggering. The annual cost to American society of Alzheimer's disease alone has been estimated at $90 billion (DHHS Advisory Panel on Alzheimer's Disease 1993).

Thus, the absolute growth of the population over the age of 65, coupled with the personal and economic significance of mental disorders for this age group, sets the stage for the evolution of a new field of clinical work and scientific inquiry—geriatric psychiatry.

◆ Growth of a Field

Although aging has always been a fact of living and although Alois Alzheimer identified the degenerative dementia that now bears his name at the turn of the century, research in the field of psychogeriatrics began in earnest only in the 1970s. This came about with the "reidentification" of Alzheimer's disease and the impetus of growing numbers of federal programs to begin to support this research field. The 1971 White House Conference on Aging made a series of recommendations to move public policy and programming into the fields of geriatric mental health care and research (White House Conference on Aging 1972). After committees deliberated and commissions contemplated, the national investment in geriatric health and mental health research began in earnest in 1975 with the establishment of entities within the Public Health Service and the Veterans Administration (now the Department of Veterans Affairs) that focus specifically on the aging population.

The National Institute on Aging, under the direction of a geriatric psychiatrist, was established as part of the National Institutes of Health. A parallel development in the same year heralded the creation of the first federal program specifically supporting geriatric mental health research—the Center for Studies of the Mental Health of the Aging within the National Institute of Mental Health. Recognizing the growing population of aging World War II veterans, the Veterans

Administration established a series of Geriatric Research, Education and Clinical Centers (GRECCs) to focus on both research and the clinical care of this population. Several GRECCs placed special emphasis on mental health and aging.

In 1978, specialized training in geriatric psychiatry was available in only one department of psychiatry in the United States (Cohen 1992). A decade later there were 30; 5 years later geriatric psychiatry became a formally recognized subspecialty of the American Board of Psychiatry and Neurology. A plethora of journals, textbooks, and specialized organizations has grown up in the field of geriatric psychiatry over the same brief period.

The emphasis has been not only on clinical training and education. Since 1975, the federal commitment to psychogeriatric research has grown commensurate with other segments of the bioscientific revolution. To some extent, the field's growth has been the result of the availability of research funds; to an equal extent, the opposite has been true: the growth of the field has leveraged increasing research dollars. The engagement of new researchers in the field has been driven both by the vigor of the science and the availability of increased support for the field. In this Decade of the Brain, the excitement and opportunity continue to grow.

◆ Research Directions

For reasons of both human suffering and economics (severely limited resources tend to fluctuate with the nation's economic vitality), geriatric research as a whole and psychogeriatrics in particular have targeted chronic diseases and disorders associated with the highest human and financial costs. Among these are Alzheimer's disease, depression, and the psychiatric sequelae of general medical illness. Although the burden of these diseases falls most heavily on the aged and their caregivers, their impact is felt by every age group. For this reason, the importance of the cost effectiveness of age-related mental health research must be acknowledged.

Cohen (1992) has suggested that in psychogeriatric research, three overarching conceptual orientations form the basis for all areas of scientific inquiry. These include 1) distinguishing between mental illness in late life and normal aging, 2) assuring and enhancing healthy aging, and 3) identifying and modifying mental disorders in late life. They crosscut the traditional areas of investigation—basic research, clinical inquiry, health services research, and epidemiological studies—and similarly span studies focusing on specific disease entities, including depression, Alzheimer's disease, anxiety, schizophrenia, and other disorders. The study of aging as a whole, whether by differentiating between pathology and normal aging processes, enhancing normal aging, or disclosing the specific psychiatric pathologies found in aging, will enhance the understanding of both mental health and mental disorders. This may happen as a result of epidemiological studies of wellness and disease or through basic molecular biological or genetics study of the normal and abnormal brain.

Research in the geriatric mental disorders has developed into a coherent and sophisticated body of knowledge. Investigators, using the best contemporary research approaches, are addressing the broad range of major mental disorders in late life. Significant research findings have grown up around questions of risk factors, etiology and pathophysiology, diagnosis, clinical course, treatment assessment, and prevention. The range of disorders under investigation includes Alzheimer's disease and related dementing disorders, depressive disorders, sleep disorders, delirium and other metabolic encephalopathologies, anxiety, and personality disorders. Methods of study employ a full range of molecular, neurobiological, neuropsychological, and psychosocial techniques of contemporary investigation.

The general orientation of geropsychiatric research has served to underscore the significance of the heterogeneity of the population, the contribution of normal age-associated changes in function, and the complex picture of comorbidity that characterizes mental disorders in late life. Each of these factors—alone and in combination—serves to complicate and enrich approaches to the diagnosis, treatment, and prevention of mental disorders.

The significance of age at first onset of the disorder is a common thread through much of psychogeriatric research. Research has disclosed that this factor may well represent an important source of the clinical and neurobiological heterogeneity of mental disorders in the aging population; moreover, age at onset may have major implications for both treatment and follow-up.

Another common thread running throughout psychogeriatric research is the significance of the family, including its contribution to the care of the older patient with a mental disorder and the stresses associated with this burden of patient care. A rich body of knowledge around the issue of caregiver burden—the chronic stress associated with caregiving—has led to important new approaches to psycho-biological investigation.

The goal of psychogeriatric research, as of all research in geriatrics, is to delay the onset of disease and to enhance the functional independence and quality of life for those experiencing the diseases of older age or the chronic diseases that extend across the lifespan. Not surprisingly, research has focused on etiology, pathogenesis, and prevention. In the area of Alzheimer's disease, for example, new research directions are attempting to identify the mechanisms that lead to the dysfunction and death of brain cells, to develop and evaluate reliable, valid multidimensional diagnostic procedures and instruments, and to discover and develop therapeutic interventions to slow, stop, or reverse the processes that lead to decreased brain functioning or neuronal death.

Another significant focus of investigation is the interaction between general medical conditions and mental disorders in later life. The critical need for this research is underscored by the finding that, by and large, clinical research has not focused its attention on the older population. Historic inattention to gender-related differences in the clinical study of mental disorders and general medical conditions has compounded the problem, since women are overrepresented in the geriatric population. Because mental disorders in the elderly frequently occur against a background of other ailments, they may remain undiagnosed or be considered a normal part of growing older.

Fruitful areas of inquiry at the interface of mental illness and general medical conditions include the recognition and treatment of psychiatric symptoms in chronically ill older people; the influence of medical conditions on psychological health and well-being; the effects of psychological states on the onset, course, and recovery from medical illness and disability; and the impact of depression and other affective states on everyday functioning and overall quality of life. Opportunity now exists to elaborate and understand the contribution of neuroimmune and neurobehavioral factors to the development, course, and outcome of mental disorders and medical conditions; to delineate the nature of and specific genetic and psychosocial vulnerabilities to acute and chronic stress; and to intervene at appropriate points to prevent the development or exacerbation of disease processes and enhance opportunities for recovery.

A growing literature is also documenting associations between a variety of psychosocial factors and clinical and quality of life outcomes in patients. Several studies have demonstrated associations between psychosocial factors such as depression, negative affect, social isolation, and stress, and morbidity and mortality. These studies suggest that a great opportunity lies in the development of rehabilitation approaches that take into account both physiological and psychosocial factors. Research is needed to identify the psychosocial and biobehavioral factors associated with increased survival, enhanced physical recovery, and positive quality of life. Investigation is also warranted to examine methods to improve the diagnosis of depressed elderly persons and develop multivariate models to identify those most likely to benefit from treatment; to identify risk factors and describe the course of depression in the elderly; and to clarify the cause-and-effect relationship between depression and general medical conditions.

The foregoing provides just a taste of the range of research opportunities in geropsychiatry. The potential for powerful new research techniques to advance knowledge of the causes, prevention, and management of age-related mental disorders is just beginning to be realized. With recent dramatic developments in several fields, from basic investigation to longitudinal epidemiologic study, the geropsychiatric community has been developing the scientific base needed to enhance the health care and quality of life for older citizens. Yet the field remains ripe for further fruitful investigation.

◆ Sources of Research Support

The growth of knowledge in the field of psychogeriatric research since the mid-1970s has both fostered and benefited from the development of an organizational structure that supports or undertakes the conduct of such research. Organizations and structures exist within federal agencies, state agencies, academic settings, nonprofit organizations, and the private sector. In geriatric psychiatry, as in all domains of mental health research, the federal government represents the single largest source of research and research training support (Pincus and Fine 1992; Martinez et al. 1993). In contrast to research areas such as heart disease and cancer, in which nearly a third of all investigation is supported by private funds, less than 5% of funding in mental disorders is derived from these sources (NIH 1992; Pincus and Fine 1992). Nonetheless, a number of outside organizations have begun to provide increasing levels of funding for mental health research in general and geropsychiatric research in particular.

In geriatric research the National Institutes of Health (NIH)—now including the National Institute of Mental Health (NIMH)—form a core resource. The focus of the research carried out by each institute varies. Grant proposals are received and revised in a central clearinghouse and are disseminated to the NIMH, the National Institute of Neurological Disorders and Stroke (NINDS), and the National Institute on Aging (NIA) on the basis of agreed-on Public Health Service protocols. Proposals may indicate a preference for referral to a particular institute. At times, institute grants managers may share proposals that overlap institute interests with grant managers from other institutes. Also at times, joint collaborative Requests for Applications (RFAs) are issued by two or more institutes.

Resources 8–1 lists the various federal agencies and other organizations that provide major support in the area of geriatric research and describes their programs. Resources 8–2 lists organizations involved in aging and psychogeriatrics.

◆ References

Alzheimer A: Uber eine eigenartige erkrankung der hirnrinde. Allg Z Psychiatrie Psychisch-Gerichtlich Med 64:146–148, 1907

Anthony JC, Aboraya A: The epidemiology of selected mental disorders in late life, in Handbook of Mental Health and Aging. Edited by Birren JE, Sloane RB, Cohen GD. San Diego, CA, Academic Press, 1992, pp 28–73

Blazer D: Depression. Generations 10:21–23, 1986

Blazer DG, Bachar JR, Manton KG: Suicide in late life: review and commentary. J Am Geriatr Soc 34:519–525, 1986

Blazer D, Hughes DC, George LK: The epidemiology of depression in an elderly community population. The Gerontologist 27:281–287, 1987

Butler RN, Lewis M, Sunderland T: Aging and Mental Health: Positive Psychosocial and Biomedical Approaches, 4th Edition. New York, Macmillan, 1992

Cohen GD: The future of mental health and aging, in Handbook of Mental Health and Aging. Edited by Birren JE, Sloane RB, Cohen GD. San Diego, CA, Academic Press, 1992, pp 894–914

Committee on a National Research Agenda on Aging, Institute of Medicine: Extending Life, Enhancing Life: A National Research Agenda on Aging. Washington, DC, National Academy Press, 1991

DHHS Advisory Panel on Alzheimer's Disease: Interim Report, 1993. Washington, DC, Department of Health and Human Services, 1993

Division of Health Promotion and Disease Prevention, Institute of Medicine: The Second 50 Years: Promoting Health and Preventing Disability. Washington, DC, National Academy Press, 1990

Manton KG, Blazer DG, Woodbury MA: Suicide in middle age and later life: sex and race specific life table and cohort analysis. J Gerontol 42:219–227, 1987

Martinez RA, Lebowitz BD, Cohen GD: Funding research structures. International Journal of Geriatric Psychiatry 8:19–24, 1993

National Center for Health Statistics: Health, United States, 1986 (DHHS Publ No PHS-87-1232). Washington, DC, Department of Health and Human Services, 1986

National Institute on Aging: Mission Statement. Bethesda, MD, National Institute on Aging, 1992

National Institutes of Health: NIH Data Book 1992 (NIH Publ No 92-1261). Bethesda, MD, National Institutes of Health, 1992

National Research Council: The Aging Population in the 21st Century: Statistics for Health Policy. Washington, DC, National Academy Press, 1991

Pincus HA, Fine T: The "anatomy" of research funding of mental illness and addictive disorders. Arch Gen Psychiatry 49:573–579, 1992

White House Conference on Aging: Toward a National Policy on Aging, Proceedings of the 1971 White House Conference on Aging. Washington, DC, U.S. Government Printing Office, 1972

Resources 8–1
Agencies Supporting Research in Geriatric Psychiatry

◆ National Institute of Mental Health (NIMH)

Division of Clinical and Treatment Research

The Mental Disorders of the Aging Research Branch, housed within the Division of Clinical Research, is under the direction of Barry Lebowitz, Ph.D. It serves as the Department of Health and Human Services focal point for research and research training centering on the nature, treatment, and prevention of major mental disorders and behavioral dysfunctions in late life. Research is supported on disorders with initial onset in early adulthood that continue into late life, as well as those with onset in later life. The substance of the research may be biological, behavioral, psychological, social, cultural, or methodological; it may include in vitro or in vivo clinical and laboratory investigations with both animals and humans. Under all circumstances, it must have direct relevance to mental disorders or mental health in older persons.

Support currently is available in nearly every area of aging research related to mental health and behavior: Alzheimer's disease and related dementias; psychotic disorders and schizophrenia; mood, anxiety, and personality disorders; sleep disorders; and the comorbidity of general medical disorders and mental disorders. Treatment of late life mental disorders is the fastest-growing area of research support, with studies evaluating somatic approaches to psychotherapy and family studies looking at risk factors, social support, stress, and adaptation, using both biological and behavioral approaches. Research to explore the utility of imaging techniques in the analysis of late life mental disorders is encouraged, as are investigations in molecular biology and molecular genetics.

The branch has recently described a series of areas for future investigation, among them expansion of current research on memory disorders, including but not limited to Alzheimer's disease; new treatment research on pathological grief; evaluation of the relationship between depression and physical disorders; efficacy studies of

ECT in the treatment of late life depression; clinical trials and observational studies in special populations, including the very old, patients in long-term care facilities, and underserved and ethnic minority communities; and the linkage between age and the onset, course, and treatment of schizophrenia, depression, and anxiety disorders.

Most grants supported by the branch are investigator-initiated. The branch supports regular research grants (R01s), First Independent Research Support and Transition Awards (R29), small grants (R03), and Specialized Mental Health Clinical Research Centers on Aging awards (P30). In addition, from time to time, the director of the NIMH announces the availability of research grant awards or cooperative agreements for collaborative research in special areas.

With the move of the NIMH to the NIH, the clinical training opportunities previously supported by the branch have moved to the Center for Mental Health Services within the Substance Abuse and Mental Health Services Administration (SAMHSA). However, the branch continues to support a number of research training and career development awards. National Research Service Awards (NRSAs), including individual fellowships and institutional awards at the predoctoral and postdoctoral levels, provide support to train scientists in the area of mental health and aging. The Clinical Mental Health Academic Award (formerly the Geriatric Mental Health Academic Awards, K07) supports an experienced clinical faculty member—who could be a psychiatrist—to develop expertise in the research aspects of aging and mental health. The award provides 5 years of salary support plus $30,000 for research and career development expenses to prepare the individual to assume a faculty leadership role in geriatric mental health. This program has become the key vehicle for geriatric research training available through the NIMH. Researchers and directors of training programs are encouraged to contact the staff to discuss ideas for new research or training projects. Concept papers, preliminary proposals, and drafts can be submitted for staff review and comment prior to formal submission of an application. For further information, contact Barry Lebowitz, Ph.D., (301) 443-1185.

◆ National Institute on Aging (NIA)

The National Institute on Aging conducts and supports "biomedical, social, and behavioral research, training, health information dissemination, and other programs with respect to the aging process and the diseases and other special problems and needs of the aged" (NIA 1992). To that end, its focus is on understanding the natural processes of aging and disease processes that interfere with natural aging. Priorities of the institute's research program include the study of Alzheimer's disease; the natural course of normal aging; health maintenance and effective functioning; frailty, disability, and rehabilitation in the aged (including such areas as perceptual and neurological aspects of falls and gait disorders); long-term care for older people; and special older populations. Four extramural programs support both research and research training.

Behavioral and Social Research Program

The Behavioral and Social Research Program supports social and behavioral research and training on aging processes and the place of older people in society, focusing on the relationship of older people to their environment, family, and other social groups. The program emphasizes demographic research and studies of healthy and productive functioning in the middle and later years, including work, health, and family responsibilities of older persons approaching retirement. Specific areas of interest include stress and coping, psychosocial factors in Alzheimer's disease and hypertension, health behaviors and attitudes, and methodologies examining linkages between psychosocial and biomedical aging processes. In the recent past, for example, the program has supported specialized research dealing with caregivers and caregiver burden, particularly for those caring for parents or spouses with Alzheimer's disease. For information about research opportunities supported by this program, contact Ronald Abeles, M.D., (301) 496-3136.

Biology of Aging Program

The Biology of Aging Program funds research and training on molecular and cell biology, genetics, immunology, endocrinology, and nutrition. It also supports facilities that provide investigators with aging animals and cell cultures for use in aging research projects. Contact Richard Sprott, Ph.D., (301) 496-4996.

Geriatrics Program

The Geriatrics Program supports research on diseases of older persons, funding investigations of physical frailty, pharmacology, rehabilitation, osteoporosis, geriatric assessment, and geriatric training. (The latter includes the Claude D. Pepper Geriatric Research and Training Centers and the Claude D. Pepper Older Americans Independence Centers.) Contact Evan Hadley, Ph.D., (301) 496-6761.

Neuroscience and Neuropsychology of Aging Program

The Neuroscience and Neuropsychology of Aging Program serves as the focal point for NIA Alzheimer's research, receiving more than 50% of the funds appropriated for the study of Alzheimer's disease and supporting investigations of the causes, diagnosis, epidemiology, treatment, and management of Alzheimer's disease and related disorders. The program also supports research on the structure and function of the aging nervous system and age-related changes in the nervous system. Further, the program is responsible for managing extramural research on psychoneuroimmunology as well as sleep and circadian rhythms in aging. It is responsible for oversight and funding of the Alzheimer's Disease Research Centers and also houses the Office of Alzheimer's Disease Research, a coordinative office that performs an information gathering and dissemination role for the NIA director. Contact Zaven Khachaturian, Ph.D., (301) 496-9350.

◆ National Institute of Neurological Disorders and Stroke (NINDS)

Division of Demyelinating, Atrophic, and Dementing Disorders

The NINDS, the third NIH institute with major interest in geriatric psychiatry, focuses generally on the basic neurobiological substrate of disease rather than on clinical research. Since nearly 25% of the funds appropriated in Alzheimer's disease flow to the NINDS, the institute is a valuable resource for psychogeriatric researchers. Of its five program areas, the Demyelinating, Atrophic, and Dementing Disorders Program places the greatest emphasis on psychiatric research in Alzheimer's disease and encourages the development of multidisciplinary team approaches to such research. Contact Carl M. Leventhal, M.D., (301) 496-5679.

◆ Public Health Service (PHS) Interrelationships

The PHS maintains a number of specific coordinating mechanisms designed to assure that areas of overlapping jurisdiction among the NIMH, the NIA, and the NINDS are complementary, not duplicative or conflicting. Regular meetings are convened to share new directions and to resolve any problems. These meetings provide the opportunity to plan joint funding opportunities supported by more than one institute and to assure that worthy research proposals can be evaluated by each of the institutes with a stake in the research area. The NIMH and the NIA in particular have moved grants between institutes on more than one occasion to enhance support for worthy applications. Among the collaborative initiatives of the NIMH, the NIA, and other institutes proposed in the past few years have been solicitations for grant applications in areas such as comparative approaches to brain and behavior; women's health over the life course (social and behavioral aspects) and the relation of gender to health and longevity; the human brain project (feasibility studies); health and effective functioning in the middle and later years; neural systems and mental, neurological, and aging disorders; human neurochronobiology; behavior change and prevention strategies to reduce transmission of HIV; issues in caregiving for patients with Alzheimer's disease and related dementias, and the diagnosis of Alzheimer's disease; and research on the interaction between mental disorders and physical illness in later life.

◆ Department of Veterans Affairs (VA)

Research related to mental illness and aging is a priority area within the Department of Veterans Affairs Medical Research Service. Several of the VA's Geriatric Research, Education, and Clinical Centers

(GRECCs) focus directly on Alzheimer's disease and other cognitive disorders. Although competition for grants remains high, the VA offers younger researchers a somewhat less financially volatile environment in which to launch a career in geropsychiatry. Yet researchers should be aware that the VA system is a closed system: VA research and research training funds flow only to researchers and trainees within the VA hospital faculty system. Those outside need not apply.

Medical Research Service (MRS)

Psychiatrist-researchers within GRECCs or affiliated with VA facilities apply and compete for VA research dollars through a number of research programs. The MRS includes five separate research programs: 1) the Merit Review System; 2) the Research Advisory Group Program for new investigators; 3) the Career Development Program; 4) the Cooperative Studies Program; and 5) the Special Research Initiatives Program, which now has a particular interest in aging, alcoholism, and schizophrenia. Contact Kari Hastings, Administrative Officer, (202) 535-7155.

Health Services Research and Development Service (HSR&D)

The HSR&D supports investigator-initiated research, service-directed research, and cooperative studies in health services. Priorities for the latter two programs are established annually by the VA Central Office and generally focus on large-scale, multisite studies. Mental health research in this service focuses predominantly on developing means to identify patient health care needs and on establishing cost-effective approaches to providing effective treatment. Areas of current emphasis that may touch on psychogeriatric topics include research on substance abuse, schizophrenia, and depression. Contact Daniel Deykin, M.D., Director, (202) 535-7156.

Rehabilitation Research and Development Service (Rehab R&D)

This service funds rehabilitation research in prosthetic/amputation/orthotics, spinal cord injury and related neurological disorders, communication, cognitive and sensory aids, and (of importance to psychogeriatric research) dementia and schizophrenia. The goal is to develop and test new techniques, concepts, or devices that can minimize disability for patients in the clinical setting. The dementia research emphasis is on management of problematic behaviors such as wandering and incontinence, with the object of identifying techniques or technologies that improve functioning and help patients better adapt to their environment. Proposals for research in this and other rehabilitation areas are presented through a VA medical center and are subject to peer review. Contact Victoria M. Mongiardo, Merit Review Office, (410) 962-2578.

◆ Nonfederal Sources of Support

As noted earlier in this chapter, nonfederal sources of support for research on aging and mental disorders are severely limited in comparison to the funds available through federal sources. The overdependence on federal funds makes mental health research particularly vulnerable to the vicissitudes of public policy decision making (Pincus and Fine 1992; Martinez et al. 1993). Today, state funds for mental health research predominantly support health services-related investigations rather than biomedical inquiry; this is not surprising given the health economics-driven nature of the 1990s. Moreover, state funding for mental and addictive disorders research weighs in at only 8% of the total from all sources of support (Pincus and Fine 1992). Nonetheless, state mental heath authorities are a potential source of support for specialized research in mental disorders and aging, particularly if it focuses on fiscal issues involving caregiving and treatment. Researchers who pay close attention to the changing winds of state government and state legislation may have a leg up in identifying the availability of such funding opportunities.

Private research funding, both industry and the nonprofit sector (predominantly foundations), provides another limited source of potential support. As reported elsewhere (Pincus and Fine 1992), the pharmaceutical industry contributes some 44% of the support for all health research, yet its contribution to research into mental and addictive disorders totals well under 20%. The new drug development initiatives within the NIMH may stimulate the growth of mental health research in the pharmaceutical industry; the involvement of geropsychiatric researchers in this initiative could leverage funds for the field of aging and mental health.

Foundation support represents less than 4% of the funds available for research on mental and addictive disorders (Pincus and Fine 1992). Interest in mental disorders is limited, and the majority of foundations that have funded mental health-related projects have placed greater emphasis on service delivery than on research. However, a small number of private foundations have been identified as interested in geriatric mental health research, among them the Klingenstein Fund, the James S. McDonnell Foundation, the American Health Assistance Foundation, the van Ameringen Foundation, the Ittleson Foundation, and the Hogg Foundation. Although foundation grant-making decisions are often the result of the personal interests of the benefactor, the growth of the geriatric population may stimulate support for the field of geriatrics in general, possibly broadening the base of support for geropsychiatric research.

Until recently, the stigma of mental illness thwarted the establishment and endowment of single-purpose nonprofit organizations to stimulate research and support for research into mental illness in general and geriatric mental disorders in particular. Over the past decade, however, two private health organizations, not unlike the American Cancer Society and the American Heart Association, have emerged as important sources of support and enlightenment for the field: the National Association for Research on Schizophrenia and Depression and the Alzheimer's Association. Both growing organizations, they provide a renewed acknowledgment of the role research plays in the identification, treatment, and ultimately prevention of mental disorders, including disorders that affect the elderly or that extend into the later years.

Resources 8–2
Organizations Involved in Aging and Psychogeriatrics

Administration on Aging
U.S. Department of Health and Human Services
330 Independence Avenue, SW
Washington, DC 20201
(202) 619-0724
(general information)

Agency for Health Care Policy and Research
2101 East Jefferson Street, Suite 501
Rockville, MD 20852
(301) 227-8372

Alliance for Aging Research
2021 K Street, NW, Suite 305
Washington, DC 20006
(202) 293-2856

Alzheimer's Association
70 East Lake Street, Suite 600
Chicago, IL 60601
(312) 853-3060

American Association for Geriatric Psychiatry
PO Box 376-A
Greenbelt, MD 20768
(301) 220-0952

American Association of Retired Persons
601 E Street, NW
Washington, DC 20049
(202) 434-2277

American Federation for Aging Research
725 Park Avenue
New York, NY 10012
(212) 570-2090

American Geriatrics Society
770 Lexington Avenue, Suite 300
New York, NY 10021
(212) 308-1414

American Psychiatric Association
Council on Aging
1400 K Street, NW
Washington, DC 20005
(202) 682-6000

American Psychological Association
Division 20 (Aging)
750 1st Street, NE
Washington, DC 20002
(202) 336-5500

American Psychological Society (Research)
100 North Carolina Avenue, SW
Washington, DC 20002
(202) 546-7724

American Society on Aging
833 Market Street, Suite 512
San Francisco, CA 94103
(415) 882-2910

Gerontological Society of America
1275 K Street, NW, Suite 350
Washington, DC 20005
(202) 842-1275

Group for the Advancement of Psychiatry
Committee on Aging
c/o Gene D. Cohen, M.D.
1915 Biltmore Street, NW
Washington, DC 20009

International Psychogeriatric Association
2530 North Crawford Avenue, Suite 314
Evanston, IL 60201-4972
(708) 866-7227

National Association of Social Workers
750 First Street, NE, Suite 700
Washington, DC 20002
(202) 408-8600

National Council on Aging
409 Third Street, SW, 2nd Floor
Washington, DC 20024
(202) 479-1200

National Institute on Aging
National Institutes of Health
Building 31, 5th Floor
9000 Rockville Pike
Bethesda, MD 20954
(301) 496-1752 (Public Information Office)

National Institute of Mental Health
Mental Disorders of Aging Research Branch
Parklawn Building, Room 18-105
5600 Fishers Lane
Rockville, MD 20857
(301) 443-1185

National Institute of Neurological Disorders and Stroke
Information Office
Building 31, Room 8A06
9000 Rockville Pike
Bethesda, MD 20892
(301) 496-5751

How to Publish in the Scientific Literature

Sandra L. Patterson

> When I divide the week's contributions into two
> piles—one that we are going to publish and the other
> that we are going to return—I wonder whether it
> would make any real difference to the journal or its
> readers if I exchanged one pile for another.
>
> Sir Theodore Fox, former editor, *The Lancet* (1965)

Scientific research, no matter how spectacular the results, is not completed until the results are published. Thus the researcher must not only "do" science, he or she must also "write" science. Publication of research findings is one of the most professionally satisfying means of both alerting your fellow researchers to your work and to advancing the cause of psychiatric research.

As the field itself has taken quantum leaps in the past two decades, the number of psychiatric journals has proliferated. Pressures for publication of one's research findings are high and unfortunately are not always grounded in the quest for knowledge alone. In the end, however, whether the author is a junior or a senior researcher, the quality of the submission will determine its likelihood to emerge as a published article.

There are a number of considerations that the researcher must take into account once his study is completed and he begins to prepare his manuscript. This chapter explores several of them, including how to decide which journal is the most appropriate one for the researcher's work, preparing the manuscript, issues relating to peer review, and some ethical problems encountered in publication.

◆ Preparing and Submitting the Manuscript

Selecting a Journal

Before preparing a manuscript for submission to a scientific publication, the researcher should select a journal that is likely to consider his or her work. Many fine papers are rejected because their message is not suitable for or targeted toward the journal's audience (e.g., too technical, too specialized). By reading recent issues of several journals, one can get a sense of topic areas that interest the editors, the level of sophistication of the readership (Are the readers researchers? specialists? general practitioners?), and the type of articles likely to be published (e.g., clinical research, basic science). If after doing some research the nature of a particular journal's mission is still unclear, a call or letter to the editorial office can help one decide whether the work would be considered by that journal. Although no guarantees of publication can be made at this early stage, the editorial office can let the author know whether the journal accepts certain types of manuscripts (e.g., reviews of the literature, case reports, commentaries) or manuscripts on certain topics.

Other important factors to consider in choosing a journal include whether the journal is peer reviewed, how long one can expect to wait for a decision, the journal's frequency, the time between manuscript acceptance and publication, the journal's circulation, and whether and where the journal is indexed. These factors help determine how quickly and thoroughly the manuscript will be considered, how soon the manuscript will appear in print, and how many colleagues will receive or have access to the published work.

A journal that is peer reviewed subjects all published manuscripts to critical evaluation by independent referees—that is, persons not affiliated with the journal, its editors, or editorial staff. Submitting the manuscript to a peer reviewed journal will invite the criticism of colleagues, subject the author and manuscript to the sometimes slow and laborious process of review, revision, and resubmission, and probably increase chances of rejection. However, should the journal eventually accept the manuscript, the work will have earned a measure of credibility by virtue of having been subjected to scientific scrutiny and deemed suitable for publication. Readers know this, as do review boards and promotion committees.

However, peer review should not be considered a stamp of authenticity. As the editors of the *The New England Journal of Medicine* stated in a 1989 editorial, peer review is not and cannot be an objective scientific process, nor can it be relied on to guarantee the validity or honesty of scientific research, despite much uninformed opinion to the contrary (Relman 1989). Its functions are more modest, but nonetheless valuable, the editors noted.

Turnaround time from submission to decision and acceptance to publication can be important, particularly if one is working in an area of fast-paced research, such as neuroscience or genetics, where delays can mean obsolescence. The peer review process—time from manuscript submission to first decision—may take a few weeks to several months. One should expect an 8- to 12-week wait for first decision, as this is considered acceptable by many journal editors. The time from acceptance to publication will depend on the journal's frequency (e.g., weekly, monthly, quarterly) and its backlog of accepted manuscripts. In general, a weekly journal will be able to publish the work more quickly after acceptance than a monthly, and a monthly more quickly than a quarterly. The publication lag for all journals, however, is a factor of the number of manuscripts received and the acceptance rate. Most journals can publish only a given number of pages per issue. A monthly journal with a large number of submissions and a high acceptance rate can find itself with a backlog of a year or more, whereas a starved quarterly may operate from issue to issue and will accept a manuscript and publish it within a month or two. Some journals publish the submission, revision received, and acceptance dates with the published article. From this information one can determine publication lag and make a guess at the time the journal will take to complete peer review. For journals that do not publish such information, contact the editorial office. Most journals are proud of their ability to produce quick reviews and try to encourage submissions by keeping their backlogs to a minimum, thereby offering authors rapid publication. For a journal that is reluctant to share this information, one should consult colleagues who have had experience with that publication.

A journal's circulation and where it is indexed provide some measure of how many colleagues will receive the journal in which one is published and whether those who do not receive it will be able to retrieve the work from one of the well-known databases.

Resources 9–1 provides information on some of these selection criteria for journals in psychiatry and the better known general medical and scientific journals. The list is not exhaustive; for journals not included, one should consult a librarian for the name and location of the publisher.

Information for Authors and the Uniform Guidelines

Once an author has decided where to submit the manuscript, he or she should obtain a copy of the journal's Information for Authors. This document is usually published at regular intervals in the journal or can be obtained from the editorial office. Information for Authors gives, at minimum, the formatting guidelines to be followed in preparing the manuscript, the number of copies required, and the address and telephone number of the office to which it should be sent. More comprehensive information, such as journal policy on prior and duplicate publication, criteria for authorship, acceptable abbreviations, and methods for statistical reporting, is provided by some journals. A new publication, *The Author's Guide to Biomedical Journals*, provides the complete Information for Authors for 185 journals in science and medicine (*The Author's Guide to Biomedical Journals* 1994).

Another good source to consult when preparing a manuscript is the *Uniform Requirements for Manuscripts Submitted to Biomedical Journals* (Resources 9–2). This document was created in 1978 by a group of biomedical editors who met in Vancouver, British Columbia, to establish guidelines for manuscripts submitted to their publications. Since then the guidelines have been revised four times, most recently in January 1993, and have grown to encompass the ethical issues authors and editors must confront. Over 500 journals now participate in this agreement. But journals that subscribe to the Uniform Requirements may set additional submission standards, and the guidelines do not set forth a uniform publication style. Therefore, authors should obtain the specific guidelines published by each journal to which they are submitting. The Information for Authors and Uniform Requirements are not intended to provide detailed instructions on how to write a scientific paper. Some useful resources for first-time authors to consult before sitting down to write are listed in Resources 9–3.

Papers that do not meet a journal's manuscript submission requirements (e.g., reference format, structured abstract, typed double-spaced text, number of copies) may be returned to the authors unreviewed. Journals vary in how strictly they adhere to their stated requirements at the submission stage, but to ensure prompt review authors should pay attention to each detail. Careless preparation of a manuscript can lead reviewers and editors to assume the conduct of the study being reported was careless also. A seemingly minor detail such as references done in the wrong style may invite editors to wonder whether their journal was the one for which the manuscript was originally prepared. While editors often consider manuscripts that have been rejected by other journals (surveys have shown that an estimated 80%–85% of papers rejected by *The New England Journal of Medicine*, *The Journal of Clinical Investigation*, and *The Journal of the American Medical Association* are eventually published somewhere [Relman 1980; Wilson 1978; Bailar 1986]), there is no need for authors to announce by shoddy preparation that their manuscript has been around the block a few times, albeit with possible improvement along the way. At some point—whether at submission, review, first decision, final decision, copy editing, or page proofs—every requirement in the Information for Authors must be fulfilled to the letter. Many delays and much frustration can be eliminated if the manuscript is prepared properly at the outset.

◆ Peer Review

Early in the review process, some journals employ a triage system. Manuscripts are reviewed by the editorial board or other in-house team of editors that determines whether the content of a manuscript is suitable for the journal. Manuscripts judged unsuitable are rejected immediately. This system works well for journals in highly specialized fields or for journals with an extensive pool of in-house review-

ers. These reviewers are capable of judging the merits and/or suit-
ability of a paper without outside consultation. The authors of a
manuscript rejected by such a triage team may learn the fate of their
work within a few weeks and can send it to another journal for
consideration more promptly than had several months elapsed before the editors arrived at the same decision.

A manuscript sent for "outside" review can go to anywhere from
one to 15 or more reviewers. Most psychiatric journals employ two
to six reviewers. Reviewers are selected based on their areas of expertise and any special clinical, research, or statistical knowledge they
may bring to a particular paper. Reviewers are asked to provide the
editor and authors with a critique of a paper's contribution to the
field, the study design and research methods, data collection and
analysis, citation of relevant literature, and overall presentation;
they are also asked to point out any ethical concerns in the conduct
or financing of the research. Reviewers are often asked to provide the
editor with a confidential recommendation regarding publishability,
based on priority (importance and timeliness) plus quality (study
design and presentation).

Statistical Review

Following the publication of several articles citing the poor quality
of study design and data interpretation in articles submitted to or
published in peer reviewed biomedical journals (Bailar 1986; Pocock
et al. 1987; Gardner and Bond 1990), many journals began reex-
amining the rigor of statistical review on manuscripts that contain
quantitative data. Statistical reviewers, used by some but not all
journals, judge whether the study design is adequate to reach the
stated objectives, the statistical methodology is appropriate, the conclusions are supported by the data, and the statistical significance has
any clinical or practical significance. In addition, statistical reviewers
are encouraging researchers to pay careful attention to study design
at the outset and to seek the advice of a statistician early on (Bailar
1986; Pocock et al. 1987). Doing so can reduce the risk of a manuscript's being returned for major revision requiring reanalysis of the
data and possible rejection of the study hypothesis. Computer software packages are available to assist in data analysis (SAS 1986; Nie
et al. 1975; Dixon et al. 1983), but seeking the advice of a statistician
is strongly recommended. Resources to consult for help with statistical analysis and presentation are given in Resources 9–3.

Reviewer Bias

Journals differ in whether manuscripts are sent to reviewers blind or nonblind. The potential for reviewer bias, and the ability to eliminate it, is germane to an editor's decision to conduct blind review. Controversy still exists within biomedical publishing as to which approach is best. Some argue that it is not possible to blind reviewers in all cases; manuscripts often reference work "previously conducted by this group" or methods "published in another report," and astute reviewers are aware of who is doing work in their areas of interest (Ingelfinger 1974). Some editors who favor blind review believe in the Matthew effect as it pertains to peer review, "to those that have will come" (Wilson 1978), which leads reviewers to look more favorably on research conducted by colleagues who are already well known or from well-respected institutions. There have been studies that support this view (McNutt et al. 1990). Others question whether the ability to successfully blind reviewers to authors' identities is worth the considerable effort involved (Relman 1990). There are also studies that support this view (Yankauer 1991).

The American Journal of Psychiatry does not blind reviewers, following a belief that maintaining a substantial cadre of good reviewers and selecting reviewers carefully can eliminate the most egregious bias. If an author feels strongly that a particular person or group should not review a paper because potential bias or conflict may render that person or group incapable of providing a balanced review, a comment explaining the circumstances in the cover letter accompanying the submission is perfectly acceptable.

Recommendations regarding who should or should not review a paper must not be made frivolously. Editors are free to use their judgment in these cases, and the paper may be sent to one of those mentioned in the cover letter (with the author's comments deleted) if the editor feels the need for that person's opinion.

Reviewers, on the other hand, are routinely asked when they sign on with a journal to identify any authors or institutions whose papers they do not wish to review because of the potential for bias, either positive (in cases of friendship or collaboration) or negative (in cases of competitive research agendas or ideological differences). In addition, reviewers are charged with disclosing any conflicts of interest that could bias their opinions of a manuscript, and they should disqualify themselves from reviewing a specific manuscript if they believe it appropriate.

Passing Peer Review

The perception among authors that manuscripts in some way "pass" peer review is common. Understandably, many authors do not readily accept an editor's negative decision about a paper that has received positive reviews. Others argue that reviews of their work vary so widely as to render the reliability of recommendations to the editor invalid.

There are two misunderstandings at work in the pass/fail approach to peer review: 1) that the primary function of the editor is to record and transmit information (Relman 1990) and 2) that the principal outcome of peer review is to achieve consensus (Wilson 1978; Relman 1990; Lock 1985). Scores are not tallied and weighed to arrive at a cutoff above or below which manuscripts pass or fail. Opposing viewpoints are welcomed, even solicited, to ensure a thorough critique. Reviewers act as consultants to the editor on a paper's technical and scientific merits. They may serve as arbitrators, if called on to do so, when conflicting reviews pose a dilemma for the editor. The final decision, however, rests with the editor alone.

Editors often must make decisions based on factors other than the scientific merit of a particular paper—factors that most reviewers cannot be expected to take into consideration when crafting their reviews. A paper may be accepted or rejected based on the interests or level of sophistication of the readership, number of papers on a particular topic already in press at the time of the decision, or the backlog of accepted manuscripts. None of these reasons for rejection may seem fair to an author whose work receives positive feedback from the reviewers, but they are an important part of an editor's calculations. Authors of rejected papers should also keep in mind that a reviewer's confidential comments to the editor can tell quite a different tale than that same reviewer's comments to the authors.

◆ The Decision

Once all assigned reviews are received (or an acceptable number of them, if many individuals have been asked to provide a review), the editor is charged with deciding the fate of the manuscript. Depending on the journal, the time from submission to first decision can be from 4 to 16 weeks or perhaps longer. Editors consider an 8- to 12-week review period acceptable.

The editor's decision usually takes one of the following forms: accept, reject, major revision, or minor revision. A lucky few—probably fewer than 2% at the journals in which publication is most coveted—receive the "accept outright" decision. Rejection rates vary widely among journals, from as low as 20%–30% in the physical sciences to 75%–80% or even higher among general medical and some medical specialty journals.

The American Journal of Psychiatry currently has a rejection rate of about 75%. Of the manuscripts destined to be accepted, most require at least one round of revisions. The editor of this journal, Nancy C. Andreasen, M.D., Ph.D., has discussed the rejection rate as well as other issues young researchers should consider before submitting their first manuscripts (PRR 1993).

Many journals have two classifications of revision: minor and major. Requests for minor revisions are varied; they may call for cosmetic changes or require some rewriting or reorganizing, but the classification "minor" usually indicates that the journal has taken a serious interest in the paper. The cover letter accompanying such a request may be encouraging: "We are interested in publishing your paper, but . . . " or more noncommittal: "If you make the suggested changes, we will review your paper again." The need for major revision indicates that the editor has spotted serious flaws in the manuscript and substantial work remains to be done, without guarantee of ultimate acceptance. Examples of problems for which major revisions may be required include insufficient review of the literature, flaws in methodology or data analysis, conclusions not supported by the data, failure to point out limitations of the study design or findings, or targeting the paper to the wrong audience. A cover letter asking for major revisions will usually not offer any hope of publication and may even recommend that the paper be submitted elsewhere.

◆ Revising the Manuscript

Reviewer comments that the editor considers important are returned to the author, sometimes with added directions from the editor. Responding to *all* reviewer comments when submitting a revised manuscript is important. It is not mandatory, and sometimes not possible, to modify a paper based on all comments received, but they should not be ignored. If a reviewer seems not to have grasped an important concept or part of the methodology of the study, this should be pointed out to the editor in the cover letter—politely. One should try to be dispassionate in responding to reviewer comments. Many journals edit out vitriolic language before sending reviews to authors, but reviewers do not always couch even astute criticisms in terms palatable to the author. Providing justification for not making a recommended change in the manuscript is far better than choosing not to address the issue, particularly if the original reviewer is asked to critique the revision. One should indicate in the cover letter exactly what changes have been made and should not make the editor hunt for them. Some journals will return a manuscript unreviewed if the cover letter does not highlight revisions.

Some journals will reconsider a rejected manuscript if substantial changes are made in line with the reviewers' comments; others have a strict policy against rereviewing rejected papers. It is necessary to check the Information for Authors or contact the editorial office to determine a particular journal's policy on rejected manuscripts.

◆ Ethical Issues

Authorship and Acknowledgments

As science has grown more complex, an ever-increasing number of investigators are called on to contribute their expertise to the design, implementation, and analysis of studies destined for publication. Large multicenter clinical trials can involve hundreds of investigators and participants. When the time comes to submit the final report for publication, investigators often find themselves in the position of having to sort out issues of authorship. Who should be included among the authors? In what order should authors be listed? Who should be given credit in the acknowledgments?

The Uniform Requirements document gives the following criteria for authorship:

All persons designated as authors should qualify for authorship. The order of authorship should be a joint decision of the coauthors. Each author should have participated sufficiently in the work to take public responsibility for the content.

Authorship credit should be based only on substantial contributions to 1) conception and design, or analysis and interpretation of data; 2) drafting the article or revising it critically for important intellectual content; and 3) final approval of the version to be published. All three conditions must be met.

On the basis of this description, general oversight of the research group, support of the departmental chair, data collection, financial support, and technical assistance are not sufficient to confer author status. These individuals may be thanked (with their written permission) in an acknowledgment section or appendix. Statistical assistance may be cited in the acknowledgments, or the statistician may be included among the authors. This decision depends on whether the statistician was called on to review the manuscript for methodology prior to submission or was involved in the study design from the outset.

In answer to critiques by authors of the authorship requirements set forth in the Uniform Requirements, journal editors have published articles explaining the criteria in detail, describing how the criteria are applied, and clarifying the editor's role in upholding the spirit of responsibility among authors (Huth 1986a; Kassirer and Angell 1991).

Redundant Publication

Redundant publication takes several forms. The most obvious is duplicate publication—publishing in more than one journal the same manuscript in identical form or with a few editorial changes. Most journals will not consider for publication a report that has already been published or that has been submitted or accepted elsewhere, including electronic journals and databases. This policy does not usually preclude consideration of a paper that follows a preliminary report in the form of an abstract of no more than 400 words. Studies that have been reported in an abbreviated format with details of the methods and results provided would most likely *not* be considered. This includes publication of preliminary results as letters to the editor, in a journal devoted to publishing brief reports such as *Psychopharmacology Bulletin*, or in journals that have special sections for preliminary reports. These types of publications may offer more rapid dissemination of results, but speed of publication must be weighed against the interests of full reporting.

Most journals will consider publishing a paper presented at a scientific meeting if the full text is not published in the proceedings, a journal supplement, or other publication. Press reports of a meeting are not usually considered prior publication provided the authors do not release the manuscript to the press or otherwise offer additional details of the methods or results. Some journals, such as *The New England Journal of Medicine*, have strict embargoes for release to the lay press of manuscripts under consideration unless there is clear evidence that the public health is at risk.

Gray areas persist in the definition of duplicate publication. Some journals will publish translations of published reports; some will consider manuscripts published elsewhere if they are aimed at a different audience. The best advice regarding what constitutes duplicate publication is to consult the journal's Information for Authors or contact the editorial office. When submitting a paper, authors should always inform the editor of all submissions and previous reports that might be considered duplicate publication. Copies of these reports, along with a description of how the reports differ, should be included.

Another type of redundant publication is known among editors as the "least publishable unit" or LPU (Broad 1981). In these instances, a larger study that would best be reported in its entirety is carved into several smaller studies for the sole purpose of adding to the list of publications in the author's curriculum vitae. Such authors will submit these smaller papers to different journals, omitting reference to the existence of the other manuscripts. The practice of such "salami science" is never acceptable to editors (Huth 1986b).

Redundant publication is a violation of editorial and scientific ethics. Multiple reports of the same study may lead readers to give the results more weight than they deserve. Alternatively, readers may see only one part of a larger study that was published in fragments and underestimate its importance. Redundant publication also wastes the resources of the peer review system and takes up valuable space in journals' limited page allowances (Angell and Relman 1989). Such abuses of scientific publication will bring the first-time offender a letter from the editor; repeat offenders may face stiffer sanctions in the form of being put on probation for a number of years or being banned from publishing in the journal entirely.

There are of course instances in which the dimensions of a project are so large and the questions under investigation so numerous and complex that a single report is not feasible or desirable. When several reports emerge from a single study, authors should inform the editors of the journals to which the reports are submitted of the existence and content of the other papers. Editors may ask the authors to submit copies of these other studies. Some journals inform authors that they must alert editors to any study published or under consideration that includes any of the subjects in the work submitted to their journals.

Scientific Misconduct

By far the most egregious of ethical breaches, and the most difficult for journal editors to detect and discipline, is scientific misconduct. Types of misconduct that find their way into the scientific literature include plagiarism—the representation of someone else's work as one's own—and fabrication or falsification—reporting on a study that was not in fact conducted or including data that were not actually obtained during the study (Woolf 1988). Detecting fraudulent research during peer review prior to publication is largely a matter of chance. A researcher may be asked to review a manuscript in which his or her ideas are presented without proper credit, or a reviewer may remark on a study in which the data look too good to be true. More often fraudulent research comes to light only after publication.

Editors began to reconsider their role in preserving the integrity of the scientific literature following several highly publicized cases of fraud in the 1980s. Fraudulent studies appeared in such journals as *The New England Journal of Medicine, The American Journal of Cardiology, Cell, The Journal of the American Medical Association,* and *The American Journal of Psychiatry.* Discovery of these cases not only ruined the careers of the scientists involved and cast doubt on their previous work but sparked congressional debate about the prevalence of scientific fraud and the measures that should be taken to police scientists and punish those found engaging in unethical behavior. Journal editors joined this debate and attempted to reach consensus on how they should respond to allegations of fraud against a published author and what they could do to help ensure that fraudulent studies do not get into the literature in the first place.

Editors' recommendations for deterring fraud include encouraging journals to set up rules for an independent audit of accepted manuscripts (Rennie 1989), changing the reward system for academic promotion to focus more on quality than quantity of publications (Angell 1986), and expanding the role of chairs and institutional review boards to include review of the results of research before a paper is submitted for publication (Angell and Relman 1989). Once an allegation of fraud is made, editors agree that the responsibility for conducting an investigation or making the final determination lies not with the journal editor but with the institution where the work was conducted or with the funding agency. Editors should be apprised of the final decision and, if the fraudulent study has been published, most journals will publish a retraction prominently within their pages and include reference to the retraction in the table of contents (International Committee of Medical Journal Editors 1988). Published retractions are picked up by the National Library of Medicine and included with the original citation on MEDLINE, the online database.

◆ Conclusion

The "publish or perish" phenomenon, which has accelerated in recent years, has brought in its wake myriad problems facing researchers seeking publication of their findings in respected journals. However, careful attention to such matters as thoughtful selection of the proper journal to which to submit, scrupulous observance of that journal's requirements, knowledge of the publication process including the strengths and weaknesses of peer review, and awareness of such ethical issues as redundant publication will aid the author. Assuming that the work being reported will make a contribution to the psychiatric literature, such attention will increase the likelihood that the submission will emerge as a published article.

◆ References

Angell M: Publish or perish: a proposal. Ann Intern Med 104:261–262, 1986
Angell M, Relman AS: Redundant publication. N Engl J Med 320:1212–1214, 1989
The Author's Guide to Biomedical Journals. New York, Mary Ann Liebert, Inc, 1994
Bailar JC: Science, statistics, and deception. Ann Intern Med 104:259–260, 1986
Broad WJ: The publishing game, getting more for less. Science 211:1137–1139, 1981
Dixon WJ, Brown MB, Engelman L, et al: BMDP Statistical Software. Berkeley, CA, University of California Press, 1983

Fox TF: Crisis in Communication. London, Athlone Press, 1965

Gardner MJ, Bond J: An exploratory study of statistical assessment of papers published in the *British Medical Journal*. JAMA 263:1355–1357, 1990

Huth EJ: Guidelines on authorship of medical papers. Ann Intern Med 104:269–274, 1986a

Huth EJ: Irresponsible authorship and wasteful publication. Ann Intern Med 104:257–259, 1986b

Ingelfinger FJ: Peer review in biomedical publication. Am J Med 56:686–692, 1974

International Committee of Medical Journal Editors: Retraction of research findings. Med J Aust 148:194, 1988

Kassirer JP, Angell M: On authorship and acknowledgments. N Engl J Med 321:1510–1512, 1991

Lock S: A Difficult Balance: Editorial Peer Review in Medicine. London, Nuffield Provincial Hospitals Trust, 1985

McNutt RA, Evans AT, Fletcher RH, et al: The effects of blinding on the quality of peer review: a randomized trial. JAMA 263:1371–1376, 1990

Nie NH, Hull CH, Jenkins JG, et al: Statistical Package for the Social Sciences, 2nd Edition. New York, McGraw-Hill, 1975

Pocock SJ, Hughes MD, Lee RJ: Statistical problems in the reporting of clinical trials: a survey of three medical journals. N Engl J Med 317:426–432, 1987

Relman AS: Are journals really quality filters? in Research on Selective Information Systems. Edited by Goffman W, Bruer JT, Warren KS. New York, Rockefeller Foundation, 1980

Relman AS: Peer review in scientific journals—what good is it? West J Med 153:520–522, 1990

Relman AS, Angell M: How good is peer review? N Engl J Med 321:827–829, 1989

Rennie D: The ethics of medical publication. Med J Aust 2:409–412, 1979

Rennie D: Editors and auditors. JAMA 261:2543–2545, 1989

SAS: Statistical Analysis System. Cary, NC, SAS Institute, 1986

Talking with the new editor of AJP: an interview with Nancy Andreasen. Psychiatric Research Report 8(2):1–18, 1993

Wilson JD: Peer review and publication. J Clin Invest 58:1697–1701, 1978

Woolf P: Deception in scientific research. Jurimetrics Journal 29(1):67–95, 1988

Yankauer A: How blind is blind review? Am J Public Health 81:843–845, 1991

Resources 9–1
Descriptions of Scientific Journals[a]

Journal	Date established	How often published	Affiliated organization	Peer reviewed	Circulation	Where indexed[b] HLI	IM	PA	EM	Where to send manuscripts	Types of papers
Academic Medicine	1926	Monthly	Association of American Medical Colleges	Yes	6,000	Yes	Yes	Yes	Yes	Addeane S. Caelleigh, Editor 2450 N St., NW Washington, DC 20037 (202) 828-0590	—[c]
Academic Psychiatry	1977	Quarterly	American Association of Directors of Psychiatric Residency Training and Association for Academic Psychiatry	Yes	1,928	No	No	Yes	Yes	Jonathan F. Borus, M.D., Editor American Psychiatric Press, Inc. 1400 K St., NW Washington, DC 20005 (202) 682-6310	Publishes "material describing educational efforts for and by psychiatrists as well as articles addressing other issues relevant to the academic missions of departments of psychiatry. The journal provides a forum for work which furthers knowledge in psychiatric education and stimulates improvements in academic psychiatry."
Acta Psychiatrica Scandinavica	1926	Monthly	—	Yes	1,400	Yes	Yes	Yes	Yes	Prof. Jan-Otto Ottosson, Editor Dept. of Psychiatry Sahlgrenska Hospital S-413 45 Gothenburg, Sweden 011-45-33-127030	Publishes "original papers in English on psychiatry and adjacent fields."

Journal	Founded	Frequency	Association		Circulation					Editor	Description
Addictive Behaviors: An International Journal	1975	Bimonthly	—	Yes	—	No	Yes	Yes	No	Dr. Howard J. Rankin, Associate Editor, Hilton Head Institute, Valencia Rd. in Shipyard Plantation, PO Box 7138, Hilton Head Island, SC 29938, (803) 785-7292	Focuses on "alcohol and drug abuse, smoking, and problems associated with eating."
Administration and Policy in Mental Health	1972	Quarterly	—	Yes	625	Yes	No	Yes	Yes	Dr. Saul Feldman, Editor, Bay Area Foundation for Human Resources, 850 California St., San Francisco, CA 94108, (415) 652-1402, ext. 219	Publishes "original articles and case reports on all aspects of the organization and administration of mental health services and on mental health policy."
American Imago: Studies in Psychoanalysis and Culture	1939	Quarterly	Association for Applied Psychoanalysis	—	1,000	No	No	Yes	No	Martin J. Gliserman, Ph.D., Editor, Dept. of English, Murray Hall, Rutgers University, PO Box 5054, New Brunswick, NJ 08903-5054, (908) 932-8094	Explores "the important role psychoanalysis plays in contemporary cultural, literary, and social theory."
American Journal of Drug and Alcohol Abuse	1974	4 times/year	—	—	1,546	No	No	Yes	Yes	Edward Kaufman, M.D., Editor-in-Chief, Dept. of Psychiatry and Human Behavior, University of California, Irvine Medical Center, 101 City Drive South, Orange, CA 92668, (714) 634-6021	Provides a "medically oriented forum for interchange of ideas between preclinical, clinical, and social modalities involved in the study and treatment of drug abuse and alcoholism."
American Journal of Forensic Psychiatry	1978	Quarterly	American College of Forensic Psychiatry	—	1,000	No	No	Yes	No	Debra Miller, Editor, PO Box 5870, Balboa Island, CA 92662, (714) 831-0236	"A quarterly professional journal for legal psychiatrists and attorneys."

Journal	Date established	How often published	Affiliated organization	Peer reviewed	Circulation	Where indexed[b] HLI	IM	PA	EM	Where to send manuscripts	Types of papers
American Journal of Geriatric Psychiatry	1992	Quarterly	American Association for Geriatric Psychiatry	Yes	2,187	No	No	Yes	No	Gene D. Cohen, M.D., Ph.D., Editor American Psychiatric Press, Inc. 1400 K St., NW Washington, DC 20005 (202) 682-6336	Publishes "articles on a variety of topics, including the diagnosis and classification of the psychiatric disorders of later life . . . epidemiology and biologic correlates of mental health problems in older adults . . . psychopharmacology and other somatic treatments in geriatric psychiatry . . . and innovative treatment strategies—including psychodynamic and other psychotherapeutic approaches—in the treatment of elderly patients."
American Journal of Law & Medicine	1975	Quarterly	American Society of Law & Medicine and Boston University School of Law	Yes	9,000	Yes	Yes	No	Yes	Frances H. Miller, J.D., Faculty Editor-in-Chief 765 Commonwealth Ave., 16th Floor Boston, MA 02215 (617) 353-2912	"Acceptable subjects include health law and policy; legal, ethical, social, and economic aspects of medical practice, education, and research; health-related insurance; and other important or interesting subjects involving the relationship of the life sciences to the social sciences and humanities."

Journal	Founded	Frequency	Sponsor		Circulation					Editor / Address	Description
American Journal of Neuroradiology	1980	Bimonthly		—	4,476	No	No	No	No	Juan M. Taveras, M.D., Editor, Dept. of Radiology, 55 Fruit St., Boston, MA 02114	Publishes "original clinical articles on imaging diagnosis of the CNS, including the spine, for radiologists, neuro-radiologists, neurosurgeons, and neurologists."
American Journal of Orthopsychiatry	1930	Quarterly	American Orthopsychiatric Association	Yes	13,000	Yes	Yes	Yes	Yes	Ellen L. Bassuk, M.D., Editor, 19 West 44th St., New York, NY 10036, (212) 354-5770	"Clinical, theoretical, research, or expository papers that are essentially synergistic and directed at concept or theory development, reconceptualization of major issues, explanation, and interpretation are especially welcomed."
American Journal of Psychiatry	1844	Monthly	American Psychiatric Association	Yes	47,013	Yes	Yes	Yes	Yes	Nancy C. Andreasen, M.D., Ph.D., Editor, 1400 K St., NW, Washington, DC 20005, (202) 682-6020	—[c]
American Journal of Psychoanalysis	1941	Quarterly	Association for the Advancement of Psychoanalysis	Yes	809	Yes	Yes	Yes	Yes	Douglas H. Ingram, Editor, 329 East 62nd St., New York, NY 10021, (212) 838-8044	Its purpose is "to communicate modern concepts of psychoanalytic theory and practice, and related investigations in allied fields. It is addressed to everyone interested in the understanding and therapy of emotional problems."
American Journal of Psychotherapy	1946	Quarterly	Association for the Advancement of Psychotherapy	Yes	5,000	Yes	Yes	Yes	Yes	T. Byram Karasu, M.D., Editor-in-Chief, Belfer Center, Rm. 402, 1300 Morris Park Ave., Bronx, NY 10461, (212) 823-7754	—[c]

Journal	Date established	How often published	Affiliated organization	Peer reviewed	Circulation	Where indexed[b] HLI	IM	PA	EM	Where to send manuscripts	Types of papers
American Journal on Addictions	1992	Quarterly	American Academy of Psychiatrists in Alcoholism and Addictions	Yes	1,333	No	No	No	No	Sheldon I. Miller, M.D., Editor American Psychiatric Press, Inc. 1400 K St., NW Washington, DC 20005 (202) 682-6310	Publishes "special overview articles, original clinical and research papers, a clinical update series, book reviews, and letters."
American Psychologist	1946	Monthly	American Psychological Association	Yes	70,000	Yes	Yes	Yes	No	Raymond D. Fowler, Editor 750 First St., NE Washington, DC 20002-4242 (202) 336-6011	Publishes "articles on current issues in psychology as well as empirical, theoretical, and practical articles on broad aspects of psychology."
Annals of Clinical Psychiatry	1989	Quarterly	American Academy of Clinical Psychiatrists	—	763	No	No	Yes	Yes	Charles L. Rich, M.D., Editor-in-Chief Dept. of Psychiatry University of South Alabama 3421 Medical Park Drive West, Suite 2 Mobile, AL 36693	Designed "to provide an audience of practicing clinical psychiatrists with up-to-date information regarding the phenomenology and/or treatment of persons with psychiatric disorders. Although the emphasis is on results of controlled clinical studies, timely and thorough review articles that present new appraisals of pertinent clinical topics are included."
Annals of Internal Medicine	1922	Twice monthly	American College of Physicians	Yes	91,000	Yes	Yes	No	Yes	Edward J. Huth, M.D., Interim Editor Independence Mall West Sixth Street at Race Philadelphia, PA 19106-1572 (215) 351-2629	Publishes "original articles, clinical conferences, editorials, book reviews, letters, and other information relevant to internal medicine and related fields."

Journal	Founded	Frequency	Publisher/Society		Circulation					Editor/Address		Description
Archives of General Psychiatry	1959	Monthly	American Medical Association	Yes	24,000	Yes	Yes	Yes	Yes	Jack D. Barchas, M.D., Chief Editor, Dept. of Psychiatry, Cornell Medical Center, 525 East 68th St., Box 171, New York, NY 10021	—c	
Archives of Neurology	1919	Monthly	American Medical Association	Yes	19,564	No	Yes	Yes	Yes	Robert J. Joynt, M.D., Editor, c/o Ann Westerbeke, 515 North State St., Chicago, IL 60610, (312) 464-4184		"Published as an editorial service for physicians who practice neurology as a primary specialty, and to physicians of other specialties who treat conditions of the central nervous system. It is oriented toward the clinician."
Australian and New Zealand Journal of Psychiatry	1967	Quarterly	Royal Australian and New Zealand College of Psychiatrists	Yes	2,500	Yes	Yes	Yes	Yes	Associate Prof. Sydney Bloch, Editor, PO Box 126, Karrinyup, Western Australia 6018, 09-447-5312		Publishes "original articles which describe research or report opinions of interest to psychiatrists."
Behavioral Science: Journal of the International Society for the Systems Sciences	1956	Quarterly	International Society for the Systems Sciences and Institute of Management Sciences	Yes	3,167	Yes	Yes	Yes	Yes	James Grier Miller, Editor, PO Box 8369, La Jolla, CA 92038-8369, (619) 450-9163		Publishes "original articles on new theories, experimental research, and applications relating to all levels of living and nonliving systems. . . . Articles should specifically indicate how they are generalizable. Generalizations of an implied nature are not acceptable."

Journal	Date established	How often published	Affiliated organization	Peer reviewed	Circulation	Where indexed[b]				Where to send manuscripts	Types of papers
						HLI	IM	PA	EM		
Biological Psychiatry: A Journal of Psychiatric Research	1969	Semi-monthly	Society of Biological Psychiatry	Yes	1,200	Yes	Yes	Yes	Yes	Wagner Bridger, M.D., Editor-in-Chief Medical College of Pennsylvania, EPPI 3200 Henry Ave. Philadelphia, PA 19129-1137 (215) 842-4146	Welcomes contributions "from all sources and from all disciplines and research areas relevant to psychiatry—pathology, pharmacology, electroencephalography, biochemistry, and genetics—including clinical, psychological, epidemiological, and normative studies. Occasional theoretical and review papers are published."
BMJ: British Medical Journal	1832	Weekly	British Medical Association	Yes	—	Yes	Yes	No	Yes	Richard Smith, Editor Tavistock Square London WC1H 9JR, UK 071-387-4499	—[c]
Brain and Cognition	1982	6 times/year	—	Yes	—	No	Yes	Yes	Yes	Harry A. Whitaker Jr., M.D., Editor 8610 Rockdale Lane Springfield, IL 22153 Jeffrey L. Cummings, M.D., Editor Brentwood VAMC Los Angeles, CA 10073	"Deals with the nonlinguistic aspects of neuropsychology during the past decade. Presenting case histories, original experimental research papers, reviews, notes, and commentaries, it provides a forum for the discussion of timely and important advances in the field."

Journal	Founded	Frequency	Organization		Circulation				Editor / Address	Description
Brain and Language	1974	8 times/ year	—	Yes	—	No	Yes	Yes	Harry A. Whitaker Jr., M.D., Editor 8610 Rockdale Lane Springfield, IL 22153 Andre Roch Lecours, M.D., Editor Centre de Recherche du Centre Hospitalier Côte-des-Neiges, Quebec, Canada	Publishes "original theoretical, clinical, and experimental papers on human language and communication; speech, hearing, reading, writing, higher language functions, and nonverbal communication as they relate to brain structure and function."
British Journal of Psychiatry	1853	Monthly	Royal College of Psychiatrists	Yes	12,000	Yes	Yes	Yes	Prof. Greg Wilkinson, Editor 17 Belgrave Square London SW1X 8PG, UK 01-235-8857	Publishes "original work in all fields of psychiatry."
Bulletin of the American Academy of Psychiatry and the Law	1973	Quarterly	American Academy of Psychiatry and the Law	Yes	2,000	Yes	Yes	Yes	Seymour L. Halleck, M.D., Editor-in-Chief Dept. of Psychiatry University of North Carolina, CB 7160 Medical School Wing D Chapel Hill, NC 27514 (410) 539-0379	Publishes "manuscripts dealing with the theory and practice of forensic, social-legal, criminology, and correctional psychiatry, psychiatric jurisprudence and related fields."
Bulletin of the History of Medicine	1933	Quarterly	American Association for the History of Medicine and Johns Hopkins Institute of the History of Medicine	Yes	2,250	Yes	No	No	Gert H. Brieger & Jerome J. Bylebyl, Editors 1900 East Monument St. Baltimore, MD 21205 (410) 955-3179	—[c]
Bulletin of the Menninger Clinic: A Journal for the Mental Health Professions	1936	Quarterly	Menninger Clinic	Yes	2,093	Yes	Yes	Yes	Philip R. Beard, M.Div., M.A., Managing Editor PO Box 829 Topeka, KS 66601-0829 (913) 273-7500	Publishes "original articles on psychiatry, psychology, psychoanalysis, neuropsychology, clinical research, and related subjects, as well as clinical reports, brief communications, and book reviews."

Journal	Date established	How often published	Affiliated organization	Peer reviewed	Circulation	Where indexed[b] HLI	IM	PA	EM	Where to send manuscripts	Types of papers
Canadian Journal of Psychiatry	1956	10 times/ year	Canadian Psychiatric Association	Yes	3,300	Yes	Yes	Yes	Yes	Edward Kingstone, Editor 237 Argyle St., Suite 200 Ottawa, Ontario K2P 1B8, Canada (613) 234-2815	—[c]
Cerebral Cortex	1991	Bimonthly	—	Yes	—	No	Yes	Yes	Yes	c/o Oxford University Press 200 Madison Ave. New York, NY 10016 (212) 679-7300	"Covers the large variety of modern neurobiological and neuropsychological techniques, including anatomy, biochemistry, molecular neurobiology, electrophysiology, behavior, artificial intelligence, and theoretical modelling."
CMAJ: Canadian Medical Association Journal	1911	Semi-monthly	Canadian Medical Association	Yes	35,800	Yes	Yes	Yes	Yes	Bruce P. Squires, M.D., Ph.D., Editor-in-Chief 1867 Alta Vista Drive Ottawa, Ontario K1G 3Y6, Canada (613) 731-9331	Publishes "original manuscripts in English or French on the basic and clinical aspects of medicine, medical education, medical economics or politics, medicolegal affairs, health care policy or delivery and the history of medicine."
Community Mental Health Journal	1965	Bimonthly	National Council of Community Mental Health Centers	Yes	1,629	Yes	Yes	Yes	Yes	David L. Cutler, M.D., Editor Dept. of Psychiatry OPO2 Oregon Health Sciences University 3181 Sam Jackson Park Rd. Portland, OR 97201 (212) 620-8461	Publishes papers in "the broad fields of community mental health theory, practice and research."

Journal	Founded	Frequency	Publisher		Circulation						Editor	Description
Comprehensive Psychiatry	1960	Bimonthly	American Psychopathological Association	Yes	1,258	Yes	Yes	Yes	Yes	Yes	Ralph A. O'Connell, M.D., Editor-in-Chief, St. Vincent's Hospital and Medical Center, 144 West 12th St., New York, NY 10011, (212) 790-8196	— [c]
Convulsive Therapy	1985	Quarterly	—	—	600	No	No	Yes	Yes	Yes	Dr. Charles H. Kellner, Editor, Dept. of Psychiatry and Behavioral Sciences, Medical University of South Carolina, 171 Ashley Ave., Charleston, SC 29425	Publishes "original scientific articles, reviews, commentaries, and letters. The scope of articles may be broad, encompassing anatomic, structural, physiologic, biochemical, psychologic, and neurophysiologic studies of the effects of seizures and of the seizure process itself. Discussions of sociologic, legal, and ethical aspects of research and clinical practice are of interest."
Corrective and Social Psychiatry and Journal of Behavior Technology Methods and Therapy	1954	Quarterly	American Association of Mental Health Professionals in Corrections	—	1,200	No	No	Yes	Yes	Yes	Clyde V. Martin, M.D., M.A., J.D., Editor, Martin Psychiatric Research Foundation, PO Box 3365, Fairfield, CA 94533, (707) 864-0910	Publishes "original papers contributing to the advancement of the therapeutic community in all its institutional settings, i.e., Correctional Institutions, Hospitals, Churches, Schools, Industry and the Family."

Journal	Date established	How often published	Affiliated organization	Peer reviewed	Circulation	Where indexed[b] HLI	IM	PA	EM	Where to send manuscripts	Types of papers
Culture, Medicine and Psychiatry	1977	Quarterly	—	Yes	800	No	Yes	Yes	Yes	Byron J. Good, Ph.D., & Mary-Jo DelVecchio Good, Ph.D., Editors-in-Chief Dept. of Social Medicine Harvard Medical School 641 Huntington Ave. Boston, MA 02115 (617) 432-0716	"Serves as an international and interdisciplinary forum for three interrelated fields: medical and psychiatric anthropology; cross-cultural psychiatry; and related cross-societal and clinical and epidemiological studies."
Depression	1993	Bimonthly	—	Yes	—	No	No	No	No	Charles B. Nemeroff, M.D. Dept. of Psychiatry Emory University School of Medicine, Box AF Atlanta, GA 30322 (404) 727-5881	"Welcomes original research and synthetic review articles on the neuropsychobiological precipitants of depression and its comorbid disorders; somatic, psychodynamic, behavioral, and cognitive aspects of the disorder; and pharmacotherapeutic and psychotherapeutic treatment techniques."
Dreaming: Journal of the Association for the Study of Dreams	1991	Quarterly	Association for the Study of Dreams	Yes	1,000	No	No	Yes	No	Ernest Hartmann, M.D., Editor Tufts University 170 Morton St. Boston, MA 02130	"An international forum for the publication of scholarly articles on various aspects of dreams and dreaming. Features biological/ physiological research, psychological studies.

Journal	Year	Frequency			Circulation					Editor / Address	Description
European Journal of Psychiatry	1987	Quarterly	—	Yes	5,000	No	Yes	Yes	Yes	Prof. A. Seva, Editor-in-Chief, PO Box 6.029, 50080 Saragosse, Spain, (976) 279402	Publishes articles in English "to bring about a greater degree of communication among European psychiatrists. This Journal will have an eclectic orientation in its scientific approach and is open to Psychiatry, Mental Health and all related fields. We invite contributions in these areas, including biological, psychological and social sciences."
Family Process	1962	Quarterly	—	Yes	10,000	No	Yes	Yes	Yes	Peter Steinglass, M.D., Editor, 149 East 79th St., New York, NY 10021	"Publishes clinical research, training, and theoretical contributions in the broad area of family therapy."
General Hospital Psychiatry; Psychiatry, Medicine and Primary Care	1979	6 times/ year	—	Yes	800	Yes	Yes	Yes	Yes	Don R. Lipsitt, M.D., Editor-in-Chief, Dept. of Psychiatry, Mount Auburn Hospital, 330 Mt. Auburn St., Cambridge, MA 02238, (617) 499-5008	Publishes "original articles on biopsychosocial approaches to medicine, liaison-consultation psychiatry; the relationship of psychiatric services to general medical systems; and new directions in medical education that stress psychiatry's role in primary care, family practice, and continuing education."

Journal	Date established	How often published	Affiliated organization	Peer reviewed	Circulation	Where indexed[b] HLI	IM	PA	EM	Where to send manuscripts	Types of papers
Harvard Review of Psychiatry	1993	Bimonthly	—	No	1,266	No	No	No	No	Katharine A. Phillips, M.D., Deputy Editor McLean Hospital 115 Mill St. Belmont, MA 02178 (617) 855-3396	"Includes review articles on a wide variety of subjects, emphasizing the integration of research findings with clinical care. Also included are original reports describing research of interest to clinicians, columns focusing on a number of subspecialty areas, and reports on challenging clinical cases."
Hastings Center Report	1971	Bimonthly	Hastings Center	Yes	11,500	No	Yes	No	Yes	Bette-Jane Crigger, Editor 255 Elm Rd. Briarcliff Manor, NY 10510 (914) 762-8500, ext. 222	—[c]
Hospital & Health Services Administration	1956	Quarterly	Foundation of the American College of Healthcare Executives	Yes	24,000	Yes	No	No	Yes	Richard S. Kurz, Editor 3663 Lindell Blvd. Saint Louis University School of Public Health St. Louis, MO 63108-8684 (314) 577-8682	Publishes "articles on health management and policy that advance understanding and have operational utility for the practicing manager."

Journal	Year	Frequency	Sponsor		Circulation					Editor	Description
Infant Mental Health Journal	1980	Quarterly	International Association for Infant Mental Health, World Association for Infant Psychiatry and Allied Disciplines, and Michigan Association for Infant Mental Health	No	650	No	No	Yes	No	Joy D. Osofsky, Ph.D., Editor Division of Child Psychiatry Louisiana State University Medical School 1542 Tulane Ave. New Orleans, LA 70112-2822 (203) 868-7585	Publishes "research articles, literature reviews, program descriptions/ evaluations, clinical studies, and book reviews that focus on infant social-emotional development, caregiver-infant interactions, contextual and cultural influences on infant and family development, and all conditions that place infants and their families at-risk for less than optimal development."
International Journal of Group Psychotherapy	1951	Quarterly	American Group Psychotherapy Association	Yes	2,000	Yes	Yes	Yes	Yes	William E. Piper, Ph.D., Editor 25 East 21st St., 6th Floor New York, NY 10010 (212) 477-2677	—[c]
International Journal of Law and Psychiatry	1978	Quarterly	International Academy of Law and Mental Health	Yes	1,100	Yes	Yes	Yes	Yes	David N. Weisstub, Editor-in-Chief Suite 2260, Place du Canada Montreal, Quebec H3B 2N2, Canada (514) 875-2620	Publishes "articles which are oriented to a comparative or international perspective. The journal will publish significant conceptual contributions on contemporary issues as well as serve in the rapid dissemination of important and relevant research findings."

Journal	Date established	How often published	Affiliated organization	Peer reviewed	Circulation	HLI	IM	PA	EM	Where to send manuscripts	Types of papers
International Journal of Psychiatry in Medicine: Biopsychosocial Aspects of Patient Care	1970	Quarterly	—	Yes	—	No	Yes	Yes	Yes	Daniel S.P. Schubert, M.D., Ph.D., Editor Dept. of Psychiatry MetroHealth Medical Center 2500 MetroHealth Center Drive Cleveland, OH 44109-1998 (516) 691-1270	Publishes "articles which apply the methods of psychiatry and psychology to the further understanding of disorders which are not primarily psychiatric; and articles which employ the methods of non-psychiatric medical subdisciplines in the attempt to specify further the psychobiological substrate of psychiatric illnesses."
International Journal of Psycho-Analysis	1920	6 times/ year	Institute of Psycho-Analysis	Yes	7,000	No	Yes	Yes	Yes	David Tuckett, Editor Institute of Psycho-Analysis 63 New Cavendish St. London W1M 7RD, UK & Arnold Cooper, M.D. 50 East 78th St., Suite 1C New York, NY 10021 (212) 879-7182	Publishes "contributions to developments in theory and technique, the analytic process, methodology, theoretical and technical concepts, classics revisited, clinical reports, infancy and child development, systematic research, psychoanalytic education, professional issues, history of psychoanalysis, psychoanalysis and other therapies, psychoanalysis and the arts and sciences."
Journal of the American Medical Association	1848	4 times/ month	American Medical Association	Yes	279,600	Yes	Yes	Yes	Yes	George D. Lundberg, M.D., Editor 515 North State St. Chicago, IL 60610 (312) 464-2400	—

Journal	Year	Frequency	Affiliation						Editor	Description
Jefferson Journal of Psychiatry: A Resident Publication	1983	Biannually	Residency Training Program of the Dept. of Psychiatry of Jefferson Medical College and the Committee of Residents and Fellows of the American Psychiatric Association	No	—	No	No	No	Mary E. Donovan, M.D., Chief Editor 1015 Walnut St., 3rd Floor Philadelphia, PA 19107	"Residents are invited to submit original manuscripts in the form of articles, literature reviews, case reports, book reviews, or letters to the editor."
Journal of Abnormal Psychology	1906	Quarterly	American Psychological Association	Yes	5,000	No	Yes	Yes	Milton E. Strauss, Incoming Editor Dept. of Psychology Case Western Reserve University 10900 Euclid Ave. Cleveland, OH 44106-7123	Publishes "articles on basic research and theory in the broad field of abnormal behavior, its determinants, and its correlates.... Each article should represent an addition to knowledge and understanding of abnormal behavior either in its etiology, description, or change."
Journal of Affective Disorders	1979	Monthly	—	Yes	—	No	Yes	Yes	Prof. George Winokur, Editor-in-Chief Dept. of Psychiatry Administration University of Iowa Hospitals and Clinics 200 Hawkins Drive, 2887 JPP Iowa City, IA 52242-1057 (319) 353-4551	Publishes "papers concerned with affective disorders in the widest sense: depression, mania, anxiety and panic.... High-quality papers will be accepted dealing with any aspect of affective disorders, including biochemistry, pharmacology, endocrinology, genetics, statistics, epidemiology, psychodynamics, classification, clinical studies and studies of all types of treatment."

Journal	Date established	How often published	Affiliated organization	Peer reviewed	Circulation	Where indexed[b]				Where to send manuscripts	Types of papers
						HLI	IM	PA	EM		
Journal of Applied Behavioral Science	1965	Quarterly	NTL Institute for Applied Behavioral Science	Yes	3,000	Yes	No	Yes	No	Catherine A. Messina, Managing Editor NTL Institute 1240 North Pitt St., Suite 100 Alexandria, VA 22314-1403	Publishes papers that advance one or more of four goals: 1) "to develop or test theoretical and conceptual approaches to planned change," 2) "to report on social inventions," 3) "to evaluate attempts at social intervention or change," and 4) "to evaluate directly and explicitly the underlying values, the implicit social models, and the unspoken assumptions and biases inherent in attempts at social change."
Journal of Behavior Therapy and Experimental Psychiatry	1970	Quarterly	Behavior Therapy and Research Society	Yes	3,100	Yes	Yes	Yes	Yes	Joseph Wolpe, M.D., Editor Dept. of Psychology Pepperdine University Graduate School of Education and Psychology 400 Corporate Pointe Culver City, CA 90230 (310) 568-5753	Publishes "in addition to original papers, . . . material intended to provide training in behavior therapy for psychiatrists, . . . case reports, and from time to time transcriptions from interviews to illustrate how target behaviors are identified and methods selected, how difficulties are handled and progress evaluated. Thus it includes descriptions of therapeutic methods, with technical details."

Journal	Year	Frequency	Society						Circulation	Editor/Address	Description
Journal of Cerebral Blood Flow and Metabolism	1981	Bimonthly	—	Yes	No	Yes	No	No	—	A. Murray Harper, Editor c/o Raven Press 1185 Avenue of the Americas, Dept. 1B New York, NY 10036 (212) 930–9500	"Gathers new information on experimental, theoretical, and clinical aspects of brain circulation and metabolism."
Journal of Child and Adolescent Psychopharmacology	1990	Quarterly	—	Yes	No	No	No	No	—	Charles W. Popper, M.D., Editor McLean Hospital 115 Mill St. Belmont, MA 02178–9106 (617) 855–2843	Publishes "articles encompassing investigative research, treatment techniques, basic sciences, health policy and education, and clinical case conferences."
Journal of Child Psychology and Psychiatry and Allied Disciplines	1960	8 times/year	Association for Child Psychology and Psychiatry	Yes	Yes	Yes	Yes	Yes	4,700	Michael Goldstein, Corresponding Editor Dept. of Psychology, UCLA Los Angeles, CA 90024 or Judith L. Rapoport, Corresponding Editor Child Psychiatry Branch NIMH, Bldg. 10, Rm. 6N240 9000 Rockville Pike Bethesda, MD 20892	Publishes "papers concerned with child and adolescent development, especially developmental psychopathology and the developmental disorders."
Journal of Clinical Psychiatry	1940	Monthly	American Academy of Clinical Psychiatrists	—	No	No	No	Yes	32,000	Alan J. Gelenberg, M.D., Editor-in-Chief Physicians Postgraduate Press PO Box 240008 Memphis, TN 38124 (901) 682–1001	Publishes articles that are "relevant and interesting to clinical psychiatrists. Whether the subject is a formal research experiment or a series of clinical experiences, reasoning should be cogent, literature reviews comprehensive, methodology sound, and analysis appropriate. Conclusions should flow logically from the data."

Journal	Date established	How often published	Affiliated organization	Peer reviewed	Circulation	Where indexed[b] HLI	IM	PA	EM	Where to send manuscripts	Types of papers
Journal of Clinical Psychoanalysis	1992	Quarterly	New York Psychoanalytic Institute and Society	Yes	1,000	Yes	Yes	Yes	No	Herbert M. Wyman, M.D., & Stephen M. Rittenberg, M.D., Co-Editors 200 East 59th St. New York, NY 10128 (212) 534-5565 or (212) 722-2525	Publishes "case studies in a breadth and depth hitherto unavailable.... We ask of future contributors that all clinical data be presented at the level of observation, in clear, readable, nonclinical prose."
Journal of Clinical Psychology	1945	Bimonthly —		Yes	2,400	Yes	Yes	Yes	Yes	Dr. Vladimir Pishkin, Editor 3113 NW 62nd St. Oklahoma City, OK 73112 (203) 567-5395	—[c]
Journal of Clinical Psychopharmacology	1981	Bimonthly —		Yes	4,300	Yes	Yes	No	Yes	Richard I. Shader, M.D., Editor-in-Chief Dept. of Pharmacology and Experimental Therapeutics Tufts University School of Medicine 136 Harrison Ave. Boston, MA 02111 (617) 956-0178	Publishes "clinical trials and studies, side effects and other undesired reactions, drug interactions, overdosage management, pharmacogenetics, pharmacokinetics, and the psychiatric effects of nonpsychiatric drugs. Problems of special populations (the elderly, children, adolescents, pregnant women, and minorities) are of particular concern."

Journal	Year	Frequency	Publisher		Circulation					Editor	Description
Journal of Consulting and Clinical Psychology	1937	Bimonthly	American Psychological Association	Yes	11,000	Yes	Yes	Yes	Yes	Larry E. Beutler Graduate School of Education University of California Santa Barbara, CA 93106 (805) 893–2923	Publishes "original contributions on the following topics: (a) the development, validity, and use of techniques of diagnosis and treatment in disordered behavior; (b) studies of populations of clinical interest, such as hospital, prison, rehabilitation, geriatric, and similar samples; (c) cross-cultural and demographic studies of interest for the behavior disorders; (d) studies of personality and its assessment and development that have a bearing on problems of clinical dysfunction; (e) studies of gender, ethnicity, or sexual orientation that have a clear bearing on diagnosis, assessment, and treatment; or (f) case studies pertinent to the preceding topics."
Journal of Contemporary Psychotherapy	1970	Quarterly	Long Island Institute for Mental Health	—	289	No	No	Yes	Yes	Erwin R. Parson, Ph.D., Editor-in-Chief PO Box 62 Perry Point, MD 21902–0062	Publishes "brief original papers on individual and group psychotherapy, psychoanalysis, and allied mental health disciplines."

Journal	Date established	How often published	Affiliated organization	Peer reviewed	Circulation	Where indexed[b] HLI	IM	PA	EM	Where to send manuscripts	Types of papers
Journal of Geriatric Psychiatry and Neurology: An Interdisciplinary Forum for Clinicians and Scientists	1988	Quarterly	Alzheimer's Foundation	Yes	1,000	Yes	Yes	Yes	Yes	Michael A. Jenike, M.D. Massachusetts General Hospital East Bldg. 149, 9th Floor, 13th St. Charlestown, MA 02129 (617) 726-2998	—[c]
Journal of Group Psychotherapy, Psychodrama and Sociometry	1947	Quarterly	American Society of Group Psychotherapy and Psychodrama	—	1,252	No	No	Yes	No	Helen Kress, Managing Editor HELDREF Publications 1319 18th St., NW Washington, DC 20036-1802 (202) 296-6267, ext. 213	Publishes "manuscripts that deal with the application of group psychotherapy, psychodrama, sociometry, role playing, life skills training, and other action methods to the fields of psychotherapy, counseling, and education. Preference is given to articles dealing with experimental research and empirical studies."
Journal of International Medical Research	1972	Bimonthly	—	Yes	4,000	No	Yes	Yes	Yes	E. Gomez, U.S. Coordinator 400 Plaza Drive, PO Box 1505 Secaucus, NJ 07094 (201) 865-7500	Publishes "original, full length papers on animal pharmacology, clinical pharmacology, pharmacokinetics and drug metabolism, toxicology, ... and clinical trials. Review articles on topics of current importance which are undergoing active medical research are also welcome."

Journal	Year	Frequency	Publisher		Circulation					Editor / Address	Description
Journal of Marital and Family Therapy	1975	Quarterly	American Association for Marriage and Family Therapy	—	16,000	No	No	Yes	Yes	Douglas H. Sprenkle, Ph.D., Editor, Purdue University Marriage and Family Therapy Program, 1268 Marriage and Family Therapy Center, West Lafayette, IN 47907-1268, (317) 494-8448	Publishes "articles on research, theory, clinical practice, and training in marital and family therapy."
Journal of Marriage and the Family	1939	Quarterly	National Council on Family Relations	Yes	6,800	No	No	Yes	No	Marilyn Coleman, Editor, Human Development and Family Studies, 27 Stanley Hall, University of Missouri—Columbia, Columbia, MO 65211, (314) 882-1835	Presents original theory, research interpretation, and critical discussion of materials related to marriage and the family.
Journal of Mental Health Administration	1972	3 times/ year	Association of Mental Health Administrators	Yes	3,000	Yes	No	Yes	Yes	Bruce Lubotsky Levin, Dr.P.H., FAMHA, Editor, Florida Mental Health Institute, University of South Florida, 13301 Bruce B. Downs Blvd., Tampa, FL 33612-3899, (813) 974-6400	Publishes "articles on new developments, innovations and trends in the management of mental health, alcohol and substance abuse, as well as related behavioral health and disability programs. The *Journal* also publishes articles on mental health planning, policy, analysis, marketing, law, financing, organizational structure and evaluation of mental health services."

Journal	Date established	How often published	Affiliated organization	Peer reviewed	Circulation	Where indexed[b] HLI	IM	PA	EM	Where to send manuscripts	Types of papers
Journal of Nervous and Mental Disease	1874	Monthly	—	Yes	2,520	Yes	Yes	Yes	Yes	Eugene B. Brody, M.D., Editor-in-Chief Sheppard and Enoch Pratt Hospital 6501 North Charles St. Baltimore, MD 21285–6815 (410) 938–3000, ext. 3182	Publishes "articles containing new data or ways of reorganizing established knowledge relevant to understanding and modifying human behavior, especially that called 'sick' or 'deviant.'"
Journal of Neurology, Neurosurgery and Psychiatry	1926	Monthly	British Medical Association	Yes	—	Yes	Yes	Yes	Yes	Prof. R.A.C. Hughes, Editor Medical School Bldg. UMDS of Guy's and St. Thomas Hospitals St. Thomas St. London SE1 9RT, UK 01–387–4499	Publishes "original papers relevant to the title of the journal."
Journal of Neuropsychiatry and Clinical Neurosciences	1989	Quarterly	American Neuro-psychiatric Association	Yes	1,702	No	No	No	Yes	Stuart C. Yudofsky, M.D., Editor American Psychiatric Press, Inc. 1400 K St., NW Washington, DC 20005 (202) 682–6310	Publishes "original research and clinical reports related to the assessment and treatment of neuropsychiatric disorders. The basic neurosciences underlying psychiatric and neuropsychiatric disorders are also considered."
Journal of Neuroscience	1981	Monthly	—	Yes	6,016	No	Yes	No	Yes	William Maxwell Cowan, M.D., Editor 660 S. Euclid Ave. Box 8057 St. Louis, MO 63110	"A broad-focus, interdisciplinary journal, bringing together findings in neural systems and all areas of neuroscience: molecular, cellular, developmental, and behavioral."

Journal	Founded	Frequency	Sponsor		Circulation					Contact	Description
Journal of Pastoral Care	1948	Quarterly	—		13,668	Yes	No	Yes	No	Orlo Strunk Jr., Managing Editor 1068 Harbor Drive, SW Calabash, NC 28467 (404) 320-1472	Publishes "concrete and detailed reports of significant items of pastoral work, with discussion; research studies of importance to the ministry and mission of the church and synagogue; articles advancing the understanding and practice of Clinical Pastoral Education and pastoral counseling; manuscripts which explore the distinctive as well as the common characteristics of ministry in relation to other helping professions or institutions."
Journal of Preventive Psychiatry and Allied Disciplines	1981	Quarterly	Center for Preventive Psychiatry	Yes	500	No	No	Yes	Yes	Gilbert W. Kliman, M.D., Editor-in-Chief Psychological Trauma Center Preventive Psychiatry Associates Medical Group, Inc. 1010 Sir Francis Drake Blvd. Kentfield, CA 94904	Publishes "operationalized approaches to the prevention of mental disorders, especially reports of interventions that can be replicated. Theoretical views of how psychopathology can be averted are welcome. . . . Points of departure for preventive work published in this journal may include data from psychoanalytic, biochemical, behavioral, family, group, network, and large group studies."

Journal	Date established	How often published	Affiliated organization	Peer reviewed	Circulation	Where indexed[b]				Where to send manuscripts	Types of papers
						HLI	IM	PA	EM		
Journal of Psychiatric Research	1961	Quarterly	—	Yes	—	No	Yes	Yes	Yes	John F. Greden, M.D., and Florian Holsboer, M.D., Ph.D., Editors-in-Chief Dept. of Psychiatry University of Michigan 1500 E. Medical Center Drive, B2964/0704 Ann Arbor, MI 48109-0704 (313) 763-9629	"Includes clinical and basic studies (with special emphasis on neuropsychopharmacology, neuroendocrinology, neuroimmunology, electrophysiology, genetics, experimental psychology, and epidemiology), laboratory markers in psychiatry, and those 'interface' studies that link preclinical and clinical neurosciences areas."
Journal of Psychiatry and Law	1973	Quarterly	—	No	1,500	No	No	Yes	Yes	Dianne Nashel, Managing Editor 149 Oak St. Tenafly, NJ 07670 (201) 569-5332	—[c]
Journal of Psychiatry & Neuroscience	1976	5 times/year	Canadian College of Neuropsychopharmacology	Yes	5,000	Yes	Yes	No	No	Y.D. Lapierre, M.D., Editor-in-Chief 237 Argyle Ave., Suite 200 Ottawa, Ontario K2P 1B8, Canada (613) 234-2815	Publishes "original research articles and review papers in clinical psychiatry (adult and child) and neuroscience which relate to major psychiatric disorders and neurodegenerative diseases."
Journal of Psychotherapy Practice and Research	1992	Quarterly	—	Yes	4,048	No	No	No	No	Jerald Kay, M.D., Editor American Psychiatric Press, Inc. 1400 K St., NW Washington, DC 20005 (202) 682-6310	Publishes "review articles; book reviews; and letters."

Journal	Year	Frequency	Affiliation		Circulation				Editor	Description
Journal of Studies on Alcohol	1940	Bimonthly	Center of Alcohol Studies, Rutgers University	Yes	3,000	Yes	Yes	Yes	John A. Carpenter, Ph.D., Interim Editor Rutgers Center of Alcohol Studies Smithers Hall—Busch Campus New Brunswick, NJ 08903 (908) 932–3510	Publishes "original research reports that contribute significantly to fundamental knowledge about alcohol, its use and misuse, and its biochemical, behavioral and sociocultural effects."
Journal of Substance Abuse Treatment	1984	Bimonthly	North Shore University Hospital–Cornell University Medical College	Yes	—	Yes	Yes	Yes	John E. Imhof, Ph.D., Editor-in-Chief Division of Addiction Treatment Services Dept. of Psychiatry North Shore University Hospital—Cornell Medical College 400 Community Drive Manhasset, NY 11030 (516) 562–3008	Publishes "original contributions and articles on the clinical treatment of substance abuse and alcoholism. . . . Articles submitted for publication should address techniques and treatment approaches directly utilized in the provision of clinical services, with the goal of helping the frontline practitioner to deal more effectively with this patient population."
Journal of the American Academy of Child and Adolescent Psychiatry	1962	Bimonthly	American Academy of Child and Adolescent Psychiatry	Yes	6,200	Yes	Yes	Yes	John F. McDermott Jr., M.D., Editor University of Hawaii School of Medicine at Kapiolani Medical Center 1319 Punahou St., Rm. 633 Honolulu, HI 96826–1032 (808) 949–8164	Publishes "manuscripts from a variety of viewpoints, including genetic, epidemiological, neurobiological, cognitive, behavioral, and psychodynamic. Studies of diagnostic reliability and validity as well as psychotherapeutic and psychopharmacological treatment efficacy are encouraged."

Journal	Date established	How often published	Affiliated organization	Peer reviewed	Circulation	Where indexed[b] HLI	IM	PA	EM	Where to send manuscripts	Types of papers
Journal of the American Academy of Psychoanalysis	1973	Quarterly	American Academy of Psychoanalysis	Yes	1,800	Yes	Yes	Yes	Yes	Jules R. Bemporad, M.D., Editor 47 East 19th St., 6th Floor New York, NY 10003 (212) 475-7980	—[c]
Journal of the American Geriatrics Society	1953	Monthly	American Geriatrics Society	Yes	9,300	Yes	Yes	Yes	Yes	Cynthia J.T. Clendenin, Managing Editor 66 North Pauline, Suite 232 Memphis, TN 38105 (901) 448-5567	Publishes "articles that are relevant in the broadest terms to the clinical care of older persons. Such articles may span a variety of disciplines and fields and may be of immediate, intermediate, or long-term potential benefit to clinical practice."
Journal of the American Medical Women's Association	1915	Bimonthly	American Medical Women's Association	Yes	11,000	Yes	Yes	No	No	Kathryn E. McGoldrick, M.D., Editor-in-Chief 186 Fairway Drive Stamford, CT 06903 (802) 878-6887	Publishes "scholarly articles dealing with professional issues facing women in medicine today. Feature articles cover a wide range of subjects and formats and might focus on personal issues, describe alternatives in health care, or interview a woman physician of interest. The Journal also provides a place for women to publish their medical research focusing on women's health care."

Journal	Year	Frequency	Sponsor		Circulation					Editor/Address	Description
Journal of the American Psychoanalytic Association	1953	Quarterly	American Psychoanalytic Association	Yes	2,000	Yes	Yes	Yes	Yes	Arnold D. Richards, M.D., Editor 309 East 49th St. New York, NY 10017 (212) 752-0450	—c
Journal of the History of the Behavioral Sciences	1965	Quarterly	—	Yes	1,000	Yes	Yes	Yes	No	Barbara Ross, Editor Psychology Dept. University of Massachusetts Boston, MA 02125-3393 (617) 287-6366	—c
Journal of the National Medical Association	1908	Monthly	National Medical Association	Yes	25,407	Yes	Yes	No	Yes	Calvin C. Sampson, M.D., Editor 1012 Tenth St., NW Washington, DC 20001 (202) 347-1895, ext. 19	Publishes articles dealing with "specialized clinical research activities related to the health problems of blacks and other minority groups in the inner cities. Special emphasis is placed on the application of medical science to improve the health care of blacks both in the United States and abroad."
Journal of the Royal Society of Medicine	1907	Monthly	Royal Society of Medicine	Yes	19,000	Yes	Yes	No	Yes	A. J. Harding Rains, Editor 1 Wimpole St. London W1M 8AE, UK 071-408-2119	—c
Lancet (North American Edition)	1823	Weekly	—	Yes	15,000	Yes	Yes	No	Yes	Robin Fox, MB, FRCPE, Editor 42 Bedford Square London WC1B 3SL, UK 071-436-4981	Publishes "any contribution that advances or illuminates medical science and practice; our territory extends to all aspects of human health."

Journal	Date established	How often published	Affiliated organization	Peer reviewed	Circulation	Where indexed[b] HLI	IM	PA	EM	Where to send manuscripts	Types of papers
Law and Human Behavior	1977	Bimonthly	American Psychology-Law Society/Division 41 of the American Psychological Association	Yes	—	No	No	Yes	Yes	Prof. Ronald Roesch, Editor 936 Peace Portal Drive PO Box 8014-153 Blaine, WA 98230 (604) 291-3370 or (604)-291-3354	Publishes "articles and discussions of issues arising out of the relationship between human behavior and the law, legal system, and legal process. The journal encourages submissions from people in the fields of law and psychology, and the related disciplines of sociology, criminology, psychiatry, political science, anthropology, philosophy, history, economics, communication, and other appropriate disciplines."
Law, Medicine, & Health Care	1973	Quarterly	American Society of Law & Medicine	—	9,000	Yes	No	No	No	Merrill Kaitz, Managing Editor 765 Commonwealth Ave. Boston, MA 02215 (617) 262-4990	Publishes "high-quality essays that critically examine major issues at the intersection of law, ethics, and policy in medicine and health care, including nursing. Submissions with the best chance of success will be vigorous, significant, well researched, and well written."

Journal	Founded	Frequency	Sponsor		Circulation				Editor/Address	Description
Mental Retardation	1963	Bimonthly	American Association on Mental Retardation	Yes	12,000	Yes	Yes	Yes	Steven J. Taylor, Editor Center on Human Policy School of Education Syracuse University 200 Huntington Hall Syracuse, NY 13244-2340	"New teaching approaches, administrative tools, program evaluation studies, new program developments, service utilization studies, community surveys, public policy issues, training studies, and case studies are welcome, as are research studies that emphasize the application of new methods. . . . State-of-the-art papers and philosophical essays are also welcome if they are well-expressed and well-documented."
Nature	1869	Weekly	—	Yes	40,000	Yes	Yes	Yes	John Maddux, Editor Macmillan Journals, Ltd. 65 Bleecker St. New York, NY 10021 (212) 477-9600	"Offering news, opinion, correspondence and original research reports."
Neuropsychiatric Genetics: A Section of the American Journal of Medical Genetics	1993	—	—	Yes	—	No	No	No	Ming T. Tsuang, M.D., Ph.D., Section Editor 1280-A Belmont St., Suite 192 Brockton, MA 02401 (508) 583-4500, ext. 729	Publishes research articles ("reports of novel research on the genetic mechanisms underlying psychiatric and neurological disorders"), review articles ("review a specific field through an appropriate literature survey"), and brief research communications ("report preliminary data or ongoing work").

Journal	Date established	How often published	Affiliated organization	Peer reviewed	Circulation	Where indexed[b] HLI	IM	PA	EM	Where to send manuscripts	Types of papers
Neuropsycho-pharmacology	1987	8 times/year	American College of Neuropsycho-pharmacology	Yes	—	No	Yes	Yes	No	Herbert Y. Meltzer, M.D., Editor Dept. of Psychiatry Case Western Reserve University 2074 Abington Rd. Cleveland, OH 44106 Roland D. Ciaranello, M.D., Editor Stanford Medical Center, Room 5253B Stanford, CA 94305	"Focuses on clinical and basic science contributions to the field, encompassing biological and psychological sciences relevant to the effects of centrally acting agents. Regular topics include the effects of these agents and the molecular, cellular, physiological, and psychological bases of their actions."
New England Journal of Medicine	1812	Weekly	Massachusetts Medical Society	Yes	225,000	Yes	Yes	Yes	Yes	Jerome D. Kassirer, M.D., Editor-in-Chief 10 Shattuck St. Boston, MA 02115–6094 (617) 734–9800	—[c]
New Trends in Experimental and Clinical Psychiatry	1985	Quarterly	—	—	—	No	No	Yes	Yes	Prof. Giordano Invernizzi Institute of Psychiatry Policlinico–Pad. Guardia 2 Via Francesco Sforza 35 20122, Milan, Italy Fax: 02–55013070	Publishes "two sections, the first dedicated to original articles of a traditional nature and the second to brief reports not exceeding 5 pages. In this section, authors will have the opportunity to publish preliminary or partial research results of scientific interest or which represent important new techniques or findings in scientific research. . . . The journal will accept original articles and short commu-

Occupational Therapy in Mental Health	1980	Quarterly	—	—	725	No	No	Yes	Diane Gibson, Editor Activity Therapy Sheppard & Enoch Pratt Hospital PO Box 6815 Towson, MD 21204	nications in camera-ready format. Reviews will be accepted only if they give a new contribution to knowledge of the specific field."
										—^c
Perspectives in Psychiatric Care	1963	Quarterly	—	No	5,000	No	No	Yes	Norine Kerr, R.N., Ph.D., Editor 1521 SW 24th St. Topeka, KS 66611 (913) 234-6439	Invites "original articles on clinical practice, education, research, and administration. . . . for nurses whose goal is to influence the standards and goals of psychiatric nursing."
Psychiatric Bulletin of the Royal College of Psychiatrists	1977	Monthly	Royal College of Psychiatrists	—	7,000	No	No	No	Dr. Alan Kerr, Editor 17 Belgrave Square London SW1X 8PG, UK 071-408-2119	Publishes "articles of a general interest to psychiatrists. . . . Concentrates on provision of services to people with mental disorders, and psychiatric training."
Psychiatric Forum	1969	Semi-annually	William S. Hall Psychiatric Institute of the South Carolina Dept. of Mental Health	—	4,000	No	Yes	No	Lucius C. Pressley, M.D., Editor PO Box 202 Hall Psychiatric Institute Columbia, SC 29202 (803) 734-7154	Publishes "papers related to neuropsychiatry."

Journal	Date established	How often published	Affiliated organization	Peer reviewed	Circulation	Where indexed[b] HLI	IM	PA	EM	Where to send manuscripts	Types of papers
Psychiatric Genetics	1990	Quarterly	International Society of Psychiatric Genetics	Yes	500	No	Yes	No	Yes	John I. Nurnberger Jr., M.D., Ph.D., Editor Institute of Psychiatric Research 791 Union Drive Indiana University Medical Center Indianapolis, IN 46202 (317) 274-8382	Publishes "original research reports dealing with inherited factors involved in psychiatric and neurological disorders. . . . [It] is also a forum for reporting new approaches to neurogenetic research utilizing novel techniques or methodologies. The journal aims to publish papers which bring together clinical observations, psychological and behavioural abnormalities and genetic data."
Psychiatric Hospital	1969	Quarterly	National Association of Private Psychiatric Hospitals	Yes	8,500	Yes	No	Yes	Yes	Frieda Eastmann, Managing Editor 1319 F St., NW, Suite 1000 Washington, DC 20004-1154 (202) 393-6700	Publishes "clinical and research papers, review articles, and evaluative studies as well as innovative treatment-program reports and reports on administrative, management, legal, economic, and other issues that affect private psychiatric hospital operation and, consequently, patient care."
Psychiatric Medicine	1983	Quarterly	—	Yes	500	Yes	Yes	Yes	No	Richard C.W. Hall, M.D., Editor-in-Chief Center for Psychiatry Florida Hospital 601 East Rollins St. Orlando, FL 32803 (407) 897-1801	—[c]

Journal	Year	Frequency	Sponsor		Circulation				Editor / Address	Description
Psychiatric Quarterly	1927	Quarterly	—	Yes	535	Yes	Yes	Yes	Stephen Rachlin, M.D., Editor-in-Chief, Dept. of Psychiatry and Psychology, Nassau County Medical Center, 2201 Hempstead Turnpike, East Meadow, NY 11554, (516) 542-0123	Publishes "original papers on care in private and public hospitals, schools, correctional facilities, etc. Care is discussed in its broadest sense, and the journal publishes papers related to any treatment of emotional disorders, including studies of other factors that influence such care, such as ecological and social factors and staff attitudes."
Psychiatric Services (formerly Hospital and Community Psychiatry)	1950	Monthly	American Psychiatric Association	Yes	23,247	Yes	Yes	Yes	John A. Talbott, M.D., Editor, 1400 K St., NW, Washington, DC 20005, (202) 682-6070	Publishes articles dealing with "all aspects of psychiatric service delivery. The journal publishes clinical and research papers, review articles, commentary, and reports on legal, judicial, and economic issues."
Psychiatry: Interpersonal and Biological Processes	1938	Quarterly	Washington School of Psychiatry	Yes	2,100	Yes	Yes	Yes	David Reiss, M.D., Editor, Dept. of Psychiatry and Behavioral Sciences, George Washington University Medical Center, 2300 Eye St., NW, Washington, DC 20037, (202) 994-2636	"Designed to present the highest quality quantitative research, vivid reports of qualitative data, illustrative case reports and clinical studies, synthetic theoretical essays, accounts of scientific meetings and colloquia, surveys and critiques of scientific literature, and reviews and commentary on published work. Focused on contributions that foster a thoughtful integration of biological and interpersonal reasoning."

Journal	Date established	How often published	Affiliated organization	Peer reviewed	Circulation	Where indexed[b] HLI	IM	PA	EM	Where to send manuscripts	Types of papers
Psychiatry Research and *Psychiatry Research: Neuroimaging*	1979	16 times/ year	—	Yes	—	Yes	Yes	Yes	Yes	Monte S. Buchsbaum, M.D., Editor-in-Chief Mount Sinai School of Medicine One Gustave L. Levy Place New York, NY 10029-6574	Provides "very rapid publication of short but complete reports in the field of psychiatry.... Encompasses: (1) biochemical, physiological, genetic, psychological, and social determinants of human behavior; (2) assessment of human behavior and subjective state; (3) evaluation of somatic and nonsomatic psychiatric treatments. In addition, reports of clinically related basic studies in the fields of neuropharmacology, neurochemistry, neuroendocrinology, electrophysiology, psychology, genetics, and brain imaging will be published. Significant methodological advances such as instrumentation, clinical scales, and assays directly applicable to psychiatric research will also be appropriate."

Journal	Year	Frequency	Affiliation		Circulation					Editor/Address		Description
Psychoanalytic Quarterly	1932	Quarterly	—	Yes	4,124	Yes	Yes	Yes	Yes	Owen Renik, M.D., Editor Room 517, 175 Fifth Ave. New York, NY 10010–7799 (212) 982–9358	— [c]	
Psychoanalytic Study of the Child	1945	Annually	—	Yes	8,000	No	Yes	Yes	Yes	Albert J. Solnit, M.D., Managing Editor Yale Child Study Center PO Box 3333 New Haven, CT 06510 (203) 785–2518	— [c]	
Psychological Medicine: A Journal for Research in Psychiatry and the Allied Sciences	1970	Quarterly	—	Yes	3,000	Yes	Yes	Yes	Yes	Prof. Eugene Paykel Dept. of Psychiatry University of Cambridge Addenbrooke's Hospital Cambridge, CB2 2QQ UK		Publishes "original research in clinical psychiatry and the basic sciences related to it. These comprise not only the several fields of biological enquiry traditionally associated with medicine but also the various psychological and social sciences."
Psychological Record	1937	Quarterly	Kenyon College	—	1,450	No	No	Yes	No	Charles E. Rice, Editor Kenyon College Gambier, OH 43022 (614) 427–5377		Publishes "theoretical and experimental articles and commentary on current developments. Papers that develop new methods are favored."
Psychoneuroendocrinology	1975	8 times/ year	—	Yes	1,000	No	Yes	Yes	Yes	Robert T. Rubin, M.D., Editor Harbor-UCLA Medical Center 1000 West Carson St. Torrance, CA 90509		Publishes "clinical research articles as well as more basic studies in the field."

Journal	Date established	How often published	Affiliated organization	Peer reviewed	Circulation	Where indexed[b] HLI	IM	PA	EM	Where to send manuscripts	Types of papers
Psychosomatic Medicine	1938	Bimonthly	American Psychosomatic Society	Yes	2,571	No	Yes	No	Yes	Joel E. Dimsdale, M.D., Editor-in-Chief University of California, San Diego 9500 Gilman Drive La Jolla, CA 92093-0804 (619) 543-5468	Publishes "original research articles, reviews, and case reports."
Psychosomatics: The Journal of Consultation and Liaison Psychiatry	1960	Quarterly	Academy of Psychosomatic Medicine	Yes	3,203	Yes	Yes	Yes	Yes	Thomas N. Wise, M.D., Editor-in-Chief American Psychiatric Press, Inc. 1400 K St., NW Washington, DC 20005 (202) 682-6336	"Criteria for publication include scientific merit, interest to clinicians, and pertinence to clinical psychiatry and to the interrelationship of psychiatry and medical practice."
Schizophrenia Bulletin	1969	Quarterly	National Institute of Mental Health	Yes	4,700	No	Yes	Yes	Yes	David Shore, M.D., Editor-in-Chief NIMH 5600 Fishers Lane, Rm. 18C-06 Rockville, MD 20857	Publishes "critical reviews of the literature, articles reporting original observations in laboratory or clinical research, short reports of preliminary or negative research results, first person accounts by patients or family members, and letters to the editors. News items describing research and training programs or reporting professional activities in schizophrenia are also welcome."

Journal	Year founded	Frequency	Publisher		Circulation					Editor	Scope
Schizophrenia Research	1991	9 times/ year	—	Yes	—	No	Yes	Yes	Yes	Prof. H.A. Nasrallah, Co-Editor, Dept. of Psychiatry, OSU College of Medicine, 473 West 12th Ave., Columbus, OH 43210–1228, (614) 293-8283 (papers from the Americas); Dr. L.E. DeLisi, Co-Editor, Dept. of Psychiatry, School of Medicine, Health Sciences Center, SUNY, Stony Brook, NY 11794 (papers not from the Americas)	Provides "rapid publication of new international research that contributes to the understanding of schizophrenic disorders. It is hoped that this journal will aid in bringing together previously separated biological, and psychological clinical research on this disorder, and stimulate the synthesis of these data into cohesive hypotheses."
Science	1880	Weekly	American Association for the Advancement of Science	Yes	154,000	Yes	Yes	Yes	Yes	Daniel E. Koshland Jr., Editor-in-Chief, 1333 H St., NW, Washington, DC 20005, (202) 326-6501	—[c]

[a] When the journal was not available or information was not given in the journal, *The Serials Directory: An International Reference Book*, 7th ed., 1993, vols. I–III, published by EBSCO Publishing Co., Birmingham, Alabama, was used.

[b] Only four indexes were considered: Hospital Literature Index (HLI), Index Medicus (IM), Psychological Abstracts (PA), and the Psychiatry Section of Excerpta Medica (EM). In many cases, the journal is listed in other indexes as well. Journals listed in Index Medicus, Psychological Abstracts, and Excerpta Medica are available in the online versions of these indexes (MEDLINE, PSYCINFO, and EMBASE).

[c] Journal does not print a statement regarding the types of papers it publishes.

Source. Prepared by Laura M. Little, *American Journal of Psychiatry*, and Sandy Ferris, APA Office of Research, April 1994.

Resources 9–2
Uniform Requirements for Manuscripts Submitted to Biomedical Journals

International Committee of Medical Journal Editors

A small group of editors of general medical journals met informally in Vancouver, British Columbia, in January 1978 to establish guidelines for the format of manuscripts submitted to their journals. The group, now expanded and known as the International Committee of Medical Journal Editors (also known as the Vancouver Group), has met annually since then and its concerns have broadened. The committee has produced four editions of the Uniform Requirements for Manuscripts Submitted to Biomedical Journals; *this fourth edition was revised slightly in January 1993. During discussions of manuscript requirements, questions have been raised about other issues surrounding publication, especially ethics. Some of these concerns are now covered in the* Uniform Requirements; *others are addressed in separate statements issued by the committee. The total content of this communication may be reproduced for educational, not-for-profit purposes without regard for copyright; the committee encourages distribution of the material, which we hope will be useful. Journals that agree to use the* Uniform Requirements *are asked to cite the document in their instructions to authors.*

Journals currently represented on the International Committee are *Annals of Internal Medicine, British Medical Journal, Canadian Medical Association Journal, The Journal of the American Medical Association, The Lancet, The Medical Journal of Australia, The New England Journal of Medicine, New Zealand Medical Journal, Tidsskrift for Den Norske Laegeforening, The Western Journal of Medicine,* and *Index Medicus.*

Inquiries and comments should be sent to Kathleen Case, Secretariat Office, *Annals of Internal Medicine,* Independence Mall West, Sixth Street at Race, Philadelphia, PA 19106-1572.

Single copies of *Uniform Requirements for Manuscripts Submitted to Biomedical Journals* are available free of charge from the Secretariat Office. The telephone number is (800) 523-1546, extension 2631. Prices for purchases of 10 or more copies are available from the Secretariat Office.

The editors of some major biomedical journals published in English decided on uniform technical requirements for manuscripts to be submitted to their journals. These requirements, including formats for bibliographic references developed for the Vancouver Group by the National Library of Medicine, were published in 1979. The Vancouver Group evolved into the International Committee of Medical Journal Editors. Over the years, the group has revised the requirements slightly.

Close to 500 journals have agreed to receive manuscripts prepared in accordance with the requirements. It is important to emphasize what these requirements imply and what they do not.

First, the requirements are instructions to authors on how to prepare manuscripts, not to editors on publication style. (But many journals have drawn on these requirements for elements of their publication styles.)

Second, if authors prepare their manuscripts in the style specified in these requirements, editors of the participating journals will not return manuscripts for changes in style before considering them for publication. Even so, in the publishing process journals may alter accepted manuscripts to conform with details of the journal's publication style.

Third, authors sending manuscripts to a participating journal should not try to prepare them in accordance with the publication style of that journal but should follow the *Uniform Requirements for Manuscripts Submitted to Biomedical Journals*.

Authors must also follow the instructions to authors in the journal as to what topics are suitable for that journal and the types of papers that may be submitted—for example, original articles, reviews, or case reports. In addition, the journal's instructions are likely to contain other requirements unique to that journal, such as number of copies of manuscripts, acceptable languages, length of articles, and approved abbreviations.

Participating journals are expected to state in their instructions to authors that their requirements are in accordance with the *Uniform Requirements for Manuscripts Submitted to Biomedical Journals* and to cite a published version. This document will be revised at intervals.

◆ Summary of Requirements

Type the manuscript double-spaced, including title page, abstract, text, acknowledgments, references, tables, and legends.

Each manuscript component should begin on a new page, in the following sequence: title page, abstract and key words, text, acknowledgments, references, tables (each table complete with title and footnotes on a separate page), and legends for illustrations.

Illustrations must be good-quality, unmounted glossy prints, usually 127 × 173 mm (5 × 7 in), but no larger than 203 × 254 mm (8 × 10 in).

Submit the required number of copies of manuscripts and illustrations (see journal's instructions) in a heavy paper envelope. The submitted manuscript should be accompanied by a covering letter, as described under "Submission of Manuscripts," and permissions to reproduce previously published material or to use illustrations that may identify human subjects.

Follow the journal's instructions for transfer of copyright. Authors should keep copies of everything submitted.

◆ Prior and Duplicate Publication

Most journals do not wish to consider for publication a paper on work that has already been reported in a published article or is described in a paper submitted or accepted for publication elsewhere, in print or in electronic media. This policy does not usually preclude consideration of a paper that has been rejected by another journal or of a complete report that follows publication of a preliminary report, usually in the form of an abstract. Nor does it prevent consideration of a paper that has been presented at a scientific meeting, if not published in full in a proceedings or similar publication. Press reports of the meeting will not usually be considered as breaches of this rule, but such reports should not be amplified by additional data or copies of tables and illustrations. When submitting a paper, an author should always make a full statement to the editor about all submissions and previous reports that might be regarded as prior or duplicate publication of the same or very similar work. Copies of such material should be included with the submitted paper to help the editor decide how to deal with the matter.

Multiple publication—that is, the publication more than once of the same study, irrespective of whether the wording is the same—is rarely justified. Secondary publication in another language is one possible justification, providing the following conditions are met.

1. The editors of both journals concerned are fully informed; the editor concerned with secondary publication should have a photocopy, reprint, or manuscript of the primary version.
2. The priority of the primary publication is respected by a publication interval of at least 2 weeks.
3. The paper for secondary publication is written for a different group of readers and is not simply a translated version of the primary paper; an abbreviated version will often be sufficient.
4. The secondary version reflects faithfully the data and interpretations of the primary version.
5. A footnote on the title page of the secondary version informs readers, peers, and documenting agencies that the paper was edited, and is being published, for a national audience in parallel with a primary version based on the same data and interpretations. A suitable footnote might read as follows: "This article is based on a study first reported in the [title of journal, with full reference]."

Multiple publication other than as defined above is not acceptable to editors. If authors violate this rule, they may expect appropriate editorial action to be taken.

Preliminary release, usually to public media, of scientific information described in a paper that has been accepted but not yet published is a violation of the policies of many journals. In a few cases, and only by arrangement with the editor, preliminary release of data may be acceptable—for example, to warn the public of health hazards.

◆ Preparation of Manuscript

Type or print out the manuscript on white bond paper, 216×279 mm (8.5×11 in), or ISO A4 (212×297 mm), with margins of at least 25 mm (1 in). Type or print on only one side of the paper. Use double-spacing throughout, including title page, abstract, text, acknowledgments, references, individual tables, and legends. Number pages consecutively, beginning with the title page. Put the page number in the upper or lower right-hand corner of each page.

Title Page

The title page should carry (a) the title of the article, which should be concise but informative; (b) first name, middle initial, and last name of each author, with highest academic degree(s) and institutional affiliations; (c) name of department(s) and institution(s) to which the work should be attributed; (d) disclaimers, if any; (e) name and address of author responsible for correspondence about the manuscript; (f) name and address of author to whom requests for reprints should be addressed or statement that reprints will not be available from the author; (g) source(s) of support in the form of grants, equipment, drugs, or all of these; and (h) a short running head or foot line of no more than 40 characters (count letters and spaces) placed at the foot of the title page and identified.

Authorship

All persons designated as authors should qualify for authorship. The order of authorship should be a joint decision of the coauthors. Each author should have participated sufficiently in the work to take public responsibility for the content.

Authorship credit should be based only on substantial contributions to (a) conception and design, or analysis and interpretation of data; and to (b) drafting the article or revising it critically for important intellectual content; and on (c) final approval of the version to be published. Conditions (a), (b), and (c) must all be met. Participation solely in the acquisition of funding or the collection of data does not justify authorship. General supervision of the research group is not sufficient for authorship. Any part of an article critical to its main conclusions must be the responsibility of at least one author.

Editors may require authors to justify the assignment of authorship.

Increasingly, multicenter trials are attributed to a corporate author. All members of the group who are named as authors, either in the authorship position below the title or in a footnote, should fully meet the criteria for authorship as defined in the *Uniform Requirements*. Group members who do not meet these criteria should be listed, with their permission, under acknowledgments or in an appendix (see "Acknowledgments").

Abstract and Key Words

The second page should carry an abstract (of no more than 150 words for unstructured abstracts or 250 words for structured abstracts). The abstract should state the purposes of the study or investigation, basic procedures (selection of study subjects or laboratory animals; observational and analytical methods), main findings (give specific data and their statistical significance, if possible), and the principal conclusions. Emphasize new and important aspects of the study or observations.

Below the abstract provide, and identify as such, three to 10 key words or short phrases that will assist indexers in cross-indexing the article and may be published with the abstract. Use terms from the Medical Subject Headings (MeSH) list of *Index Medicus*; if suitable MeSH terms are not yet available for recently introduced terms, present terms may be used.

Text

The text of observational and experimental articles is usually—but not necessarily—divided into sections with the headings Introduction, Methods, Results, and Discussion. Long articles may need subheadings within some sections to clarify their content, especially the Results and Discussion sections. Other types of articles such as case reports, reviews, and editorials are likely to need other formats. Authors should consult individual journals for further guidance.

Introduction.   State the purpose of the article. Summarize the rationale for the study or observation. Give only strictly pertinent references, and do not review the article extensively. Do not include data or conclusions from the work being reported.

Methods.   Describe your selection of the observational or experimental subjects (patients or laboratory animals, including controls) clearly. Identify the methods, apparatus (manufacturer's name and address in parentheses), and procedures in sufficient detail to allow other workers to reproduce the results. Give references to established methods, including statistical methods (see below): provide references and brief descriptions for methods that have been published but are not well known; describe new or substantially modified methods, give reasons for using them, and evaluate their limitations. Identify precisely all drugs and chemicals used, including generic name(s), dose(s), and route(s) of administration.

Ethics. When reporting experiments on human subjects, indicate whether the procedures followed were in accordance with the ethical standards of the responsible committee on human experimentation (institutional or regional) or with the Helsinki Declaration of 1975, as revised in 1983. Do not use patients' names, initials, or hospital numbers, especially in illustrative material. When reporting experiments on animals, indicate whether the institution's or the National Research Council's guide for, or any national law on, the care and use of laboratory animals was followed.

Statistics. Describe statistical methods with enough detail to enable a knowledgeable reader with access to the original data to verify the reported results. When possible, quantify findings and present them with appropriate indicators of measurement error or uncertainty (such as confidence intervals). Avoid sole reliance on statistical hypothesis testing, such as the use of P values, which fails to convey important quantitative information. Discuss eligibility of experimental subjects. Give details about randomization. Describe the methods for and success of any blinding of observations. Report treatment complications. Give numbers of observations. Report losses to observation (such as dropouts from a clinical trial). References for study design and statistical methods should be to standard works (with pages stated) when possible rather than to papers in which the designs or methods were originally reported. Specify any general-use computer programs used.

Put general description of methods in the Methods section. When data are summarized in the Results section, specify the statistical methods used to analyze them. Restrict tables and figures to those needed to explain the argument of the paper and to assess its support. Use graphs as an alternative to tables with many entries; do not duplicate data in graphs and tables. Avoid nontechnical uses of technical terms in statistics, such as "random" (which implies a randomizing device), "normal," "significant," "correlations," and "sample." Define statistical terms, abbreviations, and most symbols.

Results. Present results in logical sequence in the text, tables, and illustrations. Do not repeat in the text all the data in the tables or illustrations; emphasize or summarize only important observations.

Discussion. Emphasize the new and important aspects of the study and the conclusions that follow from them. Do not repeat in detail data or other material given in the Introduction or the Results section. Include in the Discussion section the implications of the findings and their limitations, including implications for future research. Relate the observations to other relevant studies. Link the conclusions with the goals of the study but avoid unqualified statements and conclusions not completely supported by your data. Avoid claiming priority and alluding to work that has not been completed. State new hypotheses when warranted, but clearly label them as such. Recommendations, when appropriate, may be included.

Acknowledgments

At an appropriate place in the article (title-page footnote or appendix to the text; see the journal's requirements) one or more statements should specify (a) contributions that need acknowledging but do not justify authorship, such as general support by a departmental chair; (b) acknowledgments of technical help; (c) acknowledgments of financial and material support, specifying the nature of the support; (d) financial relationships that may pose a conflict of interest.

Persons who have contributed intellectually to the paper but whose contributions do not justify authorship may be named and their function or contribution described—for example, "scientific adviser," "critical review of study proposal," "data collection," or "participation in clinical trial." Such persons must have given their permission to be named. Authors are responsible for obtaining written permission from persons acknowledged by name, because readers may infer their endorsement of the data and conclusions.

Technical help should be acknowledged in a paragraph separate from those acknowledging other contributions.

References

Number references consecutively in the order in which they are first mentioned in the text. Identify references in text, tables, and legends by Arabic numerals in parentheses. References cited only in tables or in legends to figures should be numbered in accordance with a sequence established by the first identification in the text of the particular table or figure.

Use the style of the examples below, which are based with slight modifications on the formats used by the US National Library of Medicine in *Index Medicus*. The titles of journals should be abbreviated according to the style used in *Index Medicus*. Consult *List of Journals Indexed in Index Medicus* published annually as a separate publication by the library and as a list in the January issue of *Index Medicus*.

Try to avoid using abstracts as references; "unpublished observations" and "personal communications" may not be used as references, although references to written, not oral, communications may be inserted (in parentheses) in the text. Include in the references papers accepted but not yet published; designate the journal and add "In press." Information from manuscripts submitted but not yet accepted should be cited in the text as "unpublished observations" (in parentheses).

The references must be verified by the author(s) against the original documents.

Examples of correct forms of references are given below.

Articles in Journals

1. Standard journal article (list all authors, but if the number exceeds six, give six followed by et al.):

    You CH, Lee KY, Chey RY, Menguy R. Electrogastrographic study of patients with unexplained nausea, bloating and vomiting. Gastroenterology 1980 Aug;79(2):311–4.

    As an option, if a journal carries continuous pagination throughout a volume, the month and issue number may be omitted:

    You CH, Lee KY, Chey RY, Menguy R. Electrogastrographic study of patients with unexplained nausea, bloating and vomiting. Gastroenterology 1980;79:311–4.

    Goate AM, Haynes AR, Owen MJ, Farrall M, James LA, Lai LY, et al. Predisposing locus for Alzheimer's disease on chromosome 21. Lancet 1989:1:352–5.

2. Organization as author:

    The Royal Marsden Hospital Bone-Marrow Transplantation Team. Failure of syngeneic bone-marrow graft without preconditioning in post-hepatitis marrow aplasia. Lancet 1977;2:742–4.

3. No author given:

    Coffee drinking and cancer of the pancreas [editorial]. BMJ 1981; 283:628.

4. Article not in English:

Massone L, Borghi S, Pestarino A, Piccini R, Gambini C. Localisations palmaires purpuriques de la dermatite herpetiforme. Ann Dermatol Venereol 1987;114:1545–7.

5. Volume with supplement:

Magni F, Rossoni G, Berti F. BN-52021 protects guinea-pig from heart anaphylaxis. Pharmacol Res Commun 1988;20 Suppl 5:75–8.

6. Issue with supplement:

Gardos G, Cole JO, Haskell D, Marby D, Paine SS, Moore P. The natural history of tardive dyskinesia. J Clin Psychopharmacol 1988;8(4 Suppl):31S–37S.

7. Volume with part:

Hanly C. Metaphysics and innateness: a psycho-analytic perspective. Int J Psychoanal 1988;69(Pt 3):389–99.

8. Issue with part:

Edwards L, Meyskens F, Levine N. Effect of oral isotretinoin on dysplastic nevi. J Am Acad Dermatol 1989;20(2 Pt 1):257–60.

9. Issue with no volume:

Baumeister AA. Origins and control of stereotyped movements. Monogr Am Assoc Ment Defic 1978;(3):353–84.

10. No issue or volume:

Danoek K: Skiing in and through the history of medicine. Nord Medicinhist Arsb 1982:86–100.

11. Pagination in Roman numerals:

Ronne Y. Ansvarsfall. Blodtransfusion till fel patient. Vardfacket 1989;13:XXVI–XXVII.

12. Type of article indicated as needed:

Spargo PM, Manners JM. DDAVP and open heart surgery [letter]. Anaesthesia 1989;44:363–4.

Fuhrman SA, Joiner KA. Binding of the third component of complement C3 by Toxoplasma gondii [abstract]. Clin Res 1987;35:475A.

13. Article containing retraction:

    Shishido A. Retraction notice: Effect of platinum compounds on murine lymphocyte mitogenesis [Retraction of Alsabti EA, Ghalib ON, Salem MH. In: Jpn J Med Sci Biol 1979;32:53–65]. Jpn J Med Sci Biol 1980;33:235–7.

14. Article retracted:

    Alsabti EA, Ghalib ON, Salem MH. Effect of platinum compounds on murine lymphocyte mitogenesis [Retracted by Shishido A. In: Jpn J Med Sci Biol 1980;33:235–7]. Jpn J Med Sci Biol 1979;32:53–65.

15. Article containing comment:

    Piccoli A, Bossatti A. Early steroid therapy in IgA neuropathy: still an open question [comment]. Nephron 1989;51:289–91. Comment on: Nephron 1988;48:12–7.

16. Article commented on:

    Kobayashi Y, Fujii K, Hiki Y, Tateno S, Kurokawa A, Kamiyama M. Steroid therapy in IgA nephropathy: a retrospective study in heavy proteinuric cases [see comments]. Nephron 1988;48:12–7. Comment in: Nephron 1989;51:289–91.

17. Article with published erratum:

    Schofield A. The CAGE questionnaire and psychological health [published erratum appears in Br J Addict 1989;84:701]. Br J Addict 1988;83:761–4.

Books and Other Monographs

18. Personal author(s):

    Colson JH, Armour WJ. Sports injuries and their treatment. 2nd rev. ed. London: S. Paul, 1986.

19. Editor(s), compiler as author:

    Diener HC, Wilkinson M, editors. Drug-induced headache. New York: Springer-Verlag, 1988.

20. Organization as author and publisher:

    Virginia Law Foundation. The medical and legal implications of AIDS. Charlottesville: The Foundation, 1987.

21. Chapters in a book:

    Weinstein L, Swartz MN. Pathologic properties of invading micro-organisms. In: Sodeman WA Jr, Sodeman WA, editors. Pathologic physiology: mechanisms of disease. Philadelphia: Saunders, 1974: 457–72.

22. Conference proceedings:

    Vivian VL, editor. Child abuse and neglect: a medical community response. Proceedings of the First AMA National Conference on Child Abuse and Neglect; 1984 Mar 30–31; Chicago. Chicago: American Medical Association, 1985.

23. Conference paper:

    Harley NH. Comparing radon daughter dosimetric and risk models. In: Gammage RB, Kaye SV, editors. Indoor air and human health. Proceedings of the Seventh Life Sciences Symposium; 1984 Oct 29–31; Knoxville (TN). Chelsea (MI): Lewis, 1985:69–78.

24. Scientific or technical report:

    Akutsu T. Total heart replacement device. Bethesda (MD): National Institutes of Health, National Heart and Lung Institute; 1974 Apr. Report No.: NIH-NHLI-69-2185-4.

25. Dissertation:

    Youssef NM. School adjustment of children with congenital heart disease [dissertation]. Pittsburgh (PA): Univ. of Pittsburgh, 1988.

26. Patent:

    Harred JF, Knight AR, McIntyre JS, inventors. Dow Chemical Company, assignee. Epoxidation process. US patent 3,654,317. 1972 Apr 4.

Other Published Material

27. Newspaper article:

    Rensberger B, Specter B. CFCs may be destroyed by natural process. The Washington Post 1989 Aug 7;Sect. A:2 (col. 5).

28. Audiovisual:

    AIDS epidemic: the physician's role [video-recording]. Cleveland (OH): Academy of Medicine of Cleveland, 1987.

29. Computer file:

> Renal system [computer program]. MS–DOS version. Edwardsville (KS): MediSim, 1988.

30. Legal material:

> Toxic Substances Control Act: Hearing on S. 776 Before the Subcomm. on the Environment of the Senate Comm. on Commerce. 94th Cong., 1st Sess. 343 (1975).

31. Map:

> Scotland [topographic map]. Washington: National Geographic Society (US), 1981.

32. Book of the Bible:

> Ruth 3:1–18. The Holy Bible. Authorized King James version. New York: Oxford Univ. Press, 1972.

33. Dictionary and similar references:

> Ectasia. Dorland's illustrated medical dictionary. 27th ed. Philadelphia: Saunders, 1988:527.

34. Classical material:

> The Winter's Tale: act 5, scene 1, lines 13–16. The complete works of William Shakespeare. London: Rex, 1973.

Unpublished Material

35. In press:

> Lillywhite HD, Donald JA. Pulmonary blood flow regulation in an aquatic snake. Science. In press.

Tables

Type or print out each table double-spaced on a separate sheet. Do not submit tables as photographs. Number tables consecutively in the order of their first citation in the text and supply a brief title for each. Give each column a short or abbreviated heading. Place explanatory matter in footnotes, not in the heading. Explain in footnotes all nonstandard abbreviations that are used in each table. For footnotes, use the following symbols, in this sequence: *, †, ‡, §, ‖, ¶, **, ††, ‡‡, ...

Identify statistical measures of variations such as standard deviation and standard error of the mean.

Do not use internal horizontal and vertical rules.

Be sure that each table is cited in the text.

If you use data from another published or unpublished source, obtain permission and acknowledge fully.

The use of too many tables in relation to the length of the text may produce difficulties in the layout of pages. Examine issues of the journal to which you plan to submit your paper to estimate how many tables can be used per 1000 words of text.

The editor, on accepting a paper, may recommend that additional tables containing important backup data too extensive to publish be deposited with an archival service, such as the National Auxiliary Publications Service in the United States, or made available by the authors. In that event an appropriate statement will be added to the text. Submit such tables for consideration with the paper.

Illustrations (Figures)

Submit the required number of complete sets of figures. Figures should be professionally drawn and photographed; freehand or typewritten lettering is unacceptable. Instead of original drawings, roentgenograms, and other material. send sharp, glossy black-and-white photographic prints, usually 127 × 173 mm (5 × 7 in), but no larger than 203 × 254 mm (8 × 10 in). Letters, numbers, and symbols should be clear and even throughout and of sufficient size that, when reduced for publication, each item will still be legible. Titles and detailed explanations belong in the legends for illustrations, not on the illustrations themselves.

Each figure should have a label pasted on its back indicating the number of the figure, author's name, and top of the figure. Do not write on the back of figures or scratch or mar them by using paper clips. Do not bend figures or mount them on cardboard.

Photomicrographs must have internal scale markers. Symbols, arrows, or letters used in the photomicrographs should contrast with the background.

If photographs of persons are used, either the subjects must not be identifiable or their pictures must be accompanied by written permission to use the photograph.

Figures should be numbered consecutively according to the order in which they have been first cited in the text. If a figure has been published, acknowledge the original source and submit written permission from the copyright holder to reproduce the material. Permission is required irrespective of authorship or publisher, except for documents in the public domain.

For illustrations in color, ascertain whether the journal requires color negatives, positive transparencies, or color prints. Accompanying drawings marked to indicate the region to be reproduced may be useful to the editor. Some journals publish illustrations in color only if the author pays for the extra cost.

Legends for Illustrations

Type or print out legends for illustrations double-spaced, starting on a separate page, with Arabic numerals corresponding to the illustrations. When symbols, arrows, numbers, or letters are used to identify parts of the illustrations, identify and explain each one clearly in the legend. Explain the internal scale and identify the method of staining in photomicrographs.

◆ Units of Measurement

Measurements of length, height, weight, and volume should be reported in metric units (meter, kilogram, or liter) or their decimal multiples.

Temperatures should be given in degrees Celsius. Blood pressures should be given in millimeters of mercury.

All hematologic and clinical chemistry measurements should be reported in the metric system in terms of the International System of Units (SI). Editors may request that alternative or non-SI units be added by the authors before publication.

◆ Abbreviations and Symbols

Use only standard abbreviations. Avoid abbreviations in the title and abstract. The full term for which an abbreviation stands should precede its first use in the text unless it is a standard unit of measurement.

◆ Submission of Manuscripts

Mail the required number of manuscript copies in a heavy-paper envelope, enclosing the manuscript copies and figures in cardboard, if necessary, to prevent bending of photographs during mail handling. Place photographs and transparencies in a separate heavy-paper envelope.

Manuscripts must be accompanied by a covering letter signed by all coauthors. This must include (a) information on prior or duplicate publication or submission elsewhere of any part of the work as defined earlier in this document; (b) a statement of financial or other relationships that might lead to a conflict of interest; (c) a statement that the manuscript has been read and approved by all authors, that the requirements for authorship as previously stated in this document have been met, and furthermore, that each coauthor believes that the manuscript represents honest work; and (d) the name, address, and telephone number of the corresponding author, who is responsible for communicating with the other authors about revisions and final approval of the proofs. The letter should give any additional information that may be helpful to the editor, such as the type of article in the particular journal the manuscript represents and whether the author(s) will be willing to meet the cost of reproducing color illustrations.

The manuscript must be accompanied by copies of any permissions to reproduce published material, to use illustrations or report sensitive personal information about identifiable persons, or to name persons for their contributions.

Manuscripts on Diskettes

For papers that are close to final acceptance, some journals require authors to provide manuscripts in electronic form (on diskettes) and may accept a variety of word-processing formats or text (ASCII) files.

When submitting diskettes, authors should:

1. be certain to include a printout of the manuscript version on the diskette;
2. put only the latest version of the manuscript on the diskette;
3. name the file clearly;

4. label the diskette with the file format and the file name;
5. provide information on hardware and software used.

Authors should consult the journal's information for authors for acceptable formats, file- and diskette-naming conventions, number of copies to be submitted, and other details.

◆ Participating Journals

Journals that have notified the International Committee of Medical Journal Editors of their willingness to consider for publication manuscripts prepared in accordance with earlier versions of the committee's *Uniform Requirements* identify themselves as such in their information for authors. A full list is available on request from the Secretariat Office at *Annals of Internal Medicine*.

Resources 9–3
Selected Resources on Scientific Writing and Peer Review

◆ Style and Grammar

American Medical Association: American Medical Association Manual of Style, 8th Edition. Baltimore, MD, Williams & Wilkins, 1989

American Psychological Association: Publication Manual of the American Psychological Association, 3rd Edition. Washington, DC, American Psychological Association, 1983

Council of Biology Editors: CBE Style Manual, 5th Edition. Bethesda, MD, Council of Biology Editors, 1983

Gordon KE: The Transitive Vampire: A Handbook of Grammar for the Innocent, the Eager, and the Doomed. New York, Time Books, 1984

Gordon KE: The Well-Tempered Sentence: a Punctuation Handbook for the Innocent, the Eager, and the Doomed. New Haven, CT, Ticknor & Fields, 1983

Strunk W, White EB: The Elements of Style. New York, Macmillan Publishing, 1979

◆ Preparing and Submitting a Scientific Paper

The Author's Guide to Biomedical Journals. New York, Mary Ann Liebert, Inc, 1994

Day RA: How to Write and Publish a Scientific Paper, 4th Edition. Phoenix, AZ, Oryx Press, 1994

Huth EJ: How to Write and Publish Papers in the Medical Sciences. Philadelphia, PA, ISI Press, 1982

Huth EJ: Medical Style and Format: An International Manual for Authors, Editors, and Publishers. Philadelphia, PA, ISI Press, 1987

Illustrating Science: Standards for Publication. Bethesda, MD, Council of Biology Editors, 1988

International Committee of Medical Journal Editors: Uniform Requirements for Manuscripts Submitted to Biomedical Journals. JAMA 269:2282–2286, 1993

Morgan P: An Insider's Guide for Medical Authors and Editors. Philadelphia, PA, ISI Press, 1986

Tufte ER: The Visual Display of Quantitative Information. Cheshire, CT, Graphics Press, 1983

◆ Research Design and Statistics

Bailar J, Mosteller F (eds): Medical Uses of Statistics, 2nd Edition. Boston, MA, NEJM Books, 1992
Strayhorn JM: Foundations of Clinical Psychiatry. Chicago, IL, Year Book Medical Publishers, 1982
Surwillo WW: Experimental Design in Psychiatry: Research Methods in Clinical Practice. New York, Grune & Stratton, 1980

◆ Peer Review and Ethics

Council of Biology Editors: Ethics and Policy in Scientific Publication. Bethesda, MD, Council of Biology Editors, 1990
Guarding the guardians: research on editorial peer review: selected proceedings from the First International Congress on Peer Review in Biomedical Publications, May 10–12, 1989, Chicago, IL. JAMA 263:1317–1441, 1990
International Committee of Medical Journal Editors: Uniform Requirements for Manuscripts Submitted to Biomedical Journals and Supplemental Statements from the International Committee of Medical Journal Editors (pamphlet). Philadelphia, PA, American College of Physicians, 1993
Lock S: A Difficult Balance: Editorial Peer Review in Medicine. London, England, Nuffield Provincial Hospitals Trust, 1985

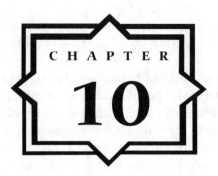

CHAPTER

10

Issues in Psychiatric Research Training

Harold Alan Pincus, M.D., and Carol A. Steele

Perhaps no other field of biomedical research offers such tremendous opportunities as the field of psychiatric and neuroscience research. Never before has the potential for influencing the clinical practice of psychiatry and the care of the mentally ill by advancing scientific knowledge been so great. Never before has public and political support of psychiatric research been so strong. Yet despite the increasing array of opportunities and support, the prospects of a research career often seem daunting to many young people entering psychiatry.

The purpose of this chapter is to demystify the prospect of a research career: to briefly lay out some of the opportunities in the field, to describe the elements that go into becoming a psychiatric researcher, and to set forth how to choose and use a research training program.

New techniques for neuroimaging and assessment of brain activity, as well as increased understanding of the processes of inter- and intracellular communication in the brain, provide powerful methods for examining how the brain functions in health and disease. New developments in molecular biology, genetics, immunology, clinical and basic pharmacology, information systems, and other areas of research have enlarged our capacity to eliminate the mysteries of mental illness.

Advances are not limited to biological areas. The development of more reliable methods for behavioral assessment, diagnosis, epidemiology, and evaluation of psychotherapy is providing the ability to more carefully assess the complex interactions between behavior and biology and to examine the developmental pathways of psychiatric illness. Relatively new areas such as mental health services research have grown tremendously and show increasing importance in influencing the field. The need to assess the outcomes of health care interventions has received a great deal of attention from health care policy makers. There are significant methodologic advances in this area, as well as large infusions of resources to better define cost-effective care.

Although the future looks bright for the psychiatric researcher, one must bear in mind that obtaining research funding remains a highly competitive process, requiring in-depth training and preparation. At the same time it represents an increasingly attractive career option. In particular, compared to the current realities of clinical practice, there is an increasingly narrow difference in both salary and "hassle" levels. While most clinical investigators in psychiatry work in academic settings, there are also opportunities in industry and in independent or government-based research institutes. In general, a career in research provides unusual flexibility, independence, collegial interaction, and the capacity to work on fascinating intellectual questions.

More specifically, with fewer medical students selecting psychiatry as a specialty and a relatively small number of residents and medical students seeking careers in psychiatric research, young minority and women researchers in the field are especially needed. Furthermore, *all* young people entering the field of psychiatric research will find themselves truly treasured commodities. But the question remains: What does it mean to be a clinical investigator in psychiatry, and how does one get there?

◆ Attributes of the Psychiatric Clinician-Researcher

Burke et al. (1986) have described five aspects of the professional role of psychiatric investigator.

The Core Identity of a Clinician

In the past, psychiatry suffered from a split between the value systems of clinical practice and scientific research—between the image of a soft-headed humanist and a biologic technocrat. Such a split implied separate lines of development, practitioner or scientist, with an inevitable tension between the two. A more desirable process is to provide clinically trained individuals with the research skills to become scientists in addition to core skills as clinicians. The psychiatric researcher is a clinician first who learns to become a scientific investigator as well.

However, major drawbacks can derive from a clinician's continuing focus on the individual patient rather than on larger groups or subgroups. The temptation to think in terms of anecdotal evidence may limit one's ability to abstract carefully from a systematic inquiry regarding a targeted problem. Although this shift may be difficult at times, it can be managed. Furthermore, consideration of the individual may also be a benefit for some issues like the calculation of risks and benefits to research subjects.

Intellectual Orientation

For highly motivated clinicians beginning careers in research, learning which questions to ask and how to ask them is much more important than mastering technical skills. In a time of high competition for research funding, not all good research is considered good enough to deserve support. So the first task is to develop a coherent intellectual framework for approaching an area of research and developing strategies to answer the essential questions.

Technical Skills

Beyond a general knowledge of research design and a workable knowledge of statistics, success as a researcher can depend on mastery of particular techniques, whether biological assays or standardized diagnostic interviews. Techniques offer good news for those who train new researchers: technical skills obviously need to be learned, training efforts are set up especially for them, and continued exercise of the skill encourages a deeper knowledge and sensitivity for it.

The problem for an eager trainee is that often technical skills seem to be all that is necessary, although they are only the tip of the training iceberg. Even more serious is the danger that commitment to just a few techniques can limit a scientist's vision. Being limited to a single approach for all purposes, no matter how focused the field of inquiry, can be another insidious restriction on the researcher's capacity to answer the questions he or she has identified.

Management Skills

The principal investigator of any grant needs to be a successful manager of a series of interrelated tasks in the project, of a variety of professional and support personnel, and of various requirements set by the local institution and the government. Professionals who manage other enterprises usually receive training in schools of business or public administration. In science, the most successful investigators must also be able to exercise a high level of administrative skill but typically are expected to pick it up without any formal training in these areas.

Consider the press of duties on a principal investigator. Besides the feverish effort to complete the application and cope with the site visit, there is a daily struggle to balance competing pressures of teaching and clinical responsibilities and often administrative duties within the department with the basic effort to conduct research projects. As in any professional career, there is a temptation to let the urgent replace the important, to let short-term demands take precedence over long-term responsibilities. Another difficult aspect of this task is to learn that successful management is more than administrative efficiency. With a variety of people involved, and often with the least-trained personnel responsible for routines of dealing with subjects and collecting important data, it is necessary for the clinician-researcher to exercise a high degree of executive leadership.

Values and Motives

With the pressure to keep the effort going, which can destroy opportunities for calm reflection, it is essential for clinician-researchers to understand their own values and motives as well as have a sense of what accomplishments are possible over the course of a career. Without a commitment to the work itself and to the ultimate goal of advancing the science of medicine, the values of an investigator facing these pressures may become distorted. In the most dramatic examples, cases of outright fraud have been found in prestigious universities. Other problems are less dramatic but also damaging to the long-term health of clinical research. The pressure to publish dominates researchers, not simply in the classic academic effort to secure promotions but also to create the image of a successful enterprise to justify continued funding. With young clinicians eager to make a name for themselves, it is of special importance to learn the value of restraint—to prepare data carefully and offer meaningful interpretations rather than rushing to get into print. These problems have been discussed within the scientific community, especially by journal editors, who lament the appearance of the "least publishable unit," which contains only portions of a study's findings or reports premature findings on portions of the sample. Other questions that investigators, and their human subjects committees, are expected to address are whether the potential benefits of the study outweigh its costs and whether informed consent has been freely given. A difficult question that has been raised at times is whether a protocol should be terminated before its anticipated completion if adverse effects become clear or a definite treatment advantage is demonstrated. The ability to consider such questions, which are likely to increase in the future, requires the researcher to have a thoughtful and balanced clinical perspective as well as an explicit ethical framework.

Ethics in research has become a focus of the National Institutes of Health (NIH). Assurance of scientific integrity and ethical conduct in science is integral to the future of all research. The NIH now reviews all training grant applications, looking for evidence of the incorporation of the principles of ethical scientific conduct into the training experience of all trainees. As more medical schools recognize that students require explicit discussion and analysis of ethical issues, future researchers are also becoming aware of this, and at an early and vital stage in their training.

◆ Choosing and Using a Research Training Program

In-depth scientific training is essential for all research, and psychiatric training is no exception. A recent study of full-time faculty in departments of internal medicine indicated that those faculty members who were most successful in a research career, as measured by grants, publications, etc., had formal training periods of at least 2 years plus 3 years of protected support as they developed their research careers (Levy et al. 1988).

Unfortunately, in psychiatry there has been a naivete about the necessity for formalized training in research. Also unfortunately, one of the distinctions between many teaching psychiatrists and other academic physicians is the lack of research training experience by potential mentors in psychiatry. Academic physicians in other specialties are likely to have completed a subspecialty fellowship (the majority of which require research experiences) and are thus more likely to be actively participating in research.

In the present day, and certainly in the future, formal research training is necessary for a successful career as a clinical investigator; it is no longer a luxury or something that can be done out of one's hip pocket. At the same time this does not necessarily imply formal training leading to a Ph.D. While in some cases such a program would be useful, the notion that a Ph.D. is necessary in order to do good research is both incorrect and unfortunate.

A number of models exist to train psychiatrists as clinician investigators. They vary in size and support but include many common features: concentrated involvement in research for at least 2 years, continuing supervision by an experienced research mentor, and the presence of an active laboratory with sufficient resources and support. In examining the possibilities for research training programs, young people need to focus on a series of questions that can aid them in evaluating the utility and fit of a particular program. There are four principal questions that need to be considered.

By Whom? The Role of the Mentor

A research training program cannot be easily reduced to a standard, *fixed* curriculum. What is needed is consistent, intense, and close observation and interaction with a senior person who can provide guidance, advice, and substantive direction. In the Odyssey, Homer gives the name Mentor (meaning steadfast and enduring) to the friend Odysseus entrusted with the guidance and education of his son Telemachus.

Anecdotes abound regarding the importance of mentor relationships in the careers of eminent people in art, literature, and sports as well as in science. In fast-moving, highly competitive fields such as scientific research, the role of the mentor can be particularly significant.

While it is easy to say that one needs a mentor, the problem facing young people is how to find one. This requires a considerable amount of effort, research, and luck. Young potential researchers should read the literature with an eye toward identifying authors of papers they find important or particularly admire, talk to people at their home institution and scientific meetings, and find out about the mentoring style of senior people in programs they might consider. It is also important to review one's own history of relationships with advisors to ascertain what kind of relationship has worked best.

Where? The Institutional Values and Resources

Personal and family issues and interests should be important considerations in deciding where one might undertake research training. From a professional perspective, however, there are three sets of questions to consider.

1. Are there the necessary resources to assist in research career development? Is there stability in the department in terms of the continuing presence of enough staff, facilities, and equipment? Is the funding base sufficiently diversified, or is there overdependence on a single source of support? One should not give too much consideration to one or two pieces of fancy equipment; on the other hand, it is important not to be working "out of the kitchen sink."
2. What is the relationship between the department of psychiatry and other departments? Are there strong collaborative research connections? Can the resources of related departments be used to augment those of the psychiatry department?
3. Probably most important, where does science stand in the value orientation of the department? Are science and scientists highly prized? Is there a tradition of excellence at the institution?

With Whom? Collegial Relationships

While there is evidence that programs with a large critical mass of faculty and trainees are most successful in producing researchers, many great scientists have come from smaller institutions. One must consider one's own stylistic and personal preference in terms of "big fish/little pond" or "little fish/big pond" issues. Many smaller programs that may not have a large critical mass within the department of psychiatry gain a critical mass of trainees by linking with other departments that maintain an extensive interdisciplinary program of research training. Also, it is important to recognize that research trainees are part of a much larger community that is connected in many ways through annual meetings and participation in scientific organizations and through the scientific literature. Nevertheless, a basic factor is whether one respects and likes the colleagues with whom one will be training. As has been clear from kindergarten through residency, much of what is learned is learned from peers.

Mentoring junior colleagues is vital to the future of psychiatry and psychiatric research. Success in the field of psychiatric research is usually preceded by a positive mentoring experience that provides a positive view of the field. Given the paucity of senior women in the field, many younger women will need to be mentored by men (Leibenluft et al. 1993). Similarly, nonminorities should be prompted to step in regardless of the race of the mentee. To foster effective communication and interaction between mentor and mentee, the special needs of the individuals involved always need to be taken into account.

How? The Training Itself

Two principal approaches to training have evolved. In what might be termed the "Ph.D. model," emphasis is on a defined curriculum that in many (but not all) cases leads to a formal degree. The "apprenticeship model" emphasizes more experiential aspects, working in close collaboration on a project with peers and mentors. Most programs are in practice combinations of these two approaches, although some are oriented more one way or the other. Some formalized instruction in research design and statistics, grant writing, technical writing, and data presentation skills and instruction in scientific ethics are generally included. Again, one must appraise his or her own stylistic preferences; balance is the key issue.

While it is essential to focus on technical aspects, at the same time there must be sufficient time spent with mentors and colleagues as well as time to develop an independent line of study. Anticipation of and preparation for life following the formal research training program are also essential. Programs should address issues related to the transition to an independent research career and incorporate the practical aspects of linking with federal and other potential funding agencies, the mechanics of applying for research grant funding, and issues of the administration of research projects.

◆ A Developmental Perspective

It is important not to fixate on just the 1- or 2-year formal training programs but instead to take a broader developmental view, emphasizing the notion of a transition to research and highlighting the changing roles from resident to research trainee to researcher, from clinician to clinician-investigator.

There are a number of points where one can intervene to encourage and develop careers of potential physician scientists. During medical school or residency they can be exposed to an intensive research experience, offering them an opportunity to assess their talent for and interest in a research career. Physicians can be provided with an uninterrupted period of basic research training and graduate to clinical training. Importantly, academic physicians need to be protected from excessive clinical duties during their first years as faculty members, to allow them to establish research programs and compete for grants. The transition from trainee to researcher usually takes 3–5 years but can be more variable; sufficient training does not necessarily occur on a fixed schedule (Pincus et al. 1993).

◆ Guide for Residents and Fellows Seeking Research Training Opportunities

Formal research training is necessary for a successful career as a clinical investigator. To ensure a high-quality experience that matches individual needs, it is essential that future researchers carefully evaluate the range of opportunities for obtaining such training. The American Psychiatric Association (APA) Committee on Research Training has developed a list of questions to help residents who are applying to psychiatric residency training and research fellowship programs (Nevin and Pincus 1992). Committee members suggest that the list be used as a guide to developing one's own questions and not as a comprehensive list. It is noted that most programs will have some but not all of the features mentioned, and some aspects of the training experience may be negotiable. It is also suggested that applicants talk to trainees and recent graduates of the programs they are considering.

Questions for Both Residency Training and Research Fellowship Programs

1. Is there an established research training program or plan for research training that residents (fellows) have completed?
2. What are the specific areas of research strength in the department of psychiatry and in the medical center/university complex?
3. Who are the potential mentors available for research training? What are the specific areas of research expertise or interest of these mentors? Are they current or past recipients of research grants? What have they published? Do these individuals regularly provide at least 1 hour per week of individual supervision to trainees? Does any of them have experience in working with minority or female research trainees? Is any of them planning on leaving the institution?
4. What time allocation is made for research and research training? Are clinical duties required during the period of research training? Are these clinical duties related to the research?
5. What salary support is available during the time of research training? What fringe benefits (e.g., health, maternity, disability, malpractice) are available? What are the sources of the salaries for trainees? What are the possibilities that these funds will be increased or decreased over the next few years?
6. What is available in the way of office space, secretarial help, copying, and library and bibliographic search support?
7. Of the following research resources, which are available to trainees?

   - Start-up funds
   - Computers
   - Laboratory measures (e.g., biochemical, psychopharmacologic, psychophysiologic, imaging, genetic)
   - Access to research subjects
   - Access to personnel (e.g., research assistants, social workers, and nurses)
   - Statistical consultation

8. With regard to the following, what type of didactic program is provided?

- Courses in research design
- Courses in statistics
- Courses or seminars in the applicant's specific area of research interest
- Courses, seminars, or conferences on research findings in psychiatry and neuroscience in general
- Training in ethics
- Opportunities to earn an academic degree (e.g., Ph.D., M.P.H., M.S.)

9. What are the current research activities of those who have completed the training program in the past 5 years?
10. To what extent have women and minorities participated in this program? What has their experience in it been? What junior and senior faculty in the institution are female or members of minority groups?
11. Is it possible to complete this program on a part-time basis?
12. What funding or other support is available so that trainees may attend regional or national conferences or meetings?

Questions for Residency Training Programs

1. Are there rotations for residents on research services? If so, do residents rotating there participate in the research? Do all residents rotate on these services?
2. Is there time for residents to pursue a research elective? If so, is this elective open to all residents?
3. How are mentors arranged?
4. Are there didactic seminars focusing on psychiatric research?
5. Is there a defined "research track"? If so, how many residents are allowed to be in the track? How and when are these selections made?
6. Is there a required research project? If so, how is the project determined and designed?

Questions for Research Fellowship Programs

1. Does the research fellowship training program have a program director? If so, how much contact does the program director have with fellows?
2. How are mentors arranged? Do fellows have a role in selecting mentors? May one change mentors during the period of research and fellowship training? Are there co-mentors?
3. Is the fellow expected and helped to develop independent research projects as well as to participate in the mentor's research? What kinds of help are there for the trainee in writing and obtaining an independent grant?
4. What is the expected length of support, and what is the potential for longer-term support in the department?
5. What collaborations exist between the fellow's mentor and other researchers, including the researchers across the clinical-basic research boundary?
6. Do fellows get to know, support, and socialize with each other?
7. Have explicit learning and performance objectives been developed?
8. Is there a payback obligation? If so, what does it involve and how is it usually fulfilled?
9. What outside activities are available to supplement the stipend? What are the restrictions on such outside activities?

To expand the number of residents and medical students seeking careers in psychiatric research and young minority and women researchers in the field, the Office of Research at the American Psychiatric Association provides information and support to assist people in taking advantage of opportunities in psychiatric research training. The *Directory of Research Fellowship Opportunities in Psychiatry 1992*, a document produced by the office, includes listings of research fellowships available. The information is compiled and updated from responses to a questionnaire about research training opportunities that is sent to residency training directors around the country. Through the Research Mentor network, mentors and mentees are matched, based on area of interest, geographic location, or any other specification requested. A more specific goal of the office is to increase the number of minorities in the field of psychiatric research; to this end, the office administers the Program for Minority Research Training in Psychiatry, a grant funded by the National Institute of Mental Health. The office also operates a Psychiatric Research Training Clearinghouse that connects medical students, psychiatric residents, and others interested in research training with resources, information, and leading programs of research training.

◆ References

Burke JB, Pincus HA, Pardes H: The clinician-researcher in psychiatry. Am J Psychiatry 143:968–975, 1986

Leibenluft E, Dial T, Haviland M, et al: Sex differences in rank attainment and research activities among academic psychiatrists. Arch Gen Psychiatry 50:896–904, 1993

Levy G, Sherman C, Gentile N, et al: Postdoctoral research training of full-time faculty in academic departments of medicine. Ann Intern Med 109:414–418, 1988

Nevin J, Pincus HA (eds): Directory of Research Fellowship Opportunities in Psychiatry 1992. Washington, DC, American Psychiatric Association, 1992

Pincus H, Dial T, Haviland M: Research activities of full-time faculty in academic departments of psychiatry. Arch Gen Psychiatry 50:657–664, 1993

CHAPTER

11

Research Ethics and
Human Subject Issues

Robert M. Wettstein, M.D.

Claims of research misconduct in biomedical research have been identified as a significant problem in recent years. In 1991–1992, for example, 55 institutions received 108 allegations of research misconduct involving U.S. Public Health Service (PHS)-supported research or related activities (ORI 1993). Such claims often evoke widespread attention in the mass media and can sully the reputation of the most accomplished investigator. Formal adjudication of research misconduct can terminate the investigator's ability to obtain research funding from an agency or even lead to loss of employment, criminal prosecution, and civil liability for damages. Available survey data reveal that ethical problems in graduate education and research activities are widespread but that many faculty and graduate students are unwilling to report these for fear of retaliation (Swazey et al. 1993).

Nevertheless, some investigators remain inattentive to ethical issues in research. Training in clinical and research ethics generally receives low priority in residency and fellowship training programs. Increasingly, however, academic medical centers are offering, if not requiring, participation in research ethics seminars, sometimes at the insistence of the federal government.

This chapter will orient the mental health investigator to some of the important issues regarding research ethics and human subjects. References at the end of this chapter and resources in Resources 11–1 provide more detailed coverage of the issues. Readers interested in ethical issues in publication and peer review are referred to Patterson (Chapter 9, this volume).

◆ Principles of Research Ethics

Basic and clinical research have become increasingly scrutinized and regulated; they are no longer private matters under the exclusive control of the investigator. Most contemporary biomedical research is conducted by interdisciplinary teams of investigators and staff, at one or multiple sites, rather than by a single investigator at a single research site. There are many interested parties in the research enterprise, and investigators have ethical obligations to more than the subjects of their research. More generally, investigators have ethical duties to their co-investigators and consultants on the project; other investigators in the field; colleagues in the department, university, or research institution where the investigators are employed; funding agency; research site; and society at large. Specific research policies, procedures, and standards are dictated by the academic department or university, Institutional Review Board (IRB), funding agency, federal and state government (Delano and Zucker 1994), and applicable professional society (e.g., American Psychiatric Association, American Psychological Association).

Research using human subjects, especially that funded by public agencies such as the federal or state governments, involves a collective partnership between the research participant, the investigator or institution, and society (Veatch 1987). Indeed, the commonly used term "research subject," as contrasted with "research participant," improperly connotes a position of inequality, inferiority, passivity, and helplessness relative to the investigator.

In 1979, the influential Belmont Report, published by the National Commission for the Protection of Human Subjects of Biomedical and Behavioral Research (1979), identified three general ethical principles for researchers: respect for persons, beneficence, and justice.

Respect for persons requires that individuals (i.e., potential or actual research subjects) should be treated with respect and that the individual's choices about research participation should be honored. Respect for persons further requires that individuals with diminished capacity for autonomous decision making about research participation (e.g., mentally retarded or demented individuals or children) be protected, even to the point of exclusion from research participation.

Beneficence obliges the investigator to attend to the subject's well-being as well as to the fruits of the research to society at large in the future. Here the investigator must recognize, and attempt to reduce, the potential risk to the subjects and maximize the potential benefits to the subjects.

The principle of justice asks who benefits from the research and who bears the burdens. This principle requires that these be distributed fairly through society. It is considered unfair, for example, to select a poor, minority, or institutionalized subject sample for research because such subjects were readily available when the benefits of the research would accrue only to another, far more advantaged group.

◆ Special Research Issues

Institutional Review Boards (IRBs)

IRBs, or Human Subjects Committees, were established in 1974 by federal law. IRBs are charged with reviewing human subjects protocols for all institutions receiving federal funding for research. IRBs review protocols prior to the investigator's beginning a project to ensure that both research ethical standards and federal and state legal research requirements have been satisfied. IRBs have the legal authority to approve, demand modifications in, or disapprove proposed research protocols within their jurisdiction. While federal and state research guidelines contain certain requirements, the IRB can apply even stricter conditions. IRBs represent a decentralized, institution-based, administrative approach to reviewing proposed research studies, informed by community standards, as opposed to having a centralized governmental agency perform this function from a distance.

The IRB review is principally oriented to human subjects issues, but it can also consider the scientific aspects of the proposed study. Scientific inquiry is relevant to the IRB review process in that research that is scientifically invalid may do more harm than good and would disrespect the subjects (Sieber 1992).

IRBs contain a diverse group of individuals with expertise in a variety of areas. In large research institutions there may be more than a single IRB, with their responsibilities divided by type of subject risk (e.g., biomedical or psychosocial) or type of subject pool (e.g., adult or child or pregnant women).

Investigators should be familiar with the policies and procedures of their local IRB. Each IRB has written guidelines, in addition to the federal and state regulations, and investigators can obtain these and relevant documents from their IRB. Investigators should view IRBs and their members as consultants and collaborators for research rather than as adversaries. Some investigators resent the IRB involvement in their protocol as a paperwork requirement and an interference with the investigator's scientific pursuit and academic freedom. Investigators must be able to anticipate human subjects issues in their protocol and can consider consulting with IRBs in advance of submission of the protocol to the IRB for approval.

IRBs operate under the jurisdiction of the Office for Protection from Research Risks (OPRR) of the National Institutes of Health (NIH), as well as the Food and Drug Administration (FDA). OPRR has published an IRB Guidebook (OPRR 1993) that thoroughly reviews IRB functions and describes human subjects issues. This excellent volume, entitled *Protecting Human Research Subjects: IRB Guidebook*, can be purchased from the U.S. Government Printing Office.

Informed Consent to Research

Federal regulations dictate when informed consent for research participation of human subjects is required or may be waived (45 CFR Part 46.116, 1991). In clinical trials using human subjects, the investigator must obtain the subject's informed consent to participate in the study: before the subject begins the study, whenever the protocol is substantially altered, and when new information (e.g., additional study risk) becomes available. Informed consent is not the consent form; the form is only the documentation that informed consent to research has been obtained. Rather, informed consent is the process of disclosing relevant information to the potential subject and obtaining consent to the study. Sometimes consent forms may be unnecessary; the IRB is authorized to determine when this is so.

There are three components to informed consent to research: information, voluntariness, and competency. Each is significant in the context of research as well as clinical work.

Information. Potential research subjects must be provided adequate information to decide whether to participate in the study. Relevant information, whether provided orally or in writing on the consent form, should be presented in readable and comprehensible terms appropriate to an eighth grader, not a graduate student. Professional jargon should be avoided.

Federal regulations specify the elements of information disclosure to human research subjects (45 CFR Part 46.116, 1991). These include 1) purposes and procedures of the study; 2) risks and discomforts of the study; 3) benefits to subject and others; 4) alternative procedures and treatments; 5) how confidentiality of research data will be protected; 6) compensation for, and treatment of, injury resulting from the research; 7) whom to contact about the research or resulting injury; and 8) statement that research participation is voluntary and consent may be revoked at any time without penalty. Other disclosures, such as the source of the research funds or the need to reveal relevant new information that becomes available during the course of the study, may be required by law or ethical codes.

Voluntariness. Research subjects must agree to participate in the study without undue influence or coercion from others (Wertheimer 1987). However, the line between acceptable persuasion of subjects and unacceptable coercion is not sharp. In the need for investigators to recruit human subjects, various pressures that may not be ethical can be brought to bear on potential subjects. For instance, Blanck et al. (1992) query whether investigators can employ young, attractive, verbal, and intelligent assistants of ethnic backgrounds similar to the target population to recruit participants. Coercion can occur when subject recruitment is conducted by the subject's attending physician, who also acts as the principal investigator. In such cases, patients may fear the loss of the physician's services should research consent be refused. Coercion can also occur when payment for research participation is excessively large, or when parents deceive or misinform their children in order to solicit their participation in a study (Parker and Lidz 1994). Subjects who are passive or emotionally dependent may be easily coerced into research participation. Also, the fact that subjects are institutionalized, although not inherently coercive, may be relevant to the voluntariness of the subjects' consent.

Competence. Research subjects must have adequate capacity to consent to the study. Among laypersons or researchers outside the mental health community, there is a widespread assumption that mentally ill individuals are unable to consent to research. However, there is no universal consensus about standards or criteria for competence for research consent; several standards exist (Appelbaum and Roth 1982). These include the requirement that the subject must clearly evidence a choice about research participation and maintain that choice over a period of time, understand the factual information about the study provided to the subject, and be able to manipulate that information to make a rational decision about research participation. A subject's capacity to consent to research can be compromised by various insults to the central nervous system as well as the context of medical crises.

In some protocols, especially those involving cognitively impaired samples, the investigator will need to specify the procedure to be used to certify that the subject meets the requisite competency threshold. Will the investigator rely on the competency assessment of the clinicians caring for the patient-subject, or will the investigator independently assess the subject's capacity to consent? Will the investigator provide for a "consent auditor" to monitor the informed consent process on a first-hand basis?

For those subjects deemed unable to consent to research participation (i.e., either clinically incapacitated or legally incompetent by court order), will substituted consent from the family or legal guardians be accepted? If so, which person in the family will be selected as the substitute decision maker? How will the substitute decision maker consent or refuse, based on the best interests of the subject, the prior statements of the subject about research participation when competent, or the decision maker's impressions of what the subject would have decided if competent (Warren et al. 1986)? Even if a substitute decision maker is authorized to decide for the potential subject, the subject may retain the right to object to research participation (Delano and Zucker 1994).

Investigators can consider using advance directives for research participation when longitudinally studying disorders such as Alzheimer's disease with a known progressive course (Fletcher et al. 1985). In such cases, subjects execute an advance directive for research before the disorder becomes incapacitating.

The need for investigators to carefully attend to the process of informed consent to research is heightened by empirical studies in this area. Such studies reveal that some subjects do not understand or appreciate that they are participants in a research study, do not understand the process or fact of randomization or placebo control, and believe that the researcher will make decisions about their care according to the subject's best interests (Lynoe et al. 1991; Riecken and Ravich 1982; Roth et al. 1987). In short, clinical research subjects often fail to understand that research differs from typical patient care (Appelbaum et al. 1987).

Privacy and Confidentiality

Privacy and confidentiality are related but distinguishable concepts. Privacy, the more basic concept, refers to a zone of psychological and physical space under the person's control; the right to privacy includes the person's right to limit access to the self by others (Warren and Brandeis 1984). Confidentiality, in contrast, involves the transfer of information from one party to another; it is only one form of privacy invasion (Everstine et al. 1980). Investigators respect the privacy of research subjects by deliberately not collecting sensitive data. Investigators respect the confidentiality of the subject's data by properly securing it. Generally, investigators promise potential research subjects that research data will be maintained in confidence or collected anonymously, if collected at all.

Establishing the subject's trust in the investigator may be indispensable to completing the research when one is obtaining sensitive behavioral or historical data such as on sexual behavior, infectious diseases, or criminal conduct (e.g., violence). The investigator's ability to safeguard confidentiality varies with the study's design and method. As in clinical work, the promise of confidentiality to subjects is likely to enhance the validity of the data and the integrity of the research since subjects are then more likely to be open and honest with research staff (Boruch and Cecil 1979).

The investigator must describe in detail who will have access to confidential information and how the confidentiality of data will be maintained. Such information should be shared with the subject and placed in the consent form. Usual methods of safeguarding confidentiality of research data include protecting computer files by single or double passwords, storing paper files and tapes in locked file cabinets, securing confidentiality statements signed by all research staff, storing the linkage between subject-identifying information and subject codes separately from the research data themselves (if not actually destroying the linkages as soon as possible), and using subject-selected aliases rather than actual names (Sieber 1992). When publishing data or sharing data sets with other researchers, investigators must be certain that no subjects can be identified from the disclosed account.

The investigator must also consider, and plan for, the limitations to the confidentiality of the data and then disclose these to potential subjects. Such limits may include child or elder abuse or imminent suicidality and homicidality (Appelbaum and Rosenbaum 1989). The investigator will find it useful to be familiar with the details of applicable confidentiality law in the jurisdiction of the study.

Some research areas (e.g., violence, drug use and abuse, perinatal injuries, toxic torts) may be of interest to outside businesses or parties (e.g., chemical or drug manufacturers or the research subjects themselves). These data may be vulnerable to legal attempts at discovery for purposes of litigation. Licensed physicians and psychologists enjoy statutory testimonial privileges that protect otherwise confidential clinical data from courtroom disclosure. Investigators, however, do not have such a testimonial privilege. The investigators and their data are especially likely to be subpoenaed if the investigators testify as expert witnesses in litigation related to their research (Holder 1985, 1986). Nevertheless, investigators can obtain federal confidentiality certificates upon request whether or not the study is federally funded. These certificates may help maintain the confidentiality of research data following subpoena of research data in litigation. Investigators using subjects with mental illness in protocols can obtain confidentiality certificates from the National Institute of Mental Health (NIMH), Division of Extramural Activities, Parklawn Building, Room 9C-04, 5600 Fishers Lane, Rockville, MD 20897, (301) 443-4673. For subjects with drug abuse, contact the National Institute on Drug Abuse (NIDA), Office of Extramural Program Review, Parklawn Building, Room 10-42, 5600 Fishers Lane, Rockville, MD 20897, (301) 443-2755. For subjects with alcohol abuse, contact the National Institute of Alcohol Abuse and Alcoholism (NIAAA), Willco Building, 6000 Executive Boulevard, Rockville, MD 20892,

(301) 443-5733. For public health studies, contact John P. Fanning, Office of the Assistant Secretary for Health, PHS, Hubert Humphrey Building, Room 737-F, 200 Independence Avenue, SW, Washington, DC, (202) 690-7100.

Other confidentiality issues relate largely to the interests of the investigator rather than those of the subject. The investigator may want, or have the right, to maintain in confidence the protocol, funding application, consent forms, or IRB application against outside special interest or advocacy groups in the community.

Assessment of Risks and Benefits

Investigators and IRBs are responsible for fully identifying the anticipated risks and benefits of a proposal and then attempting to maximize the benefits while minimizing the risks. According to federal regulations, "risks to subjects [must be] reasonable in relation to anticipated benefits, if any, to subjects, and the importance of the knowledge that may reasonably be expected to result" (45 CFR 46.111(a)(2)). Investigators must disclose to potential subjects the anticipated risks and benefits of the study, usually orally and in writing on the consent form.

Risks.   Risks vary considerably with the type of research and subject population. Even individuals in the same or similar groups often perceive an identical risk differently; of course, some subject populations are uniquely or especially vulnerable. Risks may be related to the theory and nature of the research, research procedure, study sample, study setting, or the use of the research findings (Sieber 1993). Risks to research subjects can include inconvenience, physical harm, emotional harm and distress, including breach of privacy or confidentiality, social risk, legal risk, and economic risk (Sieber 1992, 1993). When invalid research is later applied, other members of society may be harmed as well.

Performing a risk assessment for research harms is complex and often difficult. The investigator must consider the nature and type of risk, its magnitude, expected duration and reversibility, probability of occurrence, and the frequency of anticipated risks. As in clinical care, subjects conceivably may be exposed to a low probability of large-magnitude potential harms or a high probability of low-magnitude potential harms.

Investigators need to assess whether the proposed research is considered, or is greater than, minimal risk. Federal regulations define minimal risk as: "that the probability and magnitude of harm or discomfort anticipated in the research are not greater in and of themselves than those ordinarily encountered in daily life or during the performance of routine physical or psychological examinations or tests" (45 CFR 46.102(i)).

Many research risks can be minimized, avoided, or transformed into potential research benefits (Sieber 1992). To minimize potential risk to subjects, investigators must avoid exposing vulnerable subjects to research risks except when the research is directly relevant to the particular vulnerability or disability, and there are no alternative subject populations. In addition, investigators must attempt to screen out those subjects from the proposed study for whom participation would be contraindicated. The investigator carefully reviews eligibility criteria and procedures for the study to determine whether the study interventions are inappropriate for a certain potential subject pool.

Benefits.   Potential benefits to a study also vary widely with the research method and study population. As with research risks, a benefit to one person may not be a benefit to another. Even more so than risks, benefits to a research study may accrue more to other members of society than to the research subjects themselves. Others afflicted with a particular disorder or problem, the community at large, as well as the investigator and the participating research institutions also stand to gain from the proposed research.

Subjects can benefit in many ways from research participation. These include enhanced self-esteem and empowerment, altruism, favorable attention and respect from research staff, interpersonal gratification such as intimacy with others, learning or training in new skills, or enhanced services (Sieber 1992). Benefits to society, science, the investigator, and institutions may be substantive (i.e., scientific progress, economic) or psychosocial.

Investigators commonly make broad claims about the anticipated benefits of a study on the basis of the lack of knowledge in a particular area. Much research, however, never in fact provides substantial benefits in this regard since the research is never completed, does not result in statistically significant findings, or is never published. Thus, many appeals to the benefits of research are only conjectural. Investigators should therefore attempt to be precise in identifying and stating the anticipated benefits of the research, especially to the individual subject, beyond filling a gap in the literature.

Conflict of Interest

Conflict of interest issues are of increasing concern in clinical medicine (Rodwin 1993) as well as in research; they are distinct from research misconduct, although the penalties for both are similar. As noted by West et al. (Chapter 6, this volume), the growth in nongovernmental research funding, particularly by private biotechnology businesses, has fueled concern about conflict of interest. There is much controversy about the prevalence, definition, resulting harm, and approaches to regulating conflict of interest (Porter and Malone 1992). Many other issues are discussed in that chapter.

Special Populations

Some issues are unique to special populations of research subjects such as prisoners, pregnant women, minors, and fetuses and to the use of in vitro fertilization. Review of these is beyond the scope of the present chapter; the reader is referred to the ample literature in these areas (Levine 1986; OPRR 1993; Stanley and Sieber 1992).

◆ Conclusions

In human subjects research, there is a tension between the desire to conduct research and the responsibility to respect a subject's dignity and autonomy. In the past, those who sought to safeguard subjects were often seen as unnecessarily obstructing the progress of science and were shunned, although this is thankfully less so today (Katz 1994). Investigators must come to terms with the notion that respect for the subject must trump the need for scientific data. Investigators should not view IRBs and outside regulatory forces as adversaries but rather should see them, like their subjects, as collaborators in the research enterprise.

As in clinical care, standards of research practice and research ethics are not fixed over time but rather are dynamic and changing. New technologies, new diseases (e.g., AIDS), and ever-unique subject populations present challenging opportunities for researchers from both a technical and ethical standpoint (Rosnow et al. 1993). In the future, new risks for research participants will be recognized. Further regulations by government, academia, and professional societies will be developed, along with procedural mechanisms to implement them. Indeed, ethical guidelines can change even during the course of a study, so that the definition of ethical practice is not constant. Investigators must continue to be familiar with technical developments not only in their respective research areas but also in research ethics.

◆ References

American Psychological Association: Ethical Principles in the Conduct of Research With Human Participants. Washington, DC, American Psychological Association, 1982

Appelbaum PS, Rosenbaum A: *Tarasoff* and the researcher: does the duty to protect apply in the research setting? Am Psychol 44:885–894, 1989

Appelbaum PS, Roth LH: Competency to consent to research. Arch Gen Psychiatry 39:951–958, 1982

Appelbaum PS, Roth LH, Lidz CW, et al: False hopes and best data: consent to research and therapeutic misconception. Hastings Cent Rep 17:20–24, 1987

Blanck PD, Bellack AS, Rosnow RL, et al: Scientific rewards and conflicts of ethical choices in human subjects research. Am Psychol 47:959–965, 1992

Boruch RF, Cecil JS: Assuring the Confidentiality of Research Data. Philadelphia, PA, University of Pennsylvania Press, 1979

Delano SJ, Zucker JL: Protecting mental health research subjects without prohibiting progress. Hosp Community Psychiatry 45:601–603, 1994

Everstine L, Everstine DS, Heymann GM, et al: Privacy and confidentiality in psychotherapy. Am Psychol 35:828–840, 1980

Fletcher JC, Dommel FW, Cowell DD: Consent to research with impaired human subjects. IRB: A Review of Human Subjects Research 7:1–6, 1985

Holder AR: When researchers are served subpoenas. IRB: A Review of Human Subjects Research 7:5–7, 1985

Holder AR: The biomedical researcher and subpoenas: judicial protection of confidential medical data. Am J Law Med 12:405–421, 1986

Katz J: Reflections on unethical experiments and the beginnings of bioethics in the United States. Kennedy Institute of Ethics Journal 4:85–92, 1994

Levine RJ: Ethics and Regulation of Clinical Research, 2nd Edition. New Haven, CT, Yale University Press, 1986

Lynoe N, Sandlund M, Dahlqvist G, et al: Informed consent: study of quality of information given to participants in a clinical trial. BMJ 303:610–613, 1991

National Commission for the Protection of Human Subjects of Biomedical and Behavioral Research: The Belmont Report: Ethical Principles and Guidelines for the Protection of Human Subjects of Research. Washington, DC, Government Printing Office, 1979

Office for Protection From Research Risks: Protecting Human Research Subjects: IRB Guidebook. Bethesda, MD, National Institutes of Health, 1993

Office of Research Integrity: Research misconduct activities reported by institutions. ORI Newsletter 2:3, 1993

Parker LS, Lidz CW: Familial coercion to participate in genetic family studies: is there cause for IRB intervention. IRB: A Review of Human Subjects Research 16:6–12, 1994

Porter RJ, Malone TE (eds): Biomedical Research: Collaboration and Conflict of Interest. Baltimore, MD, Johns Hopkins University Press, 1992

Riecken HW, Ravich R: Informed consent to biomedical research in Veterans Administration hospitals. JAMA 248:344–348, 1982

Rodwin MA: Medicine, Money, and Morals: Physicians' Conflicts of Interest. New York, Oxford University Press, 1993

Rosnow RL, Rotheram-Borus MJ, Ceci SJ, et al: The institutional review board as a mirror of scientific and ethical standards. Am Psychol 48:821–826, 1993

Roth LH, Appelbaum PS, Lidz CW, et al: Informed consent in psychiatric research. Rutgers Law Review 39:425–441, 1987

Sieber JE: Planning Ethically Responsible Research. Newbury Park, CA, Sage, 1992

Sieber JE: Ethical considerations in planning and conducting research on human subjects. Acad Med 68:S9–S13, 1993

Stanley B, Sieber JE (eds): Social Research on Children and Adolescents. Newbury Park, CA, Sage, 1992

Swazey JP, Anderson MS, Lewis KS: Ethical problems in academic research. American Scientist 81:542–553, 1993

Veatch RM: The Patient as Partner: A Theory of Human-Experimentation Ethics. Bloomington, IN, Indiana University Press, 1987

Warren S, Brandeis L: The right to privacy, in Philosophical Dimensions of Privacy: An Anthology. Edited by Schoeman F. New York, Cambridge University Press, 1984, pp 75–103

Warren JW, Sobal J, Tenney JH, et al: Informed consent by proxy. N Engl J Med 315:1124–1128, 1986

Wertheimer A: Coercion. Princeton, NJ, Princeton University Press, 1987

Resources 11–1

Selected Resources on Research Ethics

Listed below are sources for additional information regarding ethical issues in research, especially issues involving human subjects.

American Psychological Association: Ethical Principles in the Conduct of Research With Human Participants. Washington, DC, American Psychological Association, 1982.
This work reviews and discusses ethical principles and practices regarding psychological research with human subjects.

Code of Federal Regulations: 45 CFR Part 46.101 et seq 1991, Protection of Human Subjects.
This contains the official federal rules governing research involving human subjects.

IRB: A Review of Human Subjects Research
This bimonthly journal published by the Hastings Center (255 Elm Road, Briarcliff Manor, NY 10510) contains brief articles and letters about human subjects research issues.

Levine RJ: Ethics and Regulation of Clinical Research, 2nd Edition. New Haven, CT, Yale University Press, 1986.
This book is a scholarly and detailed overview of ethical issues in clinical research.

National Commission for the Protection of Human Subjects of Biomedical and Behavioral Research: The Belmont Report: Ethical Principles and Guidelines for the Protection of Human Subjects of Research. Washington, DC, Government Printing Office, 1979.
This is a brief but influential report of a national commission. A two-volume appendix (1978) contains the full text of papers that were prepared to assist the commission.

Office for Protection from Research Risks, National Institutes of Health: Protecting Human Research Subjects: IRB Guidebook (NIH Publ No 93-3470). Bethesda, MD, National Institutes of Health, 1993.
Both a reading and reference book, this excellent volume can be purchased from the Superintendent of Documents (PO Box 371954, Pittsburgh, PA 15250-7954).

Office for Protection From Research Risks, NIH, Building 31, 9000 Rockville Pike, Bethesda, MD 20892, (301) 496-7005.
This federal office is responsible for protecting research subjects.

Office of Research Integrity, PHS, 5515 Security Lane, Rockville, MD 20852, (301) 443-3400.
A quarterly newsletter is published by the ORI.

Sieber JE: Planning Ethically Responsible Research. Newbury Park, CA, Sage, 1992.
This highly readable volume guides investigators in planning and preparing human subjects research.

Animal-Based Research and the Animal Rights Movement

Adrian R. Morrison, D.V.M., Ph.D.

Basic biological and behavioral research, much of it depending on studies using animals, has contributed the foundation of information underlying modern medical and surgical practice that has resulted in the healthiest generation in history (Paton 1993).

To give just a few examples of medical discoveries that depended on animal research, one could mention antibiotics, cancer chemotherapy, cornea transplantation, prevention of rubella, immunotherapy technology, and monoclonal antibodies. At least 25 Nobel prizes have been awarded to researchers whose work used animals; these go back to the prize to Von Behring in 1901 for the development of diphtheria antiserum to the award in 1991 to Neher and Sakmann for their work on chemical communication between cells.

Despite these achievements and the need for continuing research to understand and treat such problems as addictive disorders, Alzheimer's disease, depression, schizophrenia, and traumatic brain injury, the use of animals for research is under attack today by a well-organized, well-funded, militant movement espousing the philosophy of animal rights. Although all animal use in the United

States is now being questioned (Strand and Strand 1993), the movement first focused on medical research and, in particular, behavioral studies of the nervous system. Animal rights literature proclaimed that behavioral studies would make a particularly easy target, clearly playing on the public's wariness of studies of the brain and the stigma attached to mental illness.

The early attack on biomedical research around 1980 was not happenstance. One of the movement's major philosophers, Peter Singer (1989), observed that American animal researchers are a smaller and politically less powerful group than American farmers, and they are based in regions where animal liberationists live. They therefore make a more accessible, and slightly less formidable opponent. Indeed, a recent analysis (Russell and Nicoll 1994) of the chapter expressing concerns about biomedical research in Singer's (1990) *Animal Liberation*, the "bible" of the animal rights movement, revealed that 48% of the 37.5 pages critical of various uses of animals in research were devoted to behavioral and addiction studies. Yet the institutes of the National Institutes of Health (NIH) supporting such research received only about 11% of the total 1993 NIH budget, while those funding research on cancer, diabetes, and heart disease obtained 37% of that budget.

Furthermore, a survey of 21 books dealing with animal rights revealed an inordinate amount of attention to the use of animals in biomedical research compared with their other uses (Nicoll and Russell 1990). For example, Americans use most animals—more than 6 billion annually—for food, and animal shelters and pounds put to death 10 to 20 million dogs and cats each year. Medical research absorbs only 20 million animals annually, 90% of which are rats and mice. Yet, per animal killed, those books devoted 77 times more pages to the use of animals in medical research than to animals in our diet. One obvious interpretation is that the movement calculated that a compassionate public was more likely to contribute funds to stop activities that few engage in and few understand rather than something almost all do—eat meat. Now use of animals for food and for other purposes is receiving considerable attention from the movement.

Like all human endeavors, biomedical research has not always been done perfectly. Mistakes occur, and in the past some scientists have not kept up with the latest in veterinary practices. Some have been insensitive. However, even the most publicized "exposés" of laboratories have resorted to gross misrepresentations of the experiments or laboratories involved. Even after stricter government regulation was imposed in 1985, laboratory raids by the underground Animal Liberation Front and vilification of researchers by animal rights organizations have continued unabated. The objective of the movement, in its own words, is elimination of animal use—all animal use. For a succinct yet thorough review of the methods employed to attack the use of animals in medical research specifically, see Pardes et al. (1991).

◆ Regulation of Animal Research

It is important that physicians understand how research using animals is conducted so that they can feel comfortable supporting researchers. According to a 1990 United States Department of Agriculture (USDA) report, 58% of the animals used in experiments in 1990 experienced no pain or distress; 36% were used in a manner requiring analgesics and/or anesthetics; whereas 6% were involved in experiments where pain could not be relieved because the purpose of the experiments was to study pain itself. The development of increasingly safer analgesics and anesthetics depends on such research.

The federal government regulates animal research through two agencies, the USDA and the Department of Health and Human Services (DHHS). According to the Animal Welfare Act, USDA representatives must make annual unannounced inspections of all institutions using animals (excluding rodents) for biomedical research. Both the Animal Welfare Act and the 1985 Health Research Extension Act, which governs oversight of research funded by the Public Health Service (PHS), a branch of DHHS, require that all proposed experiments be reviewed by an institutional committee. PHS policy states that such a committee, usually referred to as the Institutional Animal Care and Use Committee (IACUC), must have at least five members, including a veterinarian experienced in laboratory animal science, a practicing scientist experienced in animal research, a person whose primary interest is nonscientific (e.g., law, ethics, theology), and an individual with no ties to the institution (Office of Protection From Research Risk 1986). Bigger institutions have much larger committees because of the numerous protocols submitted for review.

The IACUC is charged with ensuring that animals are cared for appropriately. If experimental protocols do not clearly state how various procedures will be performed to minimize discomfort and how the researcher will use appropriate numbers of animals, the application will be returned to the investigator for clarification and resubmission. IACUCs are empowered to prevent what they view as inappropriate experiments—and they do.

Although much has been made of the fact that the USDA does not inspect rodent facilities (rodents constitute 90% of the animals used in research), such facilities are covered by PHS regulations (U.S. Public Health Service 1991). Thus, every laboratory and animal holding facility in an institution must receive unannounced inspections by IACUC members twice yearly in addition to those by USDA inspectors.

An independent accrediting organization composed largely of veterinarians specializing in laboratory animal medicine, the American Association for the Accreditation of Laboratory Animal Care (AAALAC), also evaluates the programs and facilities of those who would like their highly regarded seal of approval. Their reviews, which are rigorous, cover the use of all animal species. Of the research funded by the National Institutes of Health, 80% is performed in AAALAC-accredited laboratories (AAALAC, personal communication).

It is also of interest that more than 60 national voluntary organizations, most of them focused on a single illness, have supported the use of animals in medical research (see Resources 12–1).

◆ Philosophy of Animal Rights Activists

The general concern for animal welfare shared by most people is in contrast to the philosophy that drives the militant animal rights movement: Humans deserve essentially no more consideration than other animals. Radical activists have variously translated that philosophy into terrorist acts and harassment of scientists and institutions. And even if one acknowledges that improvements in laboratory animal care have resulted from publicity about laboratories, the continued campaigns against biomedical researchers suggest that something deeper drives the movement. That something may be a mix of antiscience sentiment, distrust of established institutions, and even misanthropy (Goodwin 1992). The last of these is illustrated by a quotation from the national director of People for the Ethical Treatment of Animals, Ingrid Newkirk, in response to a question about the appropriateness of animal research if it resulted in a cure for AIDS: "We'd be against it" (Barnes 1989). Clearly, one can reach no consensus or compromise with those who hold such sentiments. Attempts to put scientists at the other extreme create a false middle ground, as Goodwin (1992) and Horton (1989) have observed.

Goodwin (1992) has also noted that the radical aim and philosophy of the movement, elimination of all animal use because such use is nothing more than "speciesism" (Singer 1990), was masked initially by an attack on biomedical research as unworthy. He enumerated the following secondary arguments of animal rightists: research is inherently cruel; research is wasteful and duplicative; research diverts funds that could go into prevention or treatment; alternative methods are available. Goodwin demonstrated that none of these claims stands up to even cursory scrutiny.

Basically, the movement depends on two different philosophical views that have led many followers to one conclusion: Harm to animals, even if it will ultimately lead to a good for humans, is morally wrong. Vance (1992) has written a critique of each of the views.

One view, espoused most prominently by Regan (1983), holds that because animals have inherent value, one is ultimately led to the conclusion that they have rights and cannot be subjected to our desires. It should be noted, however, that humans are the only species capable of adhering to this philosophy, which essentially urges us to waste our highly developed brain. One cannot imagine that more than a few would acquiesce with Regan's demands: "If that means that there are some things we cannot learn, then so be it. There are also some things we cannot learn by using humans if we respect their rights" (p. 388).

Regan's rights philosophy has given the movement its name, but Singer's (1990) book, *Animal Liberation*, in which he presents a utilitarian's view, appears to have inspired the activist element—perhaps because it is more accessible intellectually and more of a polemic. Singer argues—actually it has been suggested that each demolishes the other's argument (Vance 1992)—that one should accord animals equal consideration because they equally feel pain and that one should act to bring about the best balance of good and bad consequences. Not to do so is said to be evidence of "speciesism." Singer, too, ignores the reality of biology, but he also deviates from the norms of scholarship, according to several analyses that report out-of-context misrepresentations of the achievements of biomedical and behavioral research (Nicoll et al. 1992; Russell and Nicoll, unpublished manuscript; Verhetsel 1986).

Followers of the movement include 1) those willing to commit acts seeking to destroy buildings or reputations; 2) those who accept the tenets of the movement (Herzog 1993) but seek to live their beliefs peacefully; and 3) those willing to contribute money to organizations after having been exposed to promotional materials with lurid pictures and descriptions of research; these individuals act out of concern for animal welfare but appear to lack an understanding of science and how research is conducted. The last of these groups includes many people who, when educated about these issues, can change their view.

Animal rights activists are now directing much of their efforts toward school children. Children—and the young activists, with an average age around 30 (Jamison and Lunch 1992)—have had little contact with the medical problems that afflicted earlier generations (Paton 1993) and are much less likely to have an appreciation of the realities of animal life that an earlier, more rural population had (Strand and Strand 1993). There is concern, therefore, that coming generations will be less likely to be interested in biomedical research as a career and to be supportive of such research as voting citizens (Morrison 1992). One way for physicians to forestall these developments is to involve themselves in public education (see Resources 12–2).

◆ Some Recommendations

One errs, however, by focusing too much on the animal rights movement in addressing the public. Adults generally agree that animal research has improved their lives, but they want assurance that scientists care about and care for their animals. Further, the public needs to understand that animals are used because they are absolutely necessary to answer certain questions, that scientists have developed alternatives that better answer others, but that it is unrealistic to think that such alternatives can replace animals—and irresponsible to promote that myth. The most important message, then, is this: Well-conducted animal research, in conjunction with other methods (including human clinical trials), will continue to bring tremendous benefits. In addition, one must continue to point out the difference between animal welfare and animal rights, particularly to children, and point out the falsity of allegations against researchers when this can be documented.

Resources 12–2 includes materials that expand on the issues raised in this chapter and others that will assist in public education efforts.

◆ References

Barnes F: Interview with Ingrid Newkirk in "Politics." Vogue, September 1989, p 542

Goodwin FK: Animal rights: medical research and product testing: is this a "hang together or together we hang" issue? Contemporary Topics in Laboratory Animal Science 31:6–11, 1992

Herzog HA Jr: "The movement is my life": the psychology of animal rights activism. Journal of Social Issues 9:103–119, 1993

Horton L: The enduring animal issue. J Natl Cancer Inst 81:736–743, 1989

Jamison W, Lunch W: The rights of animals, science policy and political activism. Science, Technology and Human Values 17:438–458, 1992

Morrison AR: Biomedical research and the animal rights movement: a contrast in values. American Biology Teacher 55:204–208, 1992

Nicoll CS, Russell SM: Editorial: analysis of animal rights literature reveals the underlying motives of the movement: ammunition for counter offensive by scientists. Endocrinology 127:985–989, 1990

Nicoll CS, Russell SM, Lau A: Letter to the editor. The New York Review of Books, November 5, 1992, pp 59–60

Pardes H, West A, Pincus HA: Physicians and the animal rights movement. N Engl J Med 324:1640–1643, 1991

Paton W: Man and Mouse: Animals in Medical Research, 2nd Edition. Oxford, England, Oxford University Press, 1993

Regan T: The Case for Animal Rights. Berkeley, CA, University of California Press, 1983

Russell SM, Nicoll CS: A dissection of the chapter "Tools for Research," in Peter Singer's Animal Liberation. Proceedings of the Society for Experimental Biology and Medicine (in press)

Singer P: Unkind to animals. The New York Review of Books, February 2, 1989, p 37

Singer P: Animal Liberation, 2nd Edition. New York, Random House, 1990

Strand R, Strand P: The Hijacking of the Humane Movement. Wilsonville, OR, Doral Publishing, 1993

Office of Protection From Research Risks: Public Health Service Policy on Humane Care and Use of Laboratory Animals. Bethesda, MD, National Institutes of Health, 1986

U.S. Public Health Service: Protecting Laboratory Animals (USPHS policy statement). Bethesda, MD, Office of Laboratory Research, National Institutes of Health, 1991

Vance RP: An introduction to the philosophical presuppositions of the animal liberation/rights movement. JAMA 268:1715–1719, 1992

Verhetsel E: They Threaten Your Health: A Critique of the Antivivisection/Animal Rights (AV-AR) Movement. Tucson, AZ, Nutrition Information Center, 1986

Resources 12–1

*Organizations Supporting the
Use of Animals in Medical Research*

Acoustic Neuroma Association
American Cancer Society
American Diabetes Association
American Heart Association
American Kidney Fund
American Leprosy Foundation
American Liver Foundation
American Porphyria Foundation
Amyotrophic Lateral Sclerosis Association
Ankylosing Spondylitis Association
Arthritis Foundation
Benign Blepharospasm Research Foundation
Chronic Fatigue Immune Dysfunction Syndrome Association
Chronic Fatigue Information Institute
Chronic Fatigue Syndrome Society
Cystic Fibrosis Foundation
Dysautonomia Foundation
Dystonia Medical Research Foundation
Dystrophic Epidermolysis Bullosa Research Association of America
Ehrlers-Danlos National Foundation
Epilepsy Foundation of America
Epstein-Barr Foundation
Families of Spinal Muscular Atrophy
Guillain-Barré Syndrome Support Group International
Hemochromatosis Research Foundation
Hereditary Hemorrhagic Telangiectasia Foundation, Inc.
Huntington's Disease Society of America
Immune Deficiency Foundation
incurably ill For Animal Research
International Rett Syndrome Association
Juvenile Diabetes Foundation International
Leukemia Society of America
Lowe's Syndrome Association, Inc.
Lupus Foundation of America
Myasthenia Gravis Foundation

Narcolepsy Network
National Alliance for the Mentally Ill
National Association for Research in Schizophrenia and Depression
National Coalition for Research in Neurological and
    Communicative Disorders
National Chronic Fatigue Syndrome Association
National Depressive and Manic Depressive Association
National Foundation for Ectodermal Dysplasias
National Foundation for Ileitis and Colitis, Inc.
National Foundation for Peroneal Muscular Atrophy
National Head Injury Foundation
National Health Council
National Hydrocephalus Foundation
National Kidney Foundation
National Marfan Foundation
National Multiple Sclerosis Society
National Organization for Rare Disorders, Inc.
National Tay Sachs & Allied Diseases Association, Inc.
Parkinson's Disease Foundation, Inc.
Scleroderma Federation, Inc.
Scleroderma International Foundation
Sturge-Weber Foundation
Turners Syndrome Society
United Cerebral Palsy Research and Educational Foundation
United Leukodystrophy Foundation
United Parkinson Foundation
United Scleroderma Foundation
Wilson's Disease Association

Note. This list was provided by the National Association for Biomedical Research.

Resources 12–2

Selected Resources on Animal-Based Research

◆ Books

These books, in addition to the articles by Goodwin, Morrison, and Pardes et al. listed under References, will enrich one's understanding of the issues surrounding the use of animals in research.

Lutherer LO, Simon MS: Targeted: The Anatomy of an Animal Rights Attack. Norman, OK, University of Oklahoma Press, 1992.
This book provides a case study of what happened to Dr. John Orem at Texas Tech as an illustration of the modus operandi of some elements of the animal rights movement. Chapters on history, crisis management, IACUCs, security, legal issues, legislation, and an appendix listing many organizational contacts make this a good handbook.

Oliver DT: Animal Rights: The Inhumane Crusade (Studies in Organization Trends No. 7). Washington, DC, Capitol Research Center, 1993.
In addition to an overview of the movement's activities, there are analyses of 10 major animal rights organizations and listing of animal rights leaders and other organizations.

Paton W: Man and Mouse, 2nd Edition. Oxford, England, Oxford University Press, 1993.
This is a readable, scholarly treatise on the contributions of animal research to the conquest of disease and the ethical issues involved. Excellent figures are a good source of slides for talks to a sophisticated audience.

Strand R, Strand P: The Hijacking of the Humane Movement. Wilsonville, OR, Doral Publishers, 1993.
The Strands are dog fanciers who have frequently written for dog magazines. They analyze specific cases of attacks on animal users. Their philosophical reflections are particularly relevant.

◆ Educational Brochures

These educational brochures can be ordered from the National Institute of Mental Health (NIMH), Public Inquiries, (301) 443-4513.

Animal Research: The Search for Life-Saving Answers. (ADM) 92-1771.
Suitable for a general audience.

Animals in Medical Science—Commonly Asked Questions and Answers. (ADM) 92-1961.
Suitable for a general audience.

Animals in Science: A Student Brochure. (ADM) 92-1770.
Designed for middle and high school students.

Animals in Science: A Teacher's Guide. (ADM) 92-1769.
A companion teacher's manual.

Curiosity Is the Key to Discovery. (ADM) 92-1962.
Designed to interest middle and high school students in science.

Let's Visit a Research Laboratory. (ADM) 92-1811.
A teacher's manual and colorful poster for elementary school students.

Vital Connections. (ADM) 92-1963.
Brief descriptions of a number of mental diseases and addictive problems and the role that animal research is playing in their solution.

◆ Slide Sets

Slide sets are available for presenting the issues to the public.

Slides with talking points to be used with an adult audience and a speaker's kit for addressing school children may be requested by calling Public Inquiries, (301) 443-4513.

◆ National Organizations

These national organizations assist biomedical researchers. (There are also several state organizations.)

Americans for Medical Progress Educational Foundation, 1735 Jefferson Davis Highway, Suite 907, Arlington, VA 22202, Susan E. Paris, President, (703) 412-1111.
The Americans for Medical Progress Educational Foundation, a grass-roots advocacy group for biomedical and behavioral research, seeks to educate society's leaders, the media, and the public about the benefits of research and the role of animal research in the treatment of debilitating and deadly diseases.

Foundation for Biomedical Research (FBR), 8181 Connecticut Avenue, NW, Suite 303, Washington, DC 20006, Frankie L. Trull, President, (202) 457-0654.
The FBR has recently published the 1994 edition of the Directory of Animal Rights/Welfare Organizations, which contains information about the goals, activities, and financial status of over 175 animal rights organizations.

incurably ill For Animal Research (iiFAR), P.O. Box 27454, Lansing, MI 48909, Greg Maas, Chief Operating Officer, (517) 887-1141.
iiFAR seeks to provide the patient's perspective regarding the use of animals in biological, medical, and behavioral research and testing. iiFAR serves as a nationwide resource for those seeking information about animal use in medical research, distributes education materials, and encourages pro-animal research events.

National Animal Interest Alliance, P.O. Box 66579, Portland, OR 97290, Patti Strand, Executive Director, (503) 761-1139.
The National Animal Interest Alliance's mission is to promote a more abundant life for the people of this planet through a wise and compassionate relationship with animals and the environment.

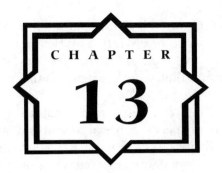

CHAPTER
13

Influencing the Political Agenda on Behalf of Psychiatric Research

Jay Cutler, J.D., and Sharon Cohen, M.A.

> The best public measures are seldom adopted from
> previous wisdom, but forced by the occasion.
>
> Benjamin Franklin

Psychiatry is a "special interest." Psychiatry's special interests range from advancing federally supported funding for psychiatric research geared toward improving our knowledge and understanding about the nature and causes of mental illness to concerns regarding the mental health benefits contained within various health care reform proposals.

While the "L" word—lobbying—for some has come to connote the undue influence of special interest groups upon America's legislative process, special interest lobbying, in fact, is nothing more than the constitutionally protected expression of your position on a particular legislative matter. In our form of representative government, the voting public elects officials to represent their views in the national legislature. Look at it this way—*if you don't look out for your*

453

own interests (and the interests of your patients), who will?

Congress is of necessity distracted by the thousands of different issues and interests that confront them every day. By lobbying, you are helping to ensure that your voice and your interests aren't lost in the shuffle.

Being a special interest doesn't mean that it's improper to lobby Congress on issues of specific concern to you and other members of the American Psychiatric Association (APA). Your interest and expertise in psychiatry—psychiatric research, the practice of psychiatry, and psychiatric education—comprise a special interest, *your* special interest. Becoming an advocate for that special interest is essential to the legislative process. It will go a long way toward broadening understanding about the needs and importance of psychiatric research. After all, who can better articulate the achievements and opportunities of psychiatric treatment than the psychiatric physician?

This chapter discusses the importance of special interest lobbying and the "dos" and "don'ts" of becoming an advocate on behalf of psychiatry and persons with mental illness.

◆ Congress: The Nature of the Beast

Knowing where to begin is half the battle in becoming an advocate/lobbyist for your cause, and the best place to start is to familiarize yourself with Congress. Congress can be intimidating. There are 100 senators (two representing each state regardless of the population of each state), who are elected to 6-year terms on a staggered basis. The House of Representatives consists of 435 members, who are elected to 2-year terms. The House membership differs from the Senate in that the entire House of Representatives is up for reelection every 2 years, and the number of representatives from any state is dependent on the number of citizens located in that state. States with large populations such as California, New York, and Texas have some of the largest state delegations.

In becoming an advocate/lobbyist you need not concern yourself with the entire Congress. Your two U.S. senators and the one U.S. representative from your congressional district should be your primary targets for lobbying purposes. Identifying your U.S. representative can sometimes be difficult if you reside in a large urban city that may have two, three, or four representatives from that one city. If you need assistance in identifying your U.S. representative, you can call your local congressional district office (usually listed in the phone book) or your local Democratic or Republican party offices.

Keep in mind that your U.S. representative is often apt to be more responsive to your advocacy efforts than your U.S. senators. This is true for two reasons. First, U.S. representatives (except for an "at-large" representative) come from a much smaller electoral base—the local district—than a U.S. senator and consequently are very concerned about the opinions of the voters from *their district*. Second, because U.S. representatives are up for reelection every 2 years, whereas senators are reelected every 6 years on a staggered basis, the pressure is always on your U.S. representative to be responsive to his or her constituents.

This doesn't mean that you would be wasting your time in lobbying your U.S. senator. It does mean, however, that you should pay attention to other considerations when "working" the Senate. U.S. senators represent the entire state, so your one voice will be better heard if you join forces with other individuals or statewide coalitions.

◆ How Congress Passes Legislation

Any member of the House of Representatives or Senate may introduce legislation while Congress is in session (not on a recess and open for business). Yearly, literally thousands of bills are introduced, ranging from legislation dealing with the federal budget, to health care reform, or to commemorative legislation marking a certain week during the year as National Ice Cream Week.

Legislation originating in the U.S. House of Representatives carries the initials H.R., followed by a number, which is the sequential order as introduced into Congress. Legislation originating in the U.S. Senate carries the initial S., followed by a sequential order number. Passage of bills requires in most cases a simple majority passage by both Houses of Congress and then a presidential signature enacting the bill into law.

The bulk of the work of Congress is handled by its numerous committees and subcommittees. There are 22 standing committees in the House and 16 in the Senate. There are also several joint standing committees. Committees have jurisdiction over measures affecting a distinct part of law. For example, the House Ways and Means Committee has jurisdiction over legislation affecting taxes and/or revenue measures; health care including Medicare, Medicaid, and national health care reform; Social Security; human resources including employee benefit issues; trade; and oversight concerns. Most committees have at least two or three subcommittees with special jurisdiction over certain aspects of legislation that falls within that full committee's jurisdiction. Each committee is provided with professional and clerical staff, who are critically important to the success or failure of moving legislation through the committee process.

Seniority plays an extremely important role in the work of congressional committees. Members rank in seniority according to the order of their appointment to the committee, with the most senior member from the party in power (majority) of that house designated as the chairman. The rules of the House require that committee chairmen be elected from nominations submitted by the majority party caucus at the commencement of each Congress.

When you become an advocate/lobbyist you need to know what committees and subcommittees your U.S. representative and senators serve on. You'll also want to know their seniority status on those committees and subcommittees. The longer your members have been on certain committees and subcommittees, the more power they can wield on your behalf.

Legislation introduced in the House generally is referred to the appropriate committee and then (usually within 2 weeks of its introduction) to the appropriate subcommittee. At the same time copies are forwarded to the agency or agencies that would be affected, to the General Accounting Office, and to the Office of Management and Budget to determine cost implications, consistency with programs of the president, and the views of the administration.

The subcommittee may decide to hold public hearings on the legislation, although from time to time such hearings are closed because of the sensitive nature of the testimony. (For example, hearings regarding military security issues are generally closed.) The best time to get your points across to your elected officials is before and during the public hearing period, when all points of view are being considered.

After hearings are held, there is a working session of the subcommittee, usually referred to as a "mark-up" session, when the members mark up or review and edit the proposed legislation. By the time the bill arrives at this stage, much behind-the-scenes lobbying has already occurred. Members come to the mark-up with amendments in mind; generally, mark-ups result in members voting on such amendments and on the final language of the bill.

Once mark-up has been successfully completed by the subcommittee, the amended legislation is forwarded to the full committee for further consideration. The full committee has a mark-up session as well, during which time the legislation may be further amended. The time between subcommittee and committee mark-up is another time for intensive lobbying since members of the full committee may bring amendments that were not successfully won in the subcommittee or address issues not considered by the subcommittee. After the full committee has completed its mark-up, the bill is voted to be reported favorably to the full house of Congress.

At this point the full committee may kill the legislation by not considering it. Legislation that is reported favorably from the full committee to the House of Representatives may be considered in several ways. The bill may be brought to the House floor on the consent calendar, which indicates that it is noncontroversial in nature. Once placed on the consent calendar for 3 days, if no objections are made, it is passed by unanimous consent without debate. Legislation may also be placed on the union calendar; this includes the vast majority of legislation and resolutions for discussion by the Committee of the Whole House.

Consideration of legislation in the Senate largely follows the pattern of the House until the legislation reaches the Senate floor. Procedural rules on the Senate floor differ significantly from those of the House. Measures may be brought to the Senate floor by a simple unanimous consent request, a consent agreement, and by motions to proceed to the consideration of legislation or to consider a measure on the calendar. A tactic used by the Senate to stall legislation is the filibuster, a delaying strategy using lengthy speeches.

Once both houses of Congress have passed a particular piece of legislation, the House and Senate versions must have their differences ironed out in conference. It is during the critical conference period when much of Congress' "horse trading" occurs. Closed-door meetings are often held in the dark of the night and often toward the end of the congressional calendar, when time pressure forces the conferees to reach a compromise over the most controversial parts of the legislation under consideration. When the conferees cannot achieve compromise and report back to their respective houses that final resolution was not achieved on certain aspects of the bill, the parts of the legislation on which the conferees could not achieve compromise are brought back to their respective houses, where they might be instructed on how to act or new conferees might be appointed.

When compromise is achieved, the conferees prepare a conference report outlining the bill as agreed upon, with sufficiently detailed information to describe its main features. This conference report and bill must then be passed by both houses of Congress; then the legislation is forwarded to the president for his approval and signing into law. If the president does not approve of the legislation, the president may choose to veto it, in which case the legislation is sent back to Congress with a veto message that may outline the president's objections. In order to override a presidential veto, both houses of Congress need to pass the legislation with a two-thirds majority.

As an advocate/lobbyist you'll need to know where in the legislative process the bill you are concerned with is. Have hearings already been held? Has the subcommittee marked up the legislation? Has the full committee reported out the legislation to the full House of Representatives? To find out this information, you can call the offices of the sponsors of the legislation—the members who introduced the bill—or you can call the committee or subcommittee to which the legislation was referred, inquiring as to what action has been taken on the bill.

◆ Becoming an Advocate/Lobbyist

All politics is local.

Tip O'Neill, former Speaker of the House

Communicating with your elected officials is the best way to get involved in advocacy/lobbying. Constituent mail is the bread and butter of every busy congressional office. Letters from the home state or congressional district provide members of Congress with an important means of assessing the views of their constituents and enable them to let their voters know of important developments in Congress.

A well-written and timely letter from home can make a real difference in the way a member of Congress looks at an important issue. Face-to-face meetings with your elected officials and their key staff aides are an extremely useful way to get to know them and to directly communicate your views on important issues. Face-to-face meetings are not restricted to Washington; visit with your member in her or her district office, or better yet, attend your member's "town hall" meeting.

Can you actually influence Congress? Certainly! Just by voting in congressional elections you help determine the shape of Congress. Your letters and personal visits are crucial in educating Congress about the nature of psychiatric illness and sensitizing its members about the needs of patients. Without your input, congressional decisions affecting psychiatry and the patients psychiatrists treat are subject to the misinformation and stigma associated with mental illness.

Have you ever written to your senators or representative on any issue? Have you ever called a congressional office? Have you ever stopped by to visit with your elected officials? If so, you have *already* become an advocate who has lobbied your federal elected officials!

One tip for getting started is to forward your senators and representative a letter of introduction telling them that you are a constituent: include your name, title, and the university you are affiliated with and highlight some new finding from the research you are involved in. Your first piece of correspondence should be kept short and written in lay language. Offer to be a resource contact if the senator or representative has questions on psychiatric illness. Close your letter with a concise message, such as "I hope you will support improved funding for psychiatric research sponsored by the National Institute of Mental Health" (NIMH). The APA would be happy to send you fact sheets on specific APA-supported positions, such as funding recommendations for the National Institutes of Health (NIH).

Once you have introduced yourself, make it a point to visit your elected officials either at their district offices or when you visit Washington. Feel free to organize a group visit. Don't be discouraged if you can only obtain a meeting with a staffer. Congressional staff play a critical role in the workings of Congress. Be brief at your meeting and address only one or two issues. Always follow up with a thank-you note. Resources 13–2 outlines the dos and don'ts when meeting with a member of Congress.

◆ The Larger Picture

> Political action is the highest responsibility of a
> citizen.
>
> John F. Kennedy

Communicating with your elected officials in only one part of becoming an advocate/lobbyist for psychiatry. Most important, *don't forget to vote on Election Day!* Voting is not only your right, it is your responsibility. Elected officials—the president, Congress, state and local representatives—are *your* elected officials. Your vote can help to put them in office or send them packing.

Also *consider the media.* If you have a particular position, consider writing a letter to the editor of your local newspaper. If it is published, make sure you send a copy to your U.S. representative, senators, and local representatives.

Use coalition building as a tactic to attract other individuals outside of psychiatry to your cause. This may include other physician groups and patient organizations. The broader your base of support for a particular view, the more credence your elected officials will give your message.

Get involved in local politics. Get involved in your local party political activities such as volunteering to serve on a campaign or re-election committee. Make it a point to attend town hall meetings that members of Congress often hold. They are usually devoted to discussion of one major issue; health care is almost certain to be on the agenda at some point. If you receive notification of such a meeting, be prepared to speak out about the need for improved access to psychiatric care. Not attending and speaking out tells the elected official one thing—your issue did not matter.

◆ Your Questions

You probably have many questions about lobbying on behalf of psychiatry. The following are some of the questions APA lobbyists are asked by APA members.

What are the major issues facing science, specifically psychiatry?

Science has been under siege for several years. Claims of scientific misconduct over fraudulent research results, conflict of interest issues between investigators and their cooperative research agreements, or last year's battle over alleged improprieties involving indirect cost accounting have all overshadowed the recent achievements won through scientific advances. But allegations of impropriety or "bad apples" in the scientific community should not lead our elected officials to quash critically important scientific research—research that may ease the suffering of millions of Americans with illnesses of all kinds.

In light of the federal budget deficit and the lack of new federal revenue sources, these threats to science could not have come at a worse time. That's why it is critically important that investigators become advocates so as to reverse the tide of bad faith.

For psychiatry, science under siege is exacerbated by the continuing stigma associated with psychiatry, mental illness, and substance abuse. There are still those in Congress who believe that mental illness is "all in one's head," or that substance abuse is merely a "character flaw." Psychiatric researchers must address both concerns head on: the more that your elected officials hear about the nature of mental illness and substance abuse and the potential for new methods of prevention, diagnosis, and treatment, the greater the likelihood that the old stereotypes will wane.

Has the APA been successful in influencing legislative initiatives and in helping secure adequate appropriations in areas important to the psychiatric research community?

Yes; the illustrations of success are numerous. One may cite a few: ending the $250 Medicare limit on reimbursement for outpatient psychiatric treatment (now there is *no* limit on dollars or number of visits, whether the treatment is psychotherapy, medication management, etc.); increasing appropriations for psychiatric research funded by the NIMH; delaying implementation of the Department of Defense psychologist prescribing program for 5 years; recapturing losses in the Resource-Based Relative Value Scale (RBRVS) by means of a nearly 50% increase in the Medicare fee schedule for a 45- to 50-minute individual psychotherapy session over the fee initially produced by the new RBRVS formula; ensuring physician consultation when a Medicare patient is treated by a psychologist; and enhancing the pay of Veterans Department psychiatrists.

In the area of appropriations, the APA has worked hard for several years to assure needed growth in NIMH, National Institute on Drug Abuse, and National Institute on Alcohol Abuse and Alcoholism (NIAAA) research funding, which was at a low level during the late 1970s and early 1980s. This effort has included making visits to members of Congress, with participation of psychiatric researchers from across the nation, building coalitions beyond the mental health community in support of improved funding, and developing important relationships with key House and Senate Appropriations Committee members who understand the need for increased federal support of mental illness and addictions research.

All of our efforts depend heavily on the work of researchers resulting in advances in understanding, diagnosing, and treating mental illness and on the advocacy of individual psychiatric physicians. Without the letter writing, congressional visits, expert testimony, and other advocacy efforts, it is less likely that APA's Division of Government Relations (DGR) would have been effective in these legislative battles.

What has been psychiatry's biggest challenge (frustration?) with respect to educating Congress about psychiatry?

Stigma is still the biggest challenge; a close second is the lack of federal dollars to do what is needed in a decade when science is advancing exponentially. Not long ago during a hearing of the House Labor, Health and Human Services Appropriations Subcommittee (the subcommittee that determines funding for the former Alcohol, Drug Abuse, and Mental Health Administration [ADAMHA] institutes), Congressman Carl Pursell (R-MI), the ranking Republican, questioned the need to spend any more federal money for NIAAA-supported research, noting, "We already know everything there is to know about alcoholism." Rep. Pursell argued that the [former] ADAMHA research budget of nearly $1 billion should be cut in half, and the saving should be used for other purposes!

In a similar vein, Senator Phil Gramm (R-TX), when questioned whether he intended to include coverage for treatment of mental and substance abuse disorders in his health care reform legislation, stated that such benefits would not be included because covering such services "would break the [health care] budget." So many in Congress are still from the "If I ignore it, it doesn't exist" school.

What issues has the APA focused on?

The APA's Division of Government Relations focuses on a wide range of issues, from Substance Abuse and Mental Health Services Administration and NIH appropriations, government agency reorganizations of concern to researchers, Medicare reimbursement and national health insurance, to scope of practice concerns, patient confidentiality, child abuse, and the insanity defense. If it affects the practice of psychiatry or psychiatric patients in any way, you can be sure your APA Division of Government Relations is involved. For a list of specific issues in which we are involved, please contact the DGR.

Research represents only a small part of the APA; how does advocacy for research help other APA objectives?

Psychiatric research stands on the threshold of new preventive, diagnostic, and treatment measures. The more Congress knows about this research, the better our chances for assuring that Congress will include mental illness and substance abuse treatment in health care reform.

Regardless of the outcome of the health care reform and its effects on academic medicine and research issues, strong, ongoing advocacy in support of nondiscriminatory mental illness and substance abuse disorder health care coverage will be necessary. Misinformation about the nature and causes of psychiatric illness and substance abuse and the perception that their treatment is either unproven or not cost effective drive their exclusion from the health care reform debate. Persons with mental illness seldom lobby Congress on their own behalf, so their voices are not heard. Advocates for research play a critical role in broadening congressional understanding about the nature of mental illness and substance abuse and the armamentarium of effective treatments that must be included in whatever health care reform package Congress finally adopts.

How can I let the APA know that I want to get involved?

The Division of Government Relations has a Grassroots Network; you can sign up to become a participant by contacting the DGR at (202) 682-6060. Once we receive your sign-up sheet, we will send a copy to your District Branch Legislative Representative so that he or she can begin to involve you in District Branch legislative affairs activities.

We'll also put you on our mailing list. You'll receive regular Legislative Newsletters and *Eco-Facts*, which will keep you up to date on the latest federal and state legislative issues affecting psychiatry.

From time to time, you will also receive APA Action Alerts, alerting you to time-sensitive issues of great concern to the APA and asking you to call or write your federal officials. These include specific information about whom to write or call and provide draft letters for you to put into your own words when writing your own elected officials.

We hope we can count on you for your help!

Resources 13–1

Selected Resources on Working With Congress

American Society of Association Executives: Beyond Washington: An Association's Guide to Shaping a State Government Affairs Program. Washington, DC, American Society of Association Executives, 1990

Birbaum JH: The Lobbyists: How Business Gets Its Way in Washington. New York, Times Books, 1992

Bohlen CC: Biologists as lobbyists. Biosci Rep, July/August 1990, p 494

Bureau of National Affairs: Federal Lobbying. Washington, DC, Bureau of National Affairs, 1989

Center for Legislative Improvement: Lobbying: A Special Report and Resource Papers on Lobbying and Its Regulation in the 50 States. Englewood, CO, Legis/50/the Center for Legislative Improvement, 1977

Cranford JR: New budget process for congress. Congressional Quarterly, November 3, 1990, p 3712

Felten E: The politics of influence peddling. Insight, September 18, 1989, p 22

Hrebenar RJ: Interest Group Politics in America. Englewood Cliffs, NJ, Prentice-Hall, 1990

Kerasote T: How to be a lobbyist: getting involved in a conservation movement is easier than you might think. Sports Afield, September 1989, p 20

Massachusetts Continuing Legal Education: How to Lobby the Government. Boston, MA, Massachusetts Continuing Legal Education, 1991

Meredith JC: Lobbying on a Shoestring. Dover, MA, Auburn Publishing, 1989

Miller C: Lobbying: Understanding and Influencing the Corridors of Power. Cambridge, MA, Blackwell, 1990

Norins L: Leading pols to the trough. Harper's Magazine, November 1991, p 33

Office of the Massachusetts Secretary of State: Lobbying: The Law, The Process and You. Boston, MA, Public Records Division, Office of the Massachusetts Secretary of State, 1990

Professional Lobbying and Consulting Center: The Lobbying Handbook. Washington, DC, Professional Lobbying & Consulting Center, 1990

Public Affairs Council: Winning at the Grassroots: How to Succeed in the Legislative Arena by Mobilizing Employees and Other Allies. Washington, DC, Public Affairs Council, 1989

Richan WC: Lobbying for Social Change. New York, Haworth Press, 1991

Smucker B: The Nonprofit Lobbying Guide: Advocating Your Cause—and Getting Results. San Francisco, CA, Jossey-Bass, 1991

Waldman M: Quid pro whoa: what your congressman shouldn't do for you. The New Republic, March 19, 1990, p 22

Wells WG Jr: Working With Congress: A Practical Guide for Scientists and Engineers. Washington, DC, American Association for the Advancement of Science, 1992

Whyte L: How to Lobby Congress. Washington, DC, Public Housing Authorities Directors Association, 1991

Wittenberg E: How to Win in Washington: Very Practical Advice about Lobbying, the Grassroots, and the Media. Cambridge, MA, Blackwell, 1989

Wolpe BC: Lobbying Congress: How the System Works. Washington, DC, Congressional Quarterly, 1990

Resources 13–2
Dos and Don'ts When Meeting
With a Member of Congress

◆ Before You Get There

Schedule your meetings in advance.   Members of Congress are very busy in Washington and at home, and their schedules fill up quickly. If you want to meet with them, you need to give them enough lead time to be able to schedule the meeting. We recommend writing or calling to book an appointment at least several weeks in advance of your desired meeting. Whether you write or call, be prepared to identify yourself as a constituent, and state the purpose of the meeting (i.e., "I'd like to meet with Representative _____ to discuss NIH funding.") Once the meeting is scheduled, it's a good idea to call to confirm the appointment a few days before arriving, just in case there's been an unavoidable change.

Don't hesitate to suggest a group meeting.   There's always strength in numbers. Bringing five or six fellow psychiatrists with you demonstrates that your concern about a specific issue is shared by many constituents. If a patient will join you or your group, all the better. Numbers do count when trying to persuade an elected official of the importance of your views.

Do your homework; be prepared.   Make it a point to know some general background information about the member of Congress you are visiting. If you have questions, your Division of Government Relations will be glad to speak with you or send you biographical information on the members you intend to visit. You'll rarely have more than 15 or 20 minutes to state your case. Your meeting may be interrupted by votes. Sometimes you may have to conduct your business while you walk with your elected official to the Capitol. So it's very important for you to be well prepared and to be able to express your views succinctly and clearly. Given the short amount of time you will have for your meeting, it's always helpful to have brief "fact sheets" or other material you can leave behind. Your Division of Government Relations will be glad to assist you with fact sheets on major issues.

◆ During the Meeting

Don't be disappointed if you meet with staff instead of the elected official. As noted, members of Congress are very busy, and last-minute changes in their schedule may force them to ask that you meet with their staff aides. Don't be upset if this happens! Key staff aides are often more familiar with specific health care or other policy issues than their busy bosses and are in the best possible position to listen to your point of view and advise the member of Congress of your concerns at precisely the right moment. Meeting with key staff is just as important as—if not more so than—meeting personally with elected officials.

Limit your agenda to no more than a few issues. Your time is limited, as is the time the member of Congress or staff member has to spend with you. So don't try to cover a large number of issues in a single meeting, even though they may all be important to you and your patients. Select one, or at most two or three, main issues to discuss. You can always bring along fact sheets that cover more than the issues you discuss during the meeting.

Be informative, be thorough, but be concise. Again, you won't have much time to present your views, so don't try to present an exhaustive history of an extremely complex issue in the 10 to 20 minutes you'll have with a member of Congress. If the issue is complicated, say so and leave behind material or offer to provide additional material that explains the problem more completely.

Try to "personalize" the issue. Rather than just asserting that such and such federal policy is "unfair to psychiatry," try to explain how the federal policy affects your practice as a psychiatrist. It's hard for elected officials to have a clear picture of how their votes on a complicated national law such as Medicare actually ends up affecting their individual constituents. By explaining in your own words how you and your patients are personally being affected, you will help the elected official better understand the consequences of the federal law to his or her constituent.

Volunteer to be a resource contact. Members of Congress and their staff aides will always welcome a constituent who is knowledgeable on specific issues and is willing to be a local resource contact who can give them advice on short notice.

◆ Protocol Concerns

Be on time.   Don't be late to a meeting. Your elected officials are very busy and may be forced to skip your meeting altogether if you're running even a few minutes late. If you're stuck in another meeting and you know you're going to be a little late, use the office phone to call ahead and let your next appointment know you may be a few minutes late. They'll try their best to accommodate you if you give them a little warning.

Bring your business cards if you have them.   Attach your business card to any written material you leave with the elected official's office.

Don't argue if there's a disagreement over policy issues.   It's fine to present your case in a straightforward and forceful manner, but don't get bogged down in an argument if the elected official or staff doesn't agree with you. "Agree to disagree" for the moment, and move on to your next topic. You can always follow up on points of disagreement with a letter explaining your views in further detail.

◆ When You Get Home

Always follow up with a "thank you."   When you get home, don't forget to send the elected official a brief thank-you note for meeting with you, and briefly restate your position or concern and requested action. If you met with staff, send the thank-you note to them (also reminding them of your position and requested action), and then send a separate letter to the elected official letting him or her know that the staff aide has ably represented his or her views.

Don't hesitate to invite your elected official to visit your practice locale.   If you are a research-based psychiatrist or run a mental health center, suggest a tour of your facility. Members of Congress will welcome the opportunity of seeing firsthand how a psychiatric facility operates. Also, don't forget to ask the elected official to speak at a district branch meeting.

Make good contacts with local congressional staff. Make it a point to get to know the key staff in your elected officials' local offices. They can be extremely helpful in helping you get access to the elected official and to the Washington, DC, staff.

Appendixes

Federal Research Contacts on Selected Issues

The appendixes provide federal contacts, organized by agency, that can provide more detailed information on current funding interests, policies, and opportunities in the following areas of research:

- ◆ Appendix A: National Institutes of Health (NIH) Extramural AIDS Contacts
- ◆ Appendix B: National Institutes of Health (NIH) Health and Behavior Coordinating Committee
- ◆ Appendix C: Federal Health Services Research Contacts
- ◆ Appendix D: Federal Sleep Research Contacts
- ◆ Appendix E: Federal Contacts on Women's Health Issues
- ◆ Appendix F: Federal Neuroscience Research Contacts

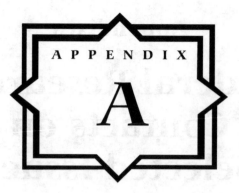

National Institutes of Health (NIH) Extramural AIDS Contacts

T he following list, reprinted from the Program Profile published in the APA Office of Research's *Psychiatric Research Report*, Vol. 9, No. 1, January 1994, provides an initial contact for fielding questions on research funding and AIDS for the NIH institutes. Unless otherwise noted, the address for the NIH institutes is on the NIH campus, 31 Center Drive, Bethesda, MD 20892.

National Institutes of Health (NIH)
Sue Ohata, Office of Director, Building 1, Room 156, (301) 496-0979

Office of AIDS Research (OAR)
Jack Whitescarver, Ph.D., Building 1, Room 201, (301) 496-0357

National Institute of Mental Health (NIMH)
Ellen Stover, Ph.D., Parklawn Building, Room 15-99, 5600 Fishers Lane, Rockville, MD 20857, (301) 443-7281

National Institute on Drug Abuse (NIDA)
Parklawn Building, 5600 Fishers Lane, Rockville, MD 20857, (301) 443-6697

National Institute on Alcohol Abuse and Alcoholism (NIAAA)
Kendall Bryant, Ph.D., Willco Building, 6000 Executive Boulevard, Bethesda, MD 20892, (301) 443-4223

National Institute on Aging (NIA)
Gail Jacoby, Building 31, Room 5C-05, (301) 496-3121

National Institute of Child Health and Human Development (NICHD)
Christine Bachrach, Ph.D., Room 8-13, 6100 Executive Boulevard, Bethesda, MD 20892, (301) 496-1174

National Institute of Neurological Disorders and Stroke (NINDS)
Carl Leventhal, M.D., Federal Building, Room 810, 7550 Rockville Pike, Bethesda, MD 20892, (301) 496-5679

National Cancer Institute (NCI)
Judith Karp, M.D., Building 31, Room 11A-27, (301) 496-3505

National Heart, Lung, and Blood Institute (NHLBI)
Elaine Sloand, M.D., Building 31, Room 5A-52, (301) 496-3245

National Institute on Deafness and Other Communication Disorders (NIDCD)
Kenneth Gruber, Ph.D., Executive Plaza South, Room 400C, 6120 Executive Boulevard, Bethesda, MD 20892, (301) 402-3458

National Institute for Nursing Research (NINR)
June Lunney, Ph.D., R.N., Westwood Building, Room 754, 5333 Westbard Avenue, Bethesda, MD 20892, (301) 594-7397

National Institute of Allergy and Infectious Diseases (NIAID)
Holly Hunter, Building 31, Room 7A-04, (301) 496-9088

National Institute of Arthritis and Musculoskeletal and Skin Diseases (NIAMS)
Stanley Pillemer, M.D., Building 31, Room 4C-13, (301) 496-0434

National Institute of Dental Research (NIDR)
Matthew Kinard, Ph.D., Westwood Building, Room 509, 5333 Westbard Avenue, Bethesda, MD 20892, (301) 594-7641

National Institute of Diabetes and Digestive and Kidney Diseases (NIDDK)
Judith Fradkin, M.D., Westwood Building, Room 621, 5333 Westbard Avenue, Bethesda, MD 20892, (301) 594-7567

National Institute of Environmental Health Sciences (NIEHS)
Ghanta Rao, Ph.D., Mail Drop AO-01, PO Box 12233, Research Triangle Park, NC 27709, (919) 541-7899

National Eye Institute (NEI)
Richard Mowery, Ph.D., Executive Plaza South, Room 350, 6120 Executive Boulevard, Bethesda, MD 20892, (301) 496-5983

National Institute of General Medical Sciences (NIGMS)
James Cassatt, Ph.D., Westwood Building, Room 907, 5333 Westbard Avenue, Bethesda, MD 20892, (301) 594-7800

National Library of Medicine (NLM)
Harold Schoolman, M.D., Building 38, Room 2E-17B, (301) 496-4725

National Center for Research Resources (NCRR)
Judith Vaitukaitis, M.D., Building 12A, Room 4007, (301) 496-5793

Fogarty International Center (FIC)
Kenneth Bridbord, M.D., Internal Studies Branch, Building 31, Room B2-C32, (301) 496-2516

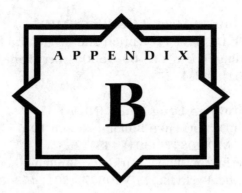

APPENDIX

B

National Institutes of Health (NIH) Health and Behavior Coordinating Committee

The following list provides a contact for fielding questions on research issues associated with health and behavior within the NIH. Unless otherwise noted, the address for the NIH institutes is on the NIH campus, 31 Center Drive, Bethesda, MD 20892.

Office of the Director
Jack Kalberer, Ph.D., Federal Building, Room 6C-10, 7550 Rockville Pike, Bethesda, MD 20892, (301) 496-6614

Office of AIDS Research (OAR)
Paul Gaist, M.P.H., Building 31, Room 5C-06, (301) 496-0358

Division of Research Grants (DRG)
Teresa Levitin, Ph.D., Westwood Building, Room 303, 5333 Westbard Avenue, Bethesda, MD 20892, (301) 594-7141

Office of Alternative Medicine (OAM)
John Spencer, Ph.D., Executive Plaza South, 6120 Executive Boulevard, Suite 450, Bethesda, MD 20892, (301) 402-2566

National Institute of Mental Health (NIMH)
Fred Altman, Ph.D., Basic Prevention and Behavioral Medicine,
Parklawn Building, Room 11C-06, 5600 Fishers Lane, Rockville,
MD 20857, (301) 443-4337

National Institute on Drug Abuse (NIDA)
Steven Gust, Ph.D., Parklawn Building, Room 10-05, 5600 Fishers
Lane, Rockville, MD 20857, (301) 443-1263
Cora Lee Wetherington, Ph.D., Parklawn Building, Room 10A-20,
5600 Fishers Lane, Rockville, MD 20857, (301) 443-1263

National Institute on Alcohol Abuse and Alcoholism (NIAAA)
Jan Howard, Ph.D., and Susan Martin, Ph.D., both at
6000 Executive Boulevard, Suite 505, Bethesda, MD 20892,
(301) 443-1677

National Institute on Aging (NIA)
Ronald P. Abeles, Ph.D., Gateway Building, Room 2C-234, 7201
Rockville Pike, Bethesda, MD 20892, (301) 496-3136
Miriam Kelty, Ph.D., Gateway Building, Room 2C-218, 7201
Rockville Pike, Bethesda, MD 20892, (301) 496-9322

**National Institute of Child Health and Human Development
  (NICHD)**
Norman Krasnegor, Ph.D., Room 4B-05, 6100 Executive
Boulevard, Bethesda, MD 20892, (301) 496-6591

National Institute of Neurological Disorders and Stroke (NINDS)
Herbert Lansdell, Ph.D., Federal Building, Room 920, 7550
Rockville Pike, Bethesda, MD 20892, (301) 496-5745
Sarah H. Broman, Ph.D., Federal Building, Room 8C-06, 7550
Rockville Pike, Bethesda, MD 20892, (301) 496-5821

National Cancer Institute (NCI)
Barry Portnoy, Ph.D., Building 31, Room 10A-49, (301) 496-1071

National Heart, Lung, and Blood Institute (NHLBI)
Sydney Parker, Ph.D., Westwood Building, Room 640C, 5333
Westbard Avenue, Bethesda, MD 20892, (301) 594-7466
Peter G. Kaufmann, Ph.D., Federal Building, Room 216B, 7550
Rockville Pike, Bethesda, MD 20892, (301) 496-9380

National Institute on Deafness and Other Communication Disorders (NIDCD)
Beth Ansel, Ph.D., Executive Plaza South, Room 400B, 6120 Executive Boulevard, Bethesda, MD 20892, (301) 496-5061

National Institute for Nursing Research (NINR)
Sharlene Weiss, Ph.D., R.N., Westwood Building, Room 757, 5333 Westbard Avenue, Bethesda, MD 20892, (301) 594-7496
Suzanne Lee Feetham, Ph.D., R.N., Building 31, Room 5B-09, (301) 402-1446

National Institute of Allergy and Infectious Diseases (NIAID)
Amy R. Sheon, M.P.H., Solar Building, 6003 Executive Boulevard, Bethesda, MD 20892, (301) 496-6177
Heather Miller, Ph.D., Solar Building, Room 3A-26, 6003 Executive Boulevard, Bethesda, MD 20892, (301) 402-0443

National Institute of Arthritis and Musculoskeletal and Skin Diseases (NIAMS)
Reva Lawrence, Ph.D., Building 31, (301) 496-0434
Julia Freeman, Ph.D., Westwood Building, Room 403, 5333 Westbard Avenue, Bethesda, MD 20892, (301) 594-9961

National Institute of Dental Research (NIDR)
Patricia Bryant, Ph.D., Westwood Building, Room 506, 5333 Westbard Avenue, Bethesda, MD 20892, (301) 594-7638
Helen Gift, Ph.D., Westwood Building, Room 525, 5333 Westbard Avenue, Bethesda, MD 20892, (301) 594-7615

National Institute of Diabetes and Digestive and Kidney Diseases (NIDDK)
Frank Hamilton, M.D., M.P.H., Westwood Building, Room 3A-15, 5333 Westbard Avenue, Bethesda, MD 20892, (301) 496-7821

National Institute of Environmental Health Sciences (NIEHS)
Sheila Newton, Building 31, Room B1-C02, (301) 496-3511

National Eye Institute (NEI)
Michael Oberdorfer, Ph.D., Executive Plaza South, 6120 Executive Boulevard, Suite 350, Bethesda, MD 20892, (301) 496-5301

National Library of Medicine (NLM)
Elliot Siegel, Ph.D., Building 38, Room 2S-20, 8600 Rockville Pike, Bethesda, MD 20892, (301) 496-8834

National Institute of General Medical Sciences (NIGMS)
James Onken, Ph.D., Westwood Building, Room 819, 5333 Westbard Avenue, Bethesda, MD 20892, (301) 594-7746

National Center for Human Genome Research (NCHGR)
Helen Simon, M.S., Building 38A, Room B2-N13, 8600 Rockville Pike, Bethesda, MD 20892, (301) 402-2205

National Center for Research Resources (NCRR)
Barbara Perrone, Building 12A, Room 4047, (301) 496-2992

Fogarty International Center (FIC)
Arlene Fonaroff, Ph.D., or Coralie Farlee, Ph.D., M.P.H., Building 31C, Room B2-C11, (301) 496-4784/1491

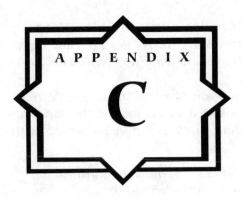

Federal Health Services Research Contacts

This listing of health services research contacts is updated from the Program Profile published in the APA Office of Research's *Psychiatric Research Report*, Vol. 8, No. 3, September 1993.

Agency for Health Care Policy and Research (AHCPR)
Unless otherwise noted, all contacts at the AHCPR are located at the Westwood Building, 5333 Westbard Avenue, Bethesda, MD 20892.

Office of the Administrator
Clifford Gaus, Ph.D., Administrator, (301) 594-6662

Center for General Health Services Extramural Research
Norman W. Weissman, Ph.D., Director, (301) 594-1349, X109
    Division of Primary Care: Carolyn Clancy, M.D., Director,
    (301) 594-1357, X137
    Division of Cost and Financing: Fred Hellinger, Ph.D., Director,
    (301) 594-1354, X121
    Division of Technology and Quality Assessment: Bertha
    Atelsek, Director, (301) 594-1352, X115

Center for Medical Effectiveness Research
Richard J. Greene, M.D., Ph.D., Director, (301) 594-1485

Center for Research Dissemination and Liaison
Allan Lazar, Acting Director, (301) 594-1360, X144

Health Care Financing Administration (HCFA)
Joseph Antos, Director, Office of Research and Demonstrations, 6325 Security Boulevard, Baltimore, MD 21207, (410) 966-6507

National Institute on Alcohol Abuse and Alcoholism (NIAAA)
Unless otherwise noted, all contacts at the NIAAA are located at the Willco Building, 6000 Executive Boulevard, Bethesda, MD 20892.

Division of Clinical and Prevention Research
Richard K. Fuller, M.D., Director, (301) 443-1206
    Homeless Demonstration and Evaluation Branch: Robert Huebner, Ph.D., Director, (301) 443-0786
    Treatment Research Branch: John P. Allen, Ph.D., Chief, (301) 443-0796

Division of Biometry and Epidemiology, Epidemiology Branch
Mary C. Dufour, M.D., M.P.H., Chief, (301) 443-4897

National Institute on Drug Abuse (NIDA)
Unless otherwise noted, all contacts at NIDA are located at the Parklawn Building, 5600 Fishers Lane, Rockville, MD 20857.

Division of Epidemiology and Prevention Research
Zili Sloboda, Sc.D., Director, (301) 443-6504
    Community Research Branch: Richard H. Needle, Ph.D., Chief, (301) 443-6720

Division of Clinical and Services Research
Robert Battjes, D.S.W., Acting Director, (301) 443-6697
    Treatment Research Branch: Jack D. Blaine, M.D., Chief, (301) 443-4060

National Institute of Mental Health (NIMH)
Unless otherwise noted, all contacts at the NIMH are located at the Parklawn Building, 5600 Fishers Lane, Rockville, MD 20857.

Division of Epidemiology and Services Research
Darrel Regier, M.D., M.P.H., Director, (301) 443-3648
Grayson Norquist, M.D., M.S.P.H., Deputy Director, (301) 443-3266
    Services Research Branch: Thomas L. Lalley, Chief; and Kathy Magruder-Habib, Ph.D., (301) 443-3364

Violence and Traumatic Stress Research Branch: Susan D. Solomon, Ph.D., (301) 443-3728
Epidemiology and Psychopathology Research Branch: Ben Z. Locke, Chief, (301) 443-3774

Department of Veterans Affairs (VA)
Daniel Deykin, M.D., Director
Ruth E. Parry, M.A., M.A.S., J.D., Health Services Research and Development Service, 810 Vermont Avenue, NW, Washington, DC 20420, (202) 535-7156

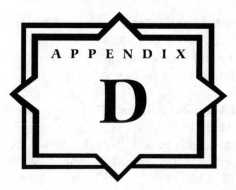

Federal Sleep Research Contacts

The following list provides a contact for fielding questions on research issues associated with sleep within the NIH. Unless otherwise noted, the address for the NIH institutes is on the NIH campus, 31 Center Drive, Bethesda, MD 20892.

National Institute of Mental Health (NIMH)
Richard Nakamura, Ph.D., Behavioral and Integrative Neuroscience Research Branch, Parklawn Building, Room 11-102, 5600 Fishers Lane, Rockville, MD 20857, (301) 443-1576

National Institute on Aging (NIA)
Andrew Monjan, Ph.D., Neurobiology and Neuropsychology Branch, Gateway Building, 7201 Rockville Pike, Suite 3C-307, Bethesda, MD 20892, (301) 496-9350

National Institute of Child Health and Human Development (NICHD)
Charlotte Catz, M.D., Pregnancy and Perinatology Branch, 6100 Executive Boulevard, Suite 4B-03, Bethesda, MD 20852, (301) 496-5575

National Institute of Neurological Disorders and Stroke (NINDS)
Floyd Brinley Jr., M.D., Ph.D., Division of Convulsive,

Developmental, and Neuromuscular Disorders, Federal Building, Room 816, 7550 Rockville Pike, Bethesda, MD 20892, (301) 496-6541

National Heart, Lung, and Blood Institute (NHLBI)
James Kiley, Ph.D., Acting Director, National Center on Sleep Disorders Research, Building 31, Room 4A-11, (301) 496-7443

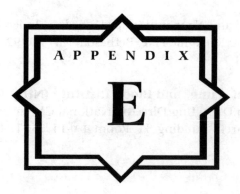

Federal Contacts on Women's Health Issues

T he following list, reprinted from the Program Profile published in the APA Office of Research's *Psychiatric Research Report*, Vol. 9, No. 2, April 1994, provides an initial contact for fielding questions on research funding and women's health issues. Unless otherwise noted, the address for the NIH institutes is on the NIH campus, 31 Center Drive, Bethesda, MD 20892.

National Institutes of Health (NIH)
Bonnie Kalberer, Office of Director, Building 1, (301) 496-0608

Office of Research on Women's Health (ORWH)
Vivian Pinn, M.D., Building 1, Room 201, (301) 402-1770

Women's Health Initiative (WHI)
Lorretta Finnegan, M.D., Federal Building, Room 6A-09, 7550
Wisconsin Avenue, Bethesda, MD 20892, (301) 402-2900

Office of AIDS Research (OAR)
Jack Whitescarver, Ph.D., Building 1, Room 201, (301) 496-0357

National Institute of Mental Health (NIMH)
Deborah Dauphinais, M.D., Parklawn Building, Room 15-99, 5600
Fishers Lane, Rockville, MD 20857, (301) 443-7281

National Institute on Drug Abuse (NIDA)
Christine Hartel, Ph.D., Parklawn Building, Room 10-A38, 5600
Fishers Lane, Rockville, MD 20857, (301) 443-6697

National Institute on Alcohol Abuse and Alcoholism (NIAAA)
Mary Dufour, Ph.D., 6000 Executive Boulevard, Bethesda, MD
20892, (301) 443-4897

National Institute on Aging (NIA)
Shirley Bagley, Building 31, Room 5C-35, (301) 496-0765

**National Institute of Child Health and Human Development
(NICHD)**
Judith Whalen, Ph.D., Building 31, Room 2A-10, (301) 496-1877

**National Institute of Neurological Disorders and Stroke
(NINDS)**
Mary Miers, Building 31, Room 8A-03, (301) 496-9271

National Cancer Institute (NCI)
Iris Schneider, Building 31, Room 11A-48, (301) 496-5534

National Heart, Lung, and Blood Institute (NHLBI)
Barbara Packard, M.D., Ph.D., Building 31, Room 5A-03,
(301) 496-6331

**National Institute on Deafness and Other Communication
Disorders (NIDCD)**
Judith Cooper, Ph.D., Executive Plaza South, Room 400B, 6120
Executive Boulevard, Bethesda, MD 20892, (301) 402-5061

National Institute for Nursing Research (NINR)
Patricia Moritz, Ph.D., Westwood Building, Room 738, 5333
Westbard Avenue, Bethesda, MD 20892, (301) 594-7496

National Institute of Allergy and Infectious Diseases (NIAID)
George Counts, M.D., Office of Research on Minority and Women's
Health, Solar Building, Room 4B-04, 6003 Executive Boulevard,
Bethesda, MD 20892, (301) 496-8697

National Institute of Arthritis and Musculoskeletal and Skin Diseases (NIAMS)
Julia Freeman, Ph.D., Westwood Building, Room 403, 5333 Westbard Avenue, Bethesda, MD 20892, (301) 594-9961

National Institute of Dental Research (NIDR)
Susan Wise, Building 31, Room 2C-34, (301) 596-6705

National Institute of Diabetes and Digestive and Kidney Diseases (NIDDK)
Nancy Cummings, M.D., Westwood Building, Room 627, 5333 Westbard Avenue, Bethesda, MD 20892, (301) 594-7599

National Institute of Environmental Health Sciences (NIEHS)
Anne Sassaman, PO Box 12233, Research Triangle Park, NC 27709, (919) 541-7723

National Eye Institute (NEI)
Richard Mowery, Ph.D., Executive Plaza South, Room 350, 6120 Executive Boulevard, Bethesda, MD 20892, (301) 496-5983

National Institute of General Medical Sciences (NIGMS)
Norka Ruiz Bravo, Ph.D., Westwood Building, Room 910, 5333 Westbard Avenue, Bethesda, MD 20892, (301) 594-7754

National Library of Medicine (NLM)
Lois Ann Colaianni, 8600 Rockville Pike, Bethesda, MD 20894, (301) 496-6921

National Center for Human Genome Research (NCHGR)
Elke Jordan, Ph.D., Building 38A, Room 605, (301) 496-0844

National Center for Research Resources (NCRR)
Harriet Gordon, M.D., Westwood Building, Room 10A-03, 5333 Westbard Avenue, Bethesda, MD 20892, (301) 594-7945

Fogarty International Center (FIC)
Josepha Ippolito-Shepherd, Ph.D., Building 31, Room B2-C08, (301) 496-1491

**Substance Abuse and Mental Health Services Administration
(SAMHSA)**
Mary Knipmeyer, Ph.D., Parklawn Building, Room 13-99, 5600
Fishers Lane, Rockville, MD 20857, (301) 443-5184

Agency for Health Care Policy and Research (AHCPR)
Ann Bavier, Westwood Building, 5333 Westbard Avenue, Bethesda,
MD 20892, (301) 594-1357, X129

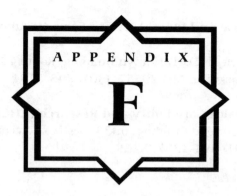

Federal Neuroscience Research Contacts

T his appendix is based on the 1994 listing of government neuroscience contacts provided by the National Institute of Mental Health (NIMH). For more detailed information, contact the NIMH, 5600 Fishers Lane, Rockville, MD 20892, (301) 443-1576.

National Institute of Mental Health (NIMH)
Unless otherwise noted, all neuroscience contacts at the NIMH are located at the Parklawn Building, 5600 Fishers Lane, Rockville, MD 20857.

Division of Neuroscience and Behavioral Science
Stephen H. Koslow, Ph.D., Director, Room 11-103, (301) 443-3563
Stanley F. Schneider, Ph.D., Associate Director for Research Training and Resources, Room 11-103, (301) 443-4347
Michael F. Huerta, Ph.D., Associate Director for Scientific Technology and Resources, Human Brain Project and SBIR/STTR Programs, Room 11-103, (301) 443-5625
Mary F. Curvey, Fellowship Program and SBIR/STTR Programs, Room 11-103, (301) 443-3107

Behavioral and Integrative Neuroscience Research Branch
Richard K. Nakamura, Ph.D., Chief and Acting Chief of the Cognitive Neuroscience Program, Room 11-102, (301) 443-1576

Dennis L. Glanzman, Ph.D., Chief, Theoretical and Computer
Neuroscience Program, Room 11-102, (301) 443-1576
Dorothy Karp, Ph.D., Chief, Behavioral Pharmacology Program,
Room 11-94, (301) 443-1576
Israel I. Lederhendler, Ph.D., Chief, Systems Neuroscience Program,
Room 11-102, (301) 443-1576

Molecular and Cellular Neuroscience Research Branch
Steven J. Zalcman, M.D., Chief and Acting Chief of the
Neuropharmacology and Drug Discovery Programs, Room 11-95,
(301) 443-3948
Henry Khachaturian, Ph.D., Chief,
Neurotransmitter–Neuroregulation Program, Room 11C-06,
(301) 443-5288
Douglas L. Meinecke, Ph.D., Chief, Developmental Neuroscience
Program, and Acting Chief of the Neuroscience Centers Program,
Room 11C-06, (301) 443-5288
Ljubisa Vitkovic, Ph.D., Chief, Neuroimmunology and
Neurovirology Program, Room 11C-06, (301) 443-5288

Behavioral, Cognitive, and Social Processes Research Branch
Mary Ellen Oliveri, Ph.D., Chief and Acting Chief of the
Sociocultural and Environmental Processes Program, Room
11C-10, (301) 443-3942
Rodney R. Cocking, Ph.D., Chief, Fundamental Cognitive
Mechanisms Program, Room 11C-16, (301) 443-9400
Della M. Hann, Ph.D., Chief, Interpersonal and Family Processes
Program, Room 11C-10, (301) 443-3942
Lynne C. Huffman, M.D., Chief, Personality and Emotion Program,
Room 11C-10, (301) 443-3942
Howard S. Kurtzman, Ph.D., Chief, Advanced Mental Processes
Program, Room 11C-16, (301) 443-9400

Division of Clinical and Treatment Research
Jane A. Steinberg, Ph.D., Acting Director, Room 18C-26,
(301) 443-3683
David Shore, M.D., Chief, Schizophrenia Research Branch, Room
18C-26, (301) 443-3266
Robert F. Prien, Ph.D., Chief, Clinical Treatment Research Branch,
Room 18-105
Mary C. Blehar, Ph.D., Acting Chief, Mood, Anxiety, and
Personality Disorders Branch, Room 10C-16, (301) 443-1636

Barry D. Lebowitz, Ph.D., Chief, Mental Disorders of Aging
Research Branch, Room 18-105
Peter S. Jensen, M.D., Chief, Child and Adolescent Disorders
Research Branch, Room 18C-17, (301) 443-5944

Office of AIDS Programs (AIDS)
Ellen L. Stover, Ph.D., Director, Room 15-99, (301) 443-7281

Division of Epidemiology and Services Research
Darrell A. Regier, M.D., M.P.H., Director, Room 10-105, (301)
443-3648

National Institute on Drug Abuse (NIDA)
Unless otherwise noted, all neuroscience contacts at NIDA are located
at the Parklawn Building, 5600 Fishers Lane, Rockville, MD 20857.

Division of Basic Research
James V. Dingell, Ph.D., Director, Room 10A-31, (301) 443-1887
Christine R. Hartel, Ph.D., Deputy Director, Room 10A-31, (301)
443-1887
Charles W. Sharp, Ph.D., AIDS, Inhalant Programs, Room 10A-31,
(301) 443-1887

Behavioral Neurobiology Research Branch
Roger M. Brown, Ph.D., Chief, Room 10A-19, (301) 443-6975
Lynda Erinoff, Ph.D., (perinatal effects of drugs), Room 10A-19,
(301) 443-6975
Jerry Frankenheim, Ph.D., (neuropsychopharmacology), Room
10A-19, (301) 443-6975
Joseph Frascella, Ph.D., (clinical neurosciences), Room 10A-19,
(301) 443-6975
Reinhard Grzanna, Ph.D., (long-term effects of drugs), Room
10A-19, (301) 443-6975

Biochemistry Branch
Karen J. Skinner, Ph.D., Chief, Room 10A-19, (301) 443-1887
Theresa N. Lee, Ph.D., Room 10A-19, (301) 443-1887
Geraldine C. Lin, Ph.D., Room 10A-19, (301) 443-1887
Pushpa V. Thadani, Ph.D., Room 10A-19, (301) 443-1887

Research Technology Branch
Rao S. Rapaka, Ph.D., Chief, Room 10A-13, (301) 443-6975
Paul S. Hillery, Ph.D., Drug Supply System and Analysis Service
Program, Room 10A-13, (301) 443-6273

Division of Epidemiology and Prevention Research, Epidemiology Research Branch
Arthur Hughes, Chief, Room 615, Rockwall Building, (301) 443-2974
Harold W. Gordon, Ph.D., Biobehavior Etiology Program, Room 615, Rockwall Building, (301) 443-2974
Jag H. Khalsa, Ph.D., Biobehavior Consequences, Room 615, Rockwall Building, (301) 443-2974

National Institute on Alcohol Abuse and Alcoholism (NIAAA)
Unless otherwise noted, all neuroscience contacts at the NIAAA are located at the Willco Building, 6000 Executive Boulevard, Bethesda, MD 20892.

Division of Basic Research
William Lands, Ph.D., Director, (301) 443-2530
Helen Chao, Ph.D., Deputy Director, (301) 443-2530
Ernestine Vanderveen, Ph.D., Associate Director, (301) 443-1273

Neurosciences and Behavioral Research Branch
Walter Hunt, Ph.D., Chief, (301) 443-4223
Ellen Witt, Ph.D., HSA (biobehavioral), (301) 443-4223
Robert Karp, Ph.D., HSA (genetics), (301) 443-4223
Francine Lancaster, Ph.D., HSA (neurochemistry), (301) 443-4223

Biomedical Research Branch
Sam Zakhari, Ph.D., Chief, (301) 443-4223
Laurie Foudin, Ph.D., HSA (pregnancy/fetal alcohol syndrome), (301) 443-4223

National Institute on Aging (NIA)
Unless otherwise noted, all neuroscience contacts at the NIA are located at the Gateway Building, 7201 Wisconsin Avenue, Bethesda, MD 20892.

Neuroscience and Neuropsychology of Aging Program
Zaven S. Khachaturian, Ph.D., Associate Director, Room 3C-307, (301) 496-9350

Dementia of Aging Branch
Neil S. Buckholtz, Ph.D., Acting Chief, Room 3C-307, (301) 496-9350
Carl D. Banner, Ph.D., Director, Alzheimer's Disease Program, Room 3C-307, (301) 496-9350

Neil S. Buckholtz, Ph.D., Director, Treatment and Management Program, Room 3C-307, (301) 496-9350
Tony Phelps, Ph.D., Director, Alzheimer's Disease Centers Program, Room 3C-307, (301) 496-9350

Neurobiology of Aging Branch
Andrew A. Monjan, Ph.D., Chief, Room 3C-307, (301) 496-9350
D. Stephen Snyder, Ph.D., Director, Fundamental Neuroscience, Room 3C-307, (301) 496-9350
Deborah L. Claman, Ph.D., Director, Sensory Processes/Motor Processes, Room 3C-307, (301) 496-9350

Neuropsychology of Aging Branch
Andrew A. Monjan, Ph.D., Acting Chief, Room 3C-307, (301) 496-9350
Deborah L. Claman, Ph.D., Director, Neuropsychology of Aging, Room 3C-307, (301) 496-9350

Office of Alzheimer's Disease Research
Zaven S. Khachaturian, Ph.D., Chief, and Director of the NIH Coordinating Committee for Alzheimer's Disease Research, Room 3C-307, (301) 496-9350

National Institute of Child Health and Human Development (NICHD)
Unless otherwise noted, all neuroscience contacts at the NICHD are located at 6100 Executive Boulevard, Rockville, MD 20892.

Center for Research for Mothers and Children
Charlotte Catz, M.D., Chief, Pregnancy and Perinatology Branch, Room 4B-03E, (301) 496-5575
Del H. Dayton, M.D., Chief, Genetics and Teratology Branch, Room 4B-01E, (301) 496-5541
Felix de la Cruz, M.D., Chief, Mental Retardation and Developmental Disability Branch, Room 4B-09E, (301) 496-1383
Norman A. Krasnegor, Ph.D., Chief, Human Learning and Behavior Branch, Room 4B-05, (301) 496-6591
Marian Willinger, Ph.D., Sudden Infant Death Syndrome, (301) 496-5575

Center for Population Research
Christine Bachrach, Ph.D., Chief, Demographic and Behavior Science Branch, (301) 496-1174

Michael E. McClure, Ph.D., Chief, Reproductive Services Branch, (301) 496-6515

National Center for Medical Rehabilitation Research
Danuta Krotoski, Ph.D., Chief, Basic Rehabilitation Medical Research Branch, Building 61E, Room 2A-03, 610 Executive Boulevard, Rockville, MD 20852, (301) 402-2242

National Institute of Neurological Disorders and Stroke (NINDS)
Unless otherwise noted, all neuroscience contacts at NINDS are located at the Federal Building, 7550 Wisconsin Avenue, Bethesda, MD 20892.

Division of Extramural Activities
Connie Atwell, Ph.D., Director, (301) 496-9248

Division of Fundamental Neurosciences
Eugene Streicher, Ph.D., Director, Room 916, (301) 496-5745
W. Watson Alberts, Ph.D., Deputy Director, Room 916, (301) 496-1447
F. Terry Hambrecht, M.D., Head, Neural Prostheses, Room 9C02, (301) 496-5745
William Heetderks, M.D., Ph.D., Neural Prostheses, Room 9C02, (301) 496-5745
Herbert C. Lansdell, Ph.D., Learning Systems, Room 920, (301) 496-5745
Alfred Weissberg, M.S., Neurochemistry, Room 916, (301) 496-5745
Novera H. Spector, Ph.D., Neuroimmunomodulation, Room 916, (301) 496-5745

Division of Convulsive, Developmental, and Neuromuscular Disorders
Floyd J. Brinley, M.D., Ph.D., Director, Room 816B, (301) 496-6541
Joseph S. Drage, M.D., Deputy Director, Room 816A, (301) 496-9022

Developmental Neurology Branch
Philip H. Sheridan, M.D., Chief, Room 8C10, (301) 496-6701
Paul L. Nichols, Ph.D., Neuromuscular Disorders, Room 8C08, (301) 496-5821
Sarah H. Broman, Ph.D., Mental Retardation and Learning Disorders, Room 8C06, (301) 496-5821

Judith A. Small, Ph.D., Neurogenetics and Birth Defects,
Room 8C04, (301) 496-5821
Giovanna Spinella, M.D., Autism, Behavioral Disorders, and
Clinical Pediatric Neurology, Room 820, (301) 496-5821

Epilepsy Branch
Walter Bell, Ph.D., Acting Chief, Room 114, (301) 496-6691
Charlotte McCutchen, M.D., Sleep Disorders and Epilepsy,
Room 114, (301) 496-1917
Harvey J. Kupferberg, Ph.D., Chief, Preclinical Pharmacology,
Room 118, (301) 496-1917

Division of Demyelinating, Atrophic, and Dementing Disorders
Carl M. Leventhal, M.D., Director, Room 810A, (301) 496-5679
A.P. Kerza-Kwiatecki, Ph.D., MS, ALS, Neuroimmunology, and
Neurovirology, Room 804A, (301) 496-1431
Eugene J. Oliver, Ph.D., Alzheimer, Huntington, and Parkinson's
Diseases, Room 806A, (301) 496-1431
Kenneth Surrey, Ph.D., Pain, Neurotoxicology, and
Neuroendocrinology, Room 802A, (301) 496-1431

Division of Stroke and Trauma
Michael D. Walker, M.D., Director, Room 8A-08A,
(301) 496-2581
George N. Eaves, Ph.D., Deputy Director, Room 8A-13A,
(301) 496-4226
Patricia A. Grady, Ph.D., Stroke and Imaging, Room 8A10,
(301) 496-4226
John R. Marler, M.D., Cerebrovascular Disease, Room 800,
(301) 496-4226
Mary Ellen Michel, Ph.D., CNS Trauma and Regeneration,
Room 8A13, (301) 496-4226

National Heart, Lung, and Blood Institute (NHLBI)
Unless otherwise noted, all neuroscience contacts with the
Divisions of Heart and Vascular Diseases and Epidemiology and
Clinical Applications of the NHLBI are located in the Federal
Building, 7550 Wisconsin Avenue, Bethesda, MD 20892; the
Division of Lung Diseases is located in the Westwood Building,
5333 Westbard Avenue, Bethesda, MD 20892.

Division of Heart and Vascular Diseases
Michael J. Horan, M.D., Director, Room 416A, (301) 496-2553

David M. Robinson, Ph.D., Associate Director, Scientific Programs, Room 416B, (301) 496-5656
Frank Altieri, Ph.D., Acting Associate Director, Cardiology, Room 320, (301) 496-5421
John L. Fakunding, Ph.D., Chief, Research Training and Development Branch, Room 3C-03, (301) 496-1724
Stephen S. Goldman, Ph.D., Cardiac Functions Branch, Room 308, (301) 496-1627
Peter M. Spooner, Ph.D., Chief, Cardiac Functions Branch, Room 304A, (301) 496-1627
Stephen C. Mockrin, Ph.D., Arteriosclerosis, Hypertension, and Lipid Metabolism, Room 4C-12B, (301) 496-1857
Constance E. Weinstein, Ph.D., Chief, Cardiac Diseases Branch, Room 3C-06, (301) 496-1081

Division of Epidemiology and Clinical Applications
Lawrence Friedman, M.D., Director, Room 212, (301) 496-2533
Gerald Payne, M.D., Associate Director, Scientific Programs, Room 220, (301) 496-2533
Peter Kaufmann, Ph.D., Chief, Behavioral Medicine Branch, Room 216, (301) 496-9380

Division of Lung Diseases
Suzanne S. Hurd, Ph.D., Director, Room 6A-16, (301) 496-7208
Carol E. Vreim, Ph.D., Associate Director, Scientific Programs, Room 6A-16, (301) 496-7208
James P. Kiley, Ph.D., Chief, Airways Diseases Branch, Room 6A15, (301) 496-7332
Sydney R. Parker, Ph.D., Chief, Prevention, Education, and Research Training Branch, Room 640C, (301) 496-7668

National Institute on Deafness and Other Communication Disorders (NIDCD)
Unless otherwise noted, all neuroscience contacts at the NIDCD are located at Executive Plaza South, 6120 Executive Boulevard, Suite 400B, Rockville, MD 20892.

Division of Communication Sciences and Disorders
Ralph F. Naunton, M.D., Director, (301) 496-1804
Judith A. Cooper, Ph.D., Deputy Director, (301) 496-5061
Beth Ansel, Ph.D., Voice and Speech, (301) 402-3461
Amy Donahue, Ph.D., Hearing, (301) 402-3458

Kenneth Gruber, Ph.D., Hearing, (301) 402-3458
Lynn Huerta, Ph.D., Hearing, (301) 402-3461
Jack Pearl, Ph.D., Chemical Senses, (301) 402-3464
Daniel Sklare, Ph.D., Balance and Vestibular, (301) 402-3461
Rochell Small, Ph.D., Chemical Senses, (301) 402-3464

National Eye Institute (NEI)
Unless otherwise noted, all neuroscience contacts at the NEI
are located at Executive Plaza South, 6120 Executive Boulevard,
Suite 350, Bethesda, MD 20892.

Extramural Research
Jack A. McLaughlin, Ph.D., Associate Director, (301) 496-9110

Strabismus, Amblyopia, and Visual Processing Branch
Michael Oberdorfer, Ph.D., Chief, (301) 496-5301

Retinal Diseases Branch
Peter A. Dudley, Ph.D., Chief, (301) 496-0484
Maria Y. Giovanni, Ph.D., Director, Fundamental Retinal Process
Program, (301) 496-0484

National Institute of Environmental Health Sciences (NIEHS)
Christopher Schonwalder, Ph.D., Chief, Scientific Programs Branch,
Division of Extramural Research and Training, (919) 541-7634,
or Annette Kirshner, Ph.D., Neuroscience and Neurobehavioral
Toxicology, (919) 541-0488, both at Building 3, Post Office Box
12233, Research Triangle Park, NC 27709

National Center for Research Resources (NCRR)
The NCRR is located in both the Westwood Building (WW),
5333 Westbard Avenue, Bethesda, MD 20892, and Building 12A,
31 Center Drive, Bethesda, MD 20892.

Extramural Research Resources
Judith L. Vaitukaitis, M.D., Acting Deputy Director,
Room 12A/4011, (301) 496-6023
Charles L. Coulter, Ph.D., Acting Director, Biomedical Research
Technology Program, Room WW/8A-15, (301) 594-7934
Richard M. Dubois, Ph.D., HSA, Biomedical Research Technology
Program, Room WW/8A-15, (301) 594-7934
Louise E. Ramm, Ph.D., Director, Biological Models and Materials
Research Program, Room WW/854, (301) 594-7906

Bernard Talbot, M.D., Ph.D., Acting Director, General Clinical Research Centers Program, Room WW/Room 10A-03, (301) 594-7945

Fogarty International Center (FIC)
David Wolff, Ph.D., Chief, International Research and Awards Branch, or Mirilee Pearl, Ph.D., Building 31, Room B2-C39, 31 Center Drive, Bethesda, MD 20892, (301) 496-1653

National Science Foundation (NSF)
Unless otherwise noted, all neuroscience contacts at the NSF are located at 4201 Wilson Boulevard, Arlington, VA 22230

Division of Integrative Biology and Neuroscience
Thomas E. Brady, Ph.D., Acting Director, Room 685, (703) 306-1420
Kathie L. Olsen, Ph.D., Acting Deputy Director, Room 685, (703) 306-1420

Neuroscience Cluster
Christopher J. Platt, Ph.D., Director, Sensory Systems, Room 685, (703) 306-1424
Christopher M. Comer, Ph.D., Director, Behavioral Neuroscience, Room 685, (703) 306-1416
Kathie L. Olsen, Ph.D., Director, Neuroendocrinology, Room 685, (703) 306-1423
Karen A. Sigvardt, Ph.D., Director, Computational Neuroscience Program, Room 685, (703) 306-1416
Felix Strumwasser, Ph.D., Director, Neuronal and Glial Mechanisms, Room 685, (703) 306-1424

Physiology and Behavior Cluster
Fred Stollnitz, Ph.D., Director, Animal Behavior, Room 685, (703) 306-1419

Division of Biological Instrumentation and Resources
Peter W. Arzberger, Ph.D., Director, Comp. Biology, Room 615, (703) 306-1469
Joanne G. Hazlett, Cross-directorate Activities, Room 615, (703) 306-1471
Charles Keith, Ph.D., Instrumentation and Instrument, (703) 306-1472
Michael K. Lamvik, Ph.D., Development Program, Room 615, (703) 306-1472

Division of Electrical and Communication Systems
Paul J. Werbos, Ph.D., Director, Neuroengineering, Room 668,
(703) 306-1339

Division of Social Behavior and Economic Research
Alan Kornberg, Ph.D., Director, Room 995, (703) 306-1766
Paul G. Chapin, Ph.D., Director, Linguistics, Room 995,
(703) 306-1731
Jean B. Intermaggio, Ph.D., Director, Social Psychology, Room 995,
(703) 306-1728
Joseph L. Young, Ph.D., Director, Human Cognition and
Perception, Room 995, (703) 306-1732
Merry Bullock, Director, Human Cognition and Perception,
Room 995, (703) 306-1732

Air Force Office of Scientific Research (AFOSR)
Unless otherwise noted, all neuroscience contacts for AFOSR are
located at Bolling Air Force Base, Office of Scientific Research,
Washington, DC 20332.

Life and Environmental Sciences Directorate
William O. Berry, Ph.D., Director, (202) 767-4278
Genevieve M. Haddad, Ph.D., Manager,
Neuroscience/Chronobiology, (202) 767-5021
John F. Tangney, Ph.D., Manager, Perception and Recognition,
Computational Neuroscience, and Cognition, (202) 767-5021
Daniel L. Collins, Ph.D., Manager, Spatial Orientation, (202) 767-5021

Math and Computer Sciences Directorate
Steven Suddarth, Ph.D., Manager, Neural Networks, (202) 767-5028

Education, Academic, and Industry Affairs Directorate
Claude Cavender Director, Training, (202) 767-4970

U.S. Army Research (ARI)
Michael Kaplan, Ph.D., Director, Office of Basic Research, Army
Research Institute for Behavioral and Social Sciences, 5001
Eisenhower Avenue, Alexandria, VA 22333, (202) 274-8641

Defense Advanced Research Projects Agency (DARPA)
Barbara Yoon, Ph.D., Manager, Neural Networks Program,
Microelectronic Technology Office, 3701 North Fairfax Drive,
Arlington, VA 22203, (703) 696-2234

Office of Naval Research (ONR)
Unless otherwise noted, all neuroscience contacts for ONR are
located 800 North Quincy Street, Arlington, VA 22217.

Life Sciences Directorate
Steven Zornetzer, Ph.D., Director, (703) 696-4501

Biological Sciences Division
Robert Newburgh, Ph.D., Director, (703) 696-4986
Jeannine Majde, Ph.D., Manager, Systems Biology, (703) 696-4055
Igor Vodyanoy, Ph.D., Science Officer, Systems Biology,
(703) 696-4056

Cognitive and Neural Sciences Division
Willard Vaughan, Ph.D., Director, (703) 696-4505
Thomas M. McKenna, Ph.D., Manager, Computational
Neuroscience Program, (703) 696-4503
Joel L. Davis, Ph.D., Science Officer, Computational Neuroscience
Program, (703) 696-4744
Harold Hawkins, Ph.D., Manager, Perceptual Sciences Program,
(703) 696-4323
Teresa McMullen, Ph.D., Science Officer, Perceptual Sciences
Program, (703) 696-3163
Susan Chipman, Ph.D., Manager, Cognitive Science Program,
(703) 696-4138
Terry Allard, Ph.D., Science Officer, Cognitive Science Program,
(703) 696-4502

Math and Physical Sciences Directorate
Michael F. Shlesinger, Ph.D., Manager, Physics Program,
(703) 696-4220

National Aeronautics and Space Administration (NASA)
Unless otherwise noted, all neuroscience contacts at NASA are
located at 300 "E" Street, SW, Mail Code UL, Washington, DC 20546.

Life Science Division
Frank Sulzman, Ph.D., Chief, Life Support Branch, (202) 358-2359
Thora Halstead, Ph.D., Manager, Space Biology, (202) 358-2359
Janice H. Stoklosa, Ph.D., Manager, Biomedical Research Program,
(202) 358-2359
Victor Schneider, Ph.D., Manager, Physiology Program,
(202) 358-2359

Index

*Page numbers printed in **boldface** type refer to tables or figures.*

BASIC ESSENTIALS™ SERIES

BASIC ✺ ESSENTIALS™

EDIBLE WILD PLANTS & USEFUL HERBS

SECOND EDITION

JIM MEUNINCK

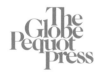

The Globe Pequot Press

Guilford, Connecticut

Acknowledgments

I owe a debt of gratitude to Laurie Kenney and Lisa Reneson, whose attention to detail and creativity assured the improvement and completion of this project.

Special thanks to my wife, Jill, and my daughter, Rebecca, for their warm companionship on our many wilderness journeys.

Copyright © 1988, 1999 by Jim Meuninck

Photographs of maples & oaks on pages 54 & 55 courtesy Fernwood Botanic Gardens, all others by Jim Meuninck.
Cover design by Lana Mullen
Cover photo of wild onion by the author.
Text design by Casey Shain
Layout design by Amy Andersen

Basic Essentials is a trademark of The Globe Pequot Press.

Library of Congress Cataloging-in-Publication Data

Meuninck, Jim, 1942-
    Basic essentials: edible wild plants & useful herbs / by
        Jim Meuninck. —2nd ed.
      p. cm. —(Basic essentials series)
    Includes bibliographical references (p.) and index.
    ISBN 0-7627-0479-9
    1. Wild plants, Edible—United States. 2. Cookery (Wild foods) 3.
Wild plants, Edible—Therapeutic use.
I. Title. II. Series.
QK98.5.U6M48 1999
581.6'32'0973—DC21   99-19357
                                        CIP

♻ Printed on recycled paper
Manufactured in Quebec, Canada
Second Edition/Second Printing

Contents

Introduction

*B*asic Essentials: Edible Wild Plants & Useful Herbs *is a record of thirty years of experience put to pen, experience I've gained foraging for edible and medicinal wildflowers in the United States, Japan, China, Europe, and Canada. This record, however, is not new. Thousands—perhaps millions—of years ago, our ancestors discovered, by trial and error, which plants were edible and which plants were poisonous.*

Today, modern studies by anthropologists around the globe suggest that eating wild plants and flowers may have numerous benefits beyond good taste. Unlike many cultivars we buy in the supermarket, these plants have not been genetically manipulated or weakened by hybridization. They are vigorous and rich in the nutrients and phytochemicals our bodies need and contain essentially complete germ plasma untampered by human hands. The more than one hundred Paleolithic plants described in this book are high in fiber, calcium, and protein, and full of vitamins and minerals. And they're low in fat, too. Many contain healthful Omega-3 essential fatty acids, which help prevent inflammatory conditions that may lead to heart disease, arthritis, and cancer.

This book is organized somewhat differently than traditional field guides. Most books are organized by season or by flower color. I have chosen to identify plants as you would stumble across them walking in a woods, trekking through a meadow, or paddling through a marsh. This practical approach begins with the familiar and progresses to the unfamiliar. All of the plants described in this book can be found in the contiguous United States, and most of the plants can also be found on my video, Jim Meuninck's Edible Wild Plants. *See Appendix 2 for information on this and other recommended videos and books.*

So let's begin our walk back through time along the tangled and twisted path of our ethnobotanical heritage. The trail will uncover authoritative, practical tips on gathering, preparing, and cultivating edible wild plants. You'll learn how to identify edible berries, and how to make berry-delicious desserts, herbal teas, and other proven recipes from my thirty years of experience and the vast human record that preceded me. Here and there along the path, modern medicinal uses will be uncovered and wildflower seed sources will be surveyed. Poisonous plants also will be attended to (see Appendix 1: Poisonous Plants & Poisonous Look-alikes).

I invite you to join me on this exciting journey. The story opens in Painter Marsh, a typical wetland harboring edible, water-loving flora.

Jim's Top Ten Edible Wild Flowers

1. Woodland Violets *(Viola* spp.*)*
2. Bee Balm *(Monarda fistulosa)*
3. Elder *(Sambucus canadensis, S. nigra)*
4. Wild Carrot, Queen Anne's Lace
   (Daucus carota)
5. Cattail *(Typha latifolia)*
6. Dandelions *(Taraxacum officinale)*
7. Mint (peppermint, spearmint, mountain mint)
   (Mentha spp.*)*
8. Garden Sorrel *(Rumex* spp.*)*
9. Hawthorn *(Crataegus* spp.*)*
10. Evening Primrose *(Oenothera biennis)*

Jim's Top Ten Favorite Edible Wild Plants
In the order I prefer, by the volume I eat.

1. Dandelions *(Taraxacum officinale)*
2. Stinging Nettle *(Urtica dioica)*
3. Violets *(Viola* spp.*)*
4. Watercress *(Nasturtium officinale)*
5. Wild Leeks *(Allium tricoccum)*
6. Wild Rice *(Zizania aquatica)*
7. Cattail (*Typha latifolia*)
8. Daylily *(Hemerocallis* spp.*)*
9. Elder *(Sambucus canadensis)*
10 Chickweed *(Stellaria* spp.*)*

Wild Plant Foraging Rules

1. It's a good idea to watch a plant through its growth cycle before eating it. This is helpful because many wild plants taste best just as they break through the ground, when they are small, furled, and difficult to identify. By watching them grow for a year, you will know what you are looking for and where to find it.

2. Before eating any wild plants, study with an expert or take the plant to an expert for positive identification. Always cross-reference with two or more field guides. Make certain you have seen color photos of the plants; Black-and-white photos or illustrations are not sufficient for positive identification.

3. After positive identification of an edible plant, taste only a very small amount of it. This precaution may protect you from an allergic reaction or misidentification.

4. Beware of the carrot family: Hemlock, water hemlock, and other members of this family are extremely poisonous. Learn to distinguish hemlock and water hemlock from elder (elderberries).

5. I do not endorse herbal medication, self-diagnosis, or self-medication. The medicinal references in this book are descriptions from what I have read. Please do not self-medicate. Consult with your physician.

6. Practice conservation. Never collect more plants than you intend to use. Do not pick rare or endangered species. Work with a professional botanist to restore wild plants from areas where they have disappeared.

7. Avoid harvesting plants from polluted ground. Plants growing along roads may be tainted with benzene, lead, oil, and other auto pollutants. Plants dwelling in streams and along fields near farms may be polluted with herbicides and pesticides. Forage carefully. Droppings from wild game may spread bacteria, viruses, worms, *Giardia,* amoebas, and other forms of contamination into water nurturing wild edible plants. Be careful! Wash and cook all plants foraged from wild lands.

8. Purchase wild plants from seed and live plant purveyors like Richter's (see Appendix 2). Grow them in your garden, close to your kitchen. Make wild foods an integral part of your diet.

Rivers, Lakes, Ponds & Swamps

Cattail *(Typha latifolia)*

Description. Long, sword-shaped leaves; green flowers on tandem spikes; lower spike female, upper spike male. Worldwide range. There are two species of cattails common to North America: broad leafed and narrow leafed.

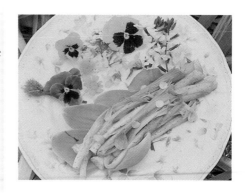

Location. Entire United States, except extreme desert climates.

Warning. *Before eating cattail shoots, learn to distinguish young shoots from their poisonous look-alike, Iris shoots (see Appendix 1). Cattail shoots are more round; Iris shoots are flat and hard. Cattail shoots are more widely spaced, while Iris shoots grow in tight clusters. If you are not certain, remember Wild Plant Foraging Rule #1.*

Cooking tips. Cattails are a versatile foodstuff. The roots, new shoots, and flowering heads are all edible. In the spring simply find the shoots, reach down into the mud, and pull. Peel off the outer leaves, and underneath is the tender tongue of cattail. Sauté this delicate core in butter for 3 to 5 minutes. Season with a few drops of soy sauce and a pinch of wild ginger.

The male flowering head (located above the female flower spike) is simple to harvest, nutritious, and freezes well. Simply strip it into a plastic bag. This high-protein flour extender will keep in your freezer for eight months. Freeze the pollen, stamens, and anthers for year-round use in baked goods.

The young female bloom spike can be cooked like corn on the cob. Simply boil or steam the spike in lightly salted water. Cook until tender, butter, and eat hot. Young spikes can be eaten uncooked. Mix five parts cattail pollen with one part honey for a quick-to-prepare high-energy food.

A bit deeper in the soil is the long root where the cattail was attached. The root core is an excellent source of starch. Eat the starch raw as quick-energy food or, better yet, crush the roots in cold water and leach out the starch. The starch can be added to soups and stews as a thickener.

Paleolithic Waffles

In a large bowl combine the following ingredients:

½ cup low-fat Bisquick
1 cup buckwheat flour
½ cup cattail pollen or male flowering parts
1 handful of chopped almonds
3 tablespoons ground flax seeds
    (best ground in a coffee mill)
⅓ cup cooked wild rice (optional)
⅓ cup cooked 12- or 20-grain cereal (optional)

Next, break in 1 egg white, pour in enough skim milk to moisten, and squeeze in the juice of half a lemon. Spray waffle iron with canola spray, pour in waffle mix, and prepare to enjoy one of the most sustaining, high-fiber, energy-rich and protein-rich breakfasts you will ever have. Makes five waffles.

Medicinal uses. Without endorsing herbal medicine, I've discovered that cattail parts have been used to treat gonorrhea, worms, and diarrhea. The chopped root is also applied to burns and minor cuts. The Chinese use the plant to stop bleeding.

Watercress *(Nasturtium officinale)*

Description. Grows along the margins of shallow, clean water. Alternate leaves to ¾-inch in width, ovate, simple, broad near base; small white flower with four petals. To avoid contamination from pesticides and herbicides, collect watercress (and, for that matter, all edible water plants) from a clean water source such as a highland stream or free-flowing spring.

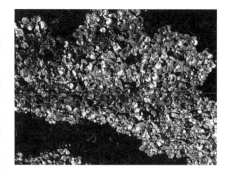

Watercress is a pungent, spicy green. It's an important ingredient in V8 cocktail juice and one of the most useful greens known to humankind. In the northern United States and Canada, watercress is available ten months a year. South of the Mason-Dixon line it's a year-round food. Watercress is high in vitamins C and A.

Location. Throughout the United States.

Warning. *It's a good idea to cook all watercress gathered from the bush to avoid possible contamination with* **Giardia** *and other waterborne parasites and contaminants.*

Cooking tips. Scramble chopped watercress with eggs, stuff a pita sandwich, add it to salads, or make watercress soup. I like to stir-fry watercress with 1 tablespoon of olive oil, 2 tablespoons of soy sauce, 1 tablespoon of lemon juice, 1 teaspoon of diced ginger root, and the juice of 1 pressed garlic clove. Cook briefly at medium heat for about 2 minutes. Your can also use watercress as a stuffing when preparing smoked or baked bass. After washing the body cavity, stuff the fish with watercress, season to taste, and bake or smoke it.

Medicinal uses. Mild diuretic. A few Indian groups used water-cress to dissolve gallstones.

Duckweed *(Lemna* spp.*)*

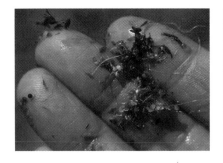

Description. Floating plant; one or two ¾₆-inch oval leaves; thread-like root hairs. You've probably seen duckweed—it's the green slime completely covering ponds, backwaters, and sloughs in midsummer. Upon closer inspection, the green water cover is one of the smallest flowering plants. This plant is hydroponic; the tiny root hairs siphon nutrients from the water.

Location. Found nationwide.

Warning. *Like all wild plants, use this plant sparingly. If you have any food allergies, be especially careful.*

Cooking tips. Duckweed is edible. Intrepid foragers can blend it into their favorite soup recipe. More conservative folks use it sparingly, as duckweed has an unusual, tough texture that is pleasing to some and distasteful to others.

Medicinal uses. The Chinese use duckweed to treat hypothermia, flatulence, and acute kidney infections.

Reed Grass
(Phragmites communis)

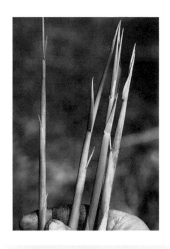

Description. Tall wetland grass; lance-shaped leaves up to 1 foot in length; flowers in tall, dense plume. Plants grow in dense cluster. Reed grass is found around the margins of streams and in wet lowlands. The root of reed grass, like cattail roots, can be harvested and leached of its starch. Note: The dried, hollow stalks of reed can be cut to 4-inch lengths and used as spigots for tapping maple trees for syrup.

Location. Throughout the United States.

Cooking tips. The first shoots of spring can be eaten raw but are best steamed until tender. Prepare the plant immediately after picking, as delays in preparation make for a tough, stringy meal. Simply chop the new shoots into a manageable size and place them in a steamer. They are ready to eat in 5 minutes. In the fall, seeds can be ground into flour or stripped, crushed, and cooked with berries. Also try reed seeds cooked in stews and soups.

Medicinal uses. The Chinese use this plant to clear fevers, quench thirst, promote diuresis, and promote salivation.

Wild Rice *(Zizania aquatica)*

Description. Tall reed-like grass; long, narrow leaf blades; flowers in tall plume; upper flowers female, lower flowers male. Wild rice is a tall grass found growing in shallow, clean water. The seeds can be harvested in August and September. Timing is critical, so check your stand of wild rice often. Mature seeds drop off easily. Return every other day to maximize the harvest.

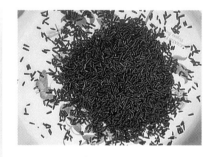

Use a rolling pin to thresh the husks from the seed. Simply roll back and forth over the grain. Use a fan or the wind to dispel the chaff.

Location. Eastern United States, roughly to the Mississippi.

Cooking tips. The simplest way to cook wild rice is to boil 2 cups of lightly salted water, add 1 cup of wild rice, and cover and simmer for 35 minutes. Makes an excellent stuffing for wild turkey. Wild rice, cooked until tender, is an excellent addition to pancake and waffle mixes. It also goes well in twelve- and twenty-grain hot cereals and is a great substitute for white rice. Extend your supply by cooking it half and half with long-grained brown rice.

Yellow Pond Lily, Spatterdock
(Nuphar variegatum, N. luteum)

Description. These two closely related species are found in ponds, shallow lakes, and streams. Their disk-shaped leaves unfurl above water. The yellow flower blooms through the summer and bears a primitive-looking fruit. The fruit pod contains numerous seeds—perhaps the only palatable part of this plant. The root stock of spatter-

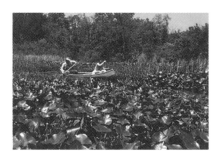

dock can be cut free and boiled. It smells sweet like an apple, but it's a bitter pill to swallow—even after cooking in two or three changes of water. Strictly a survival food, when nothing else is available.

Location. Throughout the United States, except extreme mountain and desert regions.

Cooking tips. The seeds can be dried and ground into flour or pre-pared like popcorn. Place the dried seeds in a popcorn popper. Cover the machine so the small seeds don't become airborne. The results are usually disappointing. Seeds simply pop open, but they're edible with salt and butter.

Medicinal uses. Root poulticed on wounds, swellings, boils, and inflamations. Root tea used to treat chills and fever.

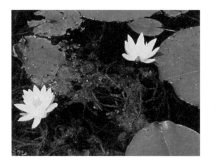

Fragrant Water Lily
(Nymphaea odorata)

Description. Large, platter-shaped leaves that float flat, 6 to 10 inches in diameter; large white flower. The fragrant water lily is edible and is also simple to trans-plant. Simply place it in a clay pot submerged in fresh water.

Location. Eastern United States, roughly to the Mississippi.

6

BASIC ESSENTIALS

Cooking tips. Pioneers ate the unfurled leaves and the unopened flower buds. The flower petals can be eaten with salad greens.

Medicinal uses. Dried root used to treat mouth sores and as an astringent.

Arrowhead, Wapato *(Saggitaria latifolia)*

Description. Arrow-shaped leaves, veins palmate; white flower, 3 platter-shaped petals. Arrowhead (also called wapato) has an edible tuber attached to its root.

Location. Found from Maine to Washington down through California.

Warning. *Arrowhead looks similar to the poisonous arrow arum (see Appendix 1). To avoid confusing the two, note that arrowhead leaves are palmate (all veins run out from a single source like fingers on the palm of a hand), whereas arrow arum has pinnate veins (veins that run out along the entire length of the mid-rib vein that dissects the leaf). Best to follow this plant through one year's growth cycle to avoid confusion.*

Cooking tips. The arrowhead tuber can be harvested in the fall, winter, or spring. Boil the tuber until tender. Remove the peel, mash the contents in a frying pan, and cook like hash browns.

Medicinal uses. Native Americans used the root to treat tuberculosis. Root used internally to treat fever.

Pickerel Weed *(Pontedera cordata)*

Description. Arrow-shaped leaf, veins spread from base, merge at tip like venation in grass leaves; blue flowers, densely clustered spikes. Young leaves and mature seeds can be eaten. Leaves most tender in spring, while unfurling beneath water.

Location. Entire United States, except extreme desert, southern California, and lower Florida.

Cooking tips. Cook leaves with dandelions and mustard greens. Season cooked greens with Italian dressing and serve hot. Add flower petals to salads. In late summer, seeds mature in tough, leathery capsules. Open capsule to get fruit. Munch as a trail food or dry and grind into flour.

Wild Rose *(Rosa* spp.*)*

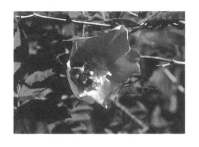

Description. Bush; spiny branches; white, pink, or red flowers; leaves alternate, compound, sharply toothed margins. Common edible flower found along the margins of waterways. Plant's autumn flowers give rise to the famous fruit, rose hip.

Location. Various species found throughout the United States, except extreme desert regions.

Cooking tips. Petals are sweet and aromatic. Rose petals and leaves can be dried and used for tea. Add to summer floral salads. Rosewater can be made by boiling aromatic rose petals in a still made with an Erlenmeyer flask, rubber stopper, copper coil, and collecting jar. Using rosewater as a marinade for skinless chicken adds both flavor and aroma.

Medicinal uses. An excellent source of vitamin C, rose hip is used to prevent scurvy. The Chinese and Native Americans used rose tea to treat worms and intestinal disorders.

American Elder, Elderberry
(Sambucus canadensis, S. racemosa, S. caerulea)

Description. Shrub; leaf feather-like, compound, leaflet number variable, 10 to 12 leaflets typical, toothed; white flowers in dense, flat, or rounded cluster; blue to black to red berries. American elder thrives along the edges of streams, bogs, and other wetlands. *S. canadensis* has black berries. *S. caerulea* has blue berries while two subspecies of *S. racemosa,* black elder and red elder, have black-to-purple and red berries, respectively.

Location. S. canadensis is found in the eastern United States, roughly to the Mississippi. *S. racemosa* and *S. caerulea* are found in the western United States.

Warning. *Learn to distinguish elder flowers from poisonous water hemlock flowers (see Appendix 1). Cross-reference with two or three field guides, and forage with a knowledgeable botanist. Make positive, expert identification. Make certain you have seen color photos of the two plants. Also, always cook red elderberries as the raw berries may cause you to vomit.*

8   B A S I C   E S S E N T I A L S

Cooking tips. Elderberry matures in late summer and can be boiled into fruit drink, made into jelly, or fermented into wine. Elderberries later in the year can be dried in a food drier or simply frozen fresh. Dried elderberries can be stirred into bread, waffle, pancake, and cookie mixes. You can eat the flower heads raw or make a rice-flour dip and deep-fry

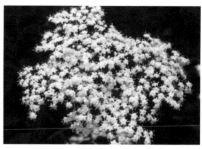

S. canadensis

them. You can make elder flower brandy by mixing the same amount of brandy by volume with the same amount of flowers by weight, i.e., 5 ounces of brandy with 5 ounces of flowers. Make certain to strip flowers off the cluster and into the brandy and keep elderberry stems out of the brew. Let the mix sit (refrigerated) for two weeks, then strain it through nylon hose and enjoy. Try this recipe with port or sherry, too.

Elderberry-Apple Pie

2 cups elderberries
1 cup blackberries or wild grapes (without seeds)
2 cups cooking apples
3 tablespoons brown sugar or maple syrup
1 teaspoon cinnamon
½ teaspoon nutmeg
1 egg
1 teaspoon flour
3 tablespoons butter
9-inch store-bought pie shell

In a bowl mix berries and apples, and stir in brown sugar or maple syrup. Add cinnamon, nutmeg, and egg. Pour contents into a 9-inch pie shell. Sprinkle a pinch of flour over each layer. Place butter over the filling. Bake pie (topless or cover with a crust) at 325° F for 45 minutes.

Medicinal uses. Elderberry extracts are antiviral. In Europe elderberry syrup (Sambucol) is used to prevent and treat colds and flu. Elder flowers contain rutin and quercitin, bioflavonoids useful in preventing heart disease. Antioxidant rich, the flowers also provide protection from cancer-causing free-radical damage.

North American Berries

Strawberry
(*Fragaria virginiana, F. vesca, F. california*)

Description. White flower; sharply toothed leaflets, in threes. Wild strawberries are found in meadows and open woods. Harvest in late May and early June. Strawberries are high in vitamin C and are fiber rich— a good choice for dieters.

Location. *F. virginiana* is found in the eastern United

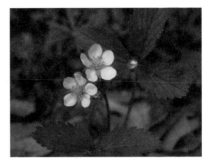

F. virginiana

Berry Good Muffins

Here's all the energy you need to kick off the day.

1 whole seedless orange
1 cup strawberries or raspberries
1 cup blackberries or mulberries (or any other berries, including rose hips)
1 egg
½ cup vegetable oil
1½ cups flour
¾ cup sugar
1 teaspoon baking powder
1 teaspoon baking soda
1 teaspoon salt
½ cup raisins
1 cup black walnuts

Combine orange—peel and all—with all berries. Add egg and vegetable oil. Blend. Mix flour, sugar, baking powder, baking soda, and salt. Add raisins and walnuts. Bake at 375° F for 20 minutes. Makes six muffins.

BASIC ESSENTIALS

States, roughly to the Mississippi; *F. vesca* is found west of the
Mississippi; and *F. california* is found in California and Baja.

Medicinal uses. Native Americans used strawberries to treat gout,
scurvy, and kidney infections. Root tannins were used to treat malaria.
The fruits contain ellagic acid.

Raspberry *(Rubus idaeus, R. occidentalis)*

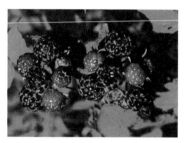
R. idaeus

Description. Shrub; spiny branches; compound leaves, three to five
leaflets, sharply toothed; white flowers,
three or more petals. Red and black
raspberries are found along the fringes
of woods, fence rows, and the margins
of fields. Berries are ready for harvest
in late spring and early summer.

Location. Throughout the
United States.

Cooking tips. Use as pie filling or stir into pancake batter and
muffin mixes. Makes excellent jam or jelly.

Medicinal uses. Leaves can be steeped in tea and used as a tonic
for pregnant women. Native Americans used root for diarrhea and
dysentery. Also used to flavor medicines. Like other berries, here's a
great dietary choice for weight watchers. High in cancer-fighting ellagic
acid. One cup of raspberries per day shows promise as an anti-cancer
agent. Nananone, the frosty appearance of wild raspberries, is an
anti-fungal agent that protects the berries from fungal infections. That's
why wild raspberries do not spoil as quickly as cultivars that have lost
their capacity to produce nananone.

Blackberry
*(Rubus allegheniensis,
R. laciniatus)*

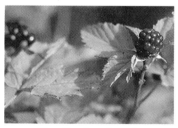
R. allegheniensis

Description. Similar to raspberry.
Shrub; spiny branches; compound
leaves, 5+/- leaflets, toothed; white
flower bloom appears after raspber-

ries. *R. laciniatus* has sharply cut leaves. Blackberries are often found near your raspberry source. There are several species. Blackberries ripen in mid- and late summer.

Location. Throughout the United States.

Cooking tips. Here's a low-calorie, high-nutrition breakfast made with raspberries, blackberries, or both. Mix 2 cups of berries with 2 cups of low-fat sweetened vanilla yogurt. Add a dash of milk and blend—a wonderful ice cream substitute with only half the sugar and fat. Also use in pies, muffins, pancakes, jellies, and jams. Make tea from the leaves.

Medicinal uses. Native Americans used roots with other herbs for eye sores, backaches, and stomachaches. Pioneers made blackberry vinegar to treat gout and arthritis. The Chinese use *Rubus* species in a tea to stimulate circulation—they claim it helps alleviate pain in muscles and bones. Blackberries also contain several cancer-fighting antioxidants.

Blueberry
(Vaccinium spp.*)*

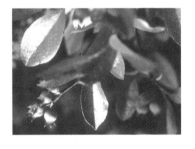

Description. Shrub; leaves alternate, simple, smooth margin; flowers white to pink, tightly clustered. Blueberries are available from early summer through early autumn. There are several species. Found in highlands, lowlands, openlands, and wooded areas.

Location. Various species found throughout the United States.

Cooking tips. For a simple blueberry treat, pour a bowl of frozen blueberries and cover them with half-and-half, whole milk, or low-fat milk. This frozen dessert sets up quickly and is ready to eat—a refreshing, cooling, low-sugar, world-class treat. Use blueberries in pies, pancakes, and other fruit recipes described in this book.

Medicinal uses. Blueberries contain anthocyanin that may protect you from *E. coli* infections. This is a fine bioflavonoid-rich food that protects you from degenerative disease. Native Americans used the antioxidant qualities of blueberries to preserve foods such as pemmican.

Gooseberry and Currant *(Ribes* spp.*)*

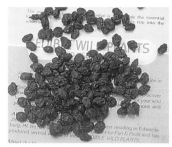

Dried currant.

Description. Shrub; spiny branches; gooseberry fruit is spined, while currant has smooth or spined fruit; deeply lobed leaves, sharply toothed; flowers yellow, purplish, or white (depending on species). You can find gooseberries and currants in woodlands and along the margins of woods. There are several species. The spiny, dangerous-looking berries are harmless and ready for harvest in midsummer.

Location. Various species found throughout the United States.

Cooking tips. Make Gooseberry-Currant Pie from Elderberry-Apple Pie recipe (see page 9). Be certain to add lemon juice to punch up the taste.

Medicinal uses. Gooseberries and currants are made into a jelly spiced with peppermint, lemon juice, and ginger, then taken as a sore throat remedy. Others claim that Gamma-Linolenic Acid (GLA), an active ingredient of currants, may prevent acne, obesity, and schizophrenia.

Mulberry *(Morus* spp.*)*

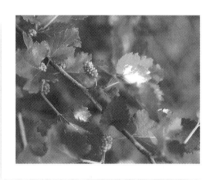

Description. Small to medium-size tree; leaves simple, alternate, toothed, round or slightly elongated, broadest near base; flowers green, tiny, clustered on spike. Not far from gooseberries are mulberries. Mulberry trees are found along roads, the fringes of woods, fence rows, and about anywhere berry-eating birds have redistributed the seeds. There are red, white, and black varieties. Ripened fruits are very edible.

Location. Eastern United States, roughly to the Mississippi.

Warning. *Do not eat the unripened fruits and leaves because they are slightly hallucinogenic.*

Cooking tips. Mulberries, gooseberries, and currants can be combined or used separately to make fudge.

Medicinal uses. White mulberry *(M. alba)* leaf extraction has shown promise as a treatment for elephantiasis. The fruits of both white and red mulberry *(M. rubra)* are said to reduce fever.

Mulberry Fudge

This candy has a taffy-like consistency and is messy to eat. Gooseberries and currants, in combination or separately, can also be used.

1 pound mulberries
2 cups sugar
5 tablespoons butter

Gently cook mulberries in ½ cup of water until hot, then mash berries through a fine sieve to separate the juice. Add sugar to mashed berries. Add butter, then reheat slowly to dissolve butter. Bring to a boil over medium heat. Do not stir. Let mix form a hot, soft ball. (This will occur at between 235° and 240° F on a candy thermometer.) Cool until warm, then whip the mixture with a wooden spoon for a few seconds. Press the mixture into a buttered 9-inch pie pan and cut into pieces. Eat immediately or cover and refrigerate.

Medicinal uses. Botanists say mulberry leaves and unripened fruits have a mild sedative effect. Ripe fruit cooked with sugar and mixed with vodka has a stimulating effect.

Wild Grape *(Vitis* spp.*)*

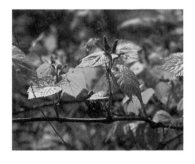

Description. Climbing vine; clinging tendrils; green flowers in a large cluster; leaves alternate, simple, round, toothed, with heart-shaped base. The young leaves and ripe fruits are edible. They are found nationwide, clinging and climbing trees, walls, and fences.

B A S I C   E S S E N T I A L S

Location. Eastern United States, roughly to the Mississippi.

Warning. *The Canadian moonseed plant looks like wild grape but is poisonous. Learn to distinguish these two plants before eating what you think are wild grapes. Get expert identification.*

Cooking tips. To make raisins, cover wild grapes with cheesecloth and dry them in the sun for three days, or dry them in a food dryer. Grape leaves can be wrapped around rice, vegetables, and meat, and steamed until tender. Add grape leaves to pickling spices when preparing dill pickles.

Medicinal uses. The fruit, leaves, and tendrils have been used by Native Americans and pioneers to treat hepatitis, diarrhea, and snakebite. Native Americans used tonic made with grape and several other herbs to increase fertility. Tannins and other phenolic compounds found in grape skins may provide protection from heart disease. Resveratrol from grapes may prevent strokes and heart attacks.

Staghorn Sumac *(Rhus typhina)*

Description. Shrub or small tree; leaves lance-shaped, alternate, compound, numerous leaflets, toothed; cone-shaped flower and berry clusters. The large berry spikes of staghorn sumac are ready to harvest in late summer.

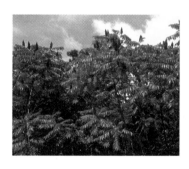

Location. Entire United States, except extreme desert, southern California, and lower Florida.

Cooking tips. Strip red staghorn sumac berries from heads. Discard stems and heads. Soak cotton-covered berries in hot water to extract a lemonade-like drink. Steep sassafras root in the tea. Add sugar and serve.

Medicinal uses. Staghorn sumac flower can be steeped into tea and taken for stomach pain. Gargles made from berries are purported to help sore throats.

Salal *(Gaultheria shallon)*

Description. Sprawling shrub forms dense thickets in pine forests. Oval, shiny, leathery, thick leaves are alternate, clinging to sturdy stems on petioles of varying lengths. Bell-shaped pink-to-white flowers, strung out like pearls near ends of stem. Dark-blue to blue-black fruit is ripe from July through September.

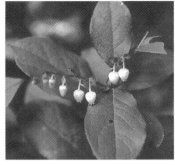

Location. Marine/seashore. West of the Cascades and coastal ranges, from California to the Alaskan peninsula.

Cooking tips. The berries can be eaten as you hike along. Take some home and blend them into jelly or maple syrup, or dry them in a food dryer and use them in muffins, waffles, and pancakes.

Medicinal uses. Native Americans chewed the leaves to stem off hunger. Dried salal berries are considered a good laxative, while the plant's dried leaves infused in water can be imbibed to treat diarrhea (the tea is astringent, thus its effectiveness). Dried leaves can also be powdered and used externally as a styptic on scrapes and abrasions. Also, dried leaf powder can be mixed with water to make a pasty poultice for wounds.

Dried Salal Berry Cakes

Salal berries were an important traditional food of Native Americans of the Northwest. They gathered the berries and prepared them in cakes.

To make a fair facsimile of a dried cake, boil the berries until they are a soft mash, and then pour them into a greased cupcake pan. Fill each cupcake holder half full and bake at 200° F until the cakes are dried (about 3½ hours). The dried cakes can be reconstituted by an overnight soak in the refrigerator.

Salmonberry *(Rubus spectabilis)*

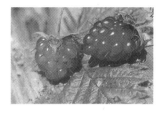

Description. Shrub 6 to 7 feet in height, found along moist slopes, sunny banks, and streams. Brown stems with yellow bark, laced with weak-to-soft thorns. Leaflets fuzzy with serrated edges, usually in threes, approximately 3 inches in length. Fuchsia flowers arrive with leaves in spring. Soft, dry fruit ranges from bright red to yellowish. Note: I find this berry on Vancouver Island along the path to Botanical Beach. To find the berries, look for bear dung.

Location. Mountain west, from Michigan to the Sierras and Rockies to Alaska.

Cooking tips. The soft (when ripe) fruit melts in your mouth and will melt in your backpack, too! Best to eat it as you hike along. Spring sprouts can be peeled, cooked, and eaten. Harvest the stems before they become hard and woody, and eat them raw, steamed, or roasted.

Thimbleberry *(Rubus parviflorus)*

Description. Found in moist places (streamside, coastal). A deciduous shrub up to 7 feet high, unbarbed, erect with shredded-to-smooth bark. Large maple-like leaves, smooth or slightly hairy on top, fuzzy underneath.

Location. Mountain west, primarily the Sierras and Rockies to Alaska.

Cooking tips. Eat the soft, ripe berries in the bush. Like salmonberry (see above), thimbleberry will turn to mush in your backpack. To eat: Apply forefinger and thumb to fruit, pull and twist, and pop in your mouth. No cooking required. Try this tart berry on cereal. Northwestern Native Americans 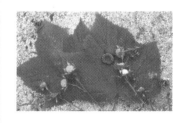 dried the berries in cakes (see page 16) or stored them in goose grease. Young shoots can be harvested, peeled, and cooked as a spring green.

Medicinal uses. Native Americans (Kwakiutls of the Northwest) made a decoction, a drink for treating bloody vomiting, with boiled blackberry roots, vines, and thimbleberry.

Yards & Meadows

Dandelion *(Taraxacum officinale)*

Description. Flower heads yellow; leaves irregular, sharply lobed, in basal whorl; large taproot. Leaves, crown, roots, and flower petals are edible. The seeds are a favorite food of goldfinch.

Location. Throughout the United States.

Cooking tips. Dandelion leaves are high in vitamins A, C, and B1. They are best in early spring, before they flower. Bitter older leaves can be improved by soaking them for an hour or so in a bowl of water mixed with a teaspoon of baking soda.

My favorite dandelion recipe goes like this. Chop two handfuls of dandelion leaves. Mix this with ¼ cup of the chopped nuts of your choice. Add the juice of ½ lemon or lime. Blend in 3 tablespoons of honey and 1 teaspoon of olive oil. Mix well. Here's a meal full of vitamins and quick energy.

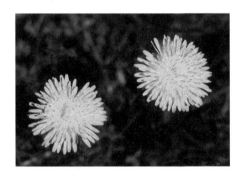

You can also use dandelion flowers in tossed salads. The crown of the plant—the whitish area just below the leaves and above the roots—can be deep-fried. Coat the crowns in tempura batter, then deep-fry. I pluck the flower petals and sprinkle them on any food that needs color. Beta-carotene rich, here is potential cancer-fighting nutrition that is free, grows everywhere, and provides for you year-round. When serving a rice dish, use dandelion petals like confetti over the rice.

From the plant's root, you can make dandelion coffee. Let the root dry in a warm, dry place. Then lightly roast the root and grind it to a powder. Add 1 teaspoon of the powder to 1 cup of hot water. Here's a bitter tonic that may be good for the liver.

Japanese Sauce

....

2 tablespoons soy sauce
1 tablespoons sesame seed oil
1 heaping teaspoon chopped ginger root
2 tablespoons lemon juice
1 clove garlic (diced)
1 mushroom (coarsely chopped)
**2 cups each dandelion leaves, watercress, and stinging
  nettles**
pinch of wasabe (Japanese hot mustard)

Combine the soy sauce, sesame seed oil, chopped ginger root, lemon, garlic, and wasabe. Stir. Add mushroom, dandelion leaves, watercress, and stinging nettles. Sauté in a wok at 375° to 400° F for 2 to 3 minutes and serve.

Medicinal uses. Dandelion tea (made from roots) was used as a laxative, blood purifier, and diuretic. For 5,000 years dandelion parts have been used to clear fevers, break up congestion, and stimulate milk flow in nursing mothers. Recent evidence suggests dandelion tea may rejuvenate alcoholics' livers. Bitter root teas from dandelions, chicory, gentian, and the like may stimulate appetite and improve digestion. Plant bitters are being used experimentally to treat anorexia.

Chickweed *(Stellaria* spp.*)*

Description. Leaves oval, ¼ inch to ½ inch; stem weak, hairy, prostrate, ½ inch; flower white, lance-shaped petals. A common ground cover.

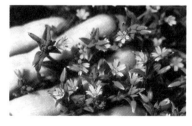

Location. Eastern United States, roughly to the Mississippi.

Cooking tips. Can be eaten raw or cooked. Sprinkle chickweed flowers in with leaves when preparing a salad. A handful on a sandwich is a good substitute for alfalfa sprouts.

Chopped in a stir-fry they add bulk, fiber, and a decent amount of vitamins A and C. Stew chickweed with rabbit, chicken, or beef. Add 4 cups of flowers, leaves, and stems to a pot. Mix in favorite stewing herbs. Enter bird, bunny, or beef. Then brace yourself for a magnificent feast. Later in the year, the mature seeds can be used to thicken soup. Seeds also make an excellent birdseed.

For chickweed pancakes, blanch 1 cup of chickweed for 3 minutes, chop in a blender, and add blended greens to pancake batter.

Medicinal uses. Chickweed is eaten as a diuretic. Leaf tea is used as a cold-relieving expectorant.

Violets *(Viola* spp.*)*

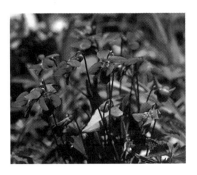

Description. Flower irregular; leaves vary, usually ovate; common blue violet has heart-shaped, serrated leaves. Found in shady areas along fringes of lawn. Violets are cultivated in France for perfume. This incredible edible is high in vitamins C, A, and E.

Location. Eastern United States, roughly to the Mississippi.

Warning. *Late-season plants without flowers can be confused with inedible greens. Forage this plant only when in bloom.*

Cooking tips. Use both the leaves and flowers in salads. Flowers can also be candied (see Candied Primrose, page 51). Experiment. Put them over finished meat dishes as a garnish and color contrast that invites eating.

Medicinal uses. Violet roots consumed in large amounts are emetic and purgative. Plant used as poultice over skin abrasions. In China indigenous health care givers use one species, *Viola diffusa,* to treat aplastic anemia, leukemia, mastitis, mumps, and poisonous snakebites. The violet's color suggests the presence of anthocyanin, secondary metabolites that give off a blue hue. Anthocyanin also provides protection from *E. coli* infection.

Bull Thistle *(Cirsium vulgare)*

Description. Thorny biennial; purple flower rises from spiny bract. Barbed leaves of the first year's growth can be eaten after the spines have been stripped away with a knife. Wear gloves when harvesting roots and leaves.

Location. Eastern United States, roughly to the Mississippi.

Cooking tips. Use a knife to strip thorny armor away from leaves. Eat raw or cooked. Flavor similar to celery. Harvest leaves in the spring and fall. In summer, flower petals can be sprinkled over salads. Roots can be boiled, sliced, and stir-fried. Some folks steam outer green bract around flower heads and eat it like an artichoke.

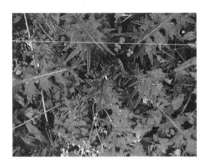

Medicinal uses. The Chinese use thistle teas and decoctions to treat appendicitis, internal bleeding, and inflammations.

Plantain, Buckhorn
(Plantago major, P. lanceolata)

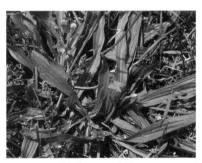

P. lanceolata

Description. Flowers green, tiny, numerous on spike; ovate leaf with pointed tip. *Lanceolata* has lance-like leaves, longer spike. Plantain is best harvested before this flower stalk appears. New leaves keep coming all year.

Location. *P. lanceolata* is found in the eastern United States, roughly to the Mississippi. *P. macrocarpa* and *P. maritima* are found in the western United States.

Cooking tips. Use tender young leaves in salads. Soak older leaves in diluted saltwater for 10 minutes, then steam until tender. Dried seeds can be eaten whole or ground into flour.

Medicinal uses. One over-the-counter laxative uses seeds from the *psyllium* species of plantain. For more than a thousand years people have chewed plantain leaves and applied them over burns, cuts, and scrapes. In China indigenous health care givers use whole plant as tea to clear fever and promote healing

Lamb's-Quarters *(Chenopodium album)*

Description. Lamb's-quarters (various herbs of the goosefoot family) can be found in fields, on waste ground, and in just about everyone's garden. A healthy lamb's-quarters plant can climb 3 feet tall, with leaves the shape of a lamb's hind quarter.

Location. Eastern United States, roughly to the Mississippi, and more rarely in the western United States.

Cooking tips. As a potherb, boil lamb's-quarters for 5 minutes with mustard greens and dandelion leaves. For a nutritious snack add seeds to your favorite bread or muffin mix. The young tender leaves and tips produce the best salad greens.

Gill-over-Ground, Ground Ivy
(Glechoma hederacea)

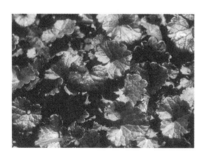

Description. Creeping plant; purple stems; roundish, lobed, violet flowers in whorls. Gill-over-ground, or ground ivy, is available year-round.

Location. Eastern United States, roughly to the Mississippi.

Cooking tips. Inedible except as strong-tasting, harshly aromatic medicinal tea made by drying leaves and steeping them in hot water for about 10 minutes.

Medicinal uses. Tea used to treat measles. The Chinese use it to clear fever, dissolve stones in urinary tract, stimulate circulation, reduce inflammation, treat influenza, and alleviate pain.

Pokeweed *(Phytolacca americana)*

Description. Large leaves; reddish, coarse stems; greenish-white flowers in clusters; purple-black berries on stalk. Pokeweed, or poke, is found growing on waste ground almost anywhere in the United States. Very young leaves, as they first emerge, are edible after cooking in at least two changes of water.

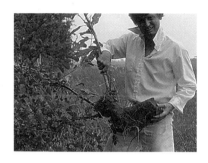

Location. Entire United States, except extreme desert, southern California, and lower Florida.

Warning. *Don't eat pokeweed unless foraging with a botanist. Root, stems, and berries of plant are poisonous. See also Appendix 1.*

Medicinal uses. Slightly narcotic, emetic, and purgative. Berries used as poultice on wounds and sores. Seeds and fruits steeped in water used to treat arthritis. Use only under medical supervision.

Peppergrass *(Lepidium virginicum)*

Description. Flat seed pods, peppery taste; leaf lance-shaped, toothed.

Location. Eastern United States, roughly to the Mississippi.

Cooking tips. Add seeds to salads. Young leaves are edible but bitter; use sparingly.

Medicinal uses. Tea from leaves and seeds is said to restore sex drive. Native Americans used plant as general medicinal.

Wild Asparagus *(Asparagus officinalis)*

Description. Green spike when first emerges. Found along roadsides and fence rows. Locate asparagus in the fall, when large, feathery adult plants are easiest to see. Mark spot. Harvest the following spring.

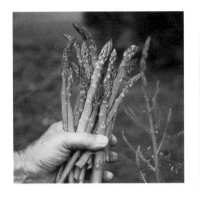

Location. Entire United States, except extreme desert, southern California, and lower Florida.

Warning. *Remember Wild Plant Foraging Rule #7: Roadside plants might be tainted with benzene, lead, oil, and other auto pollutants.*

Cooking tips. One favorite is asparagus roll-ups. Place three spears of asparagus on a flour tortilla. Cover asparagus with cheddar cheese, Miracle Whip, and bean sprouts. Roll up tortilla and microwave 35 seconds on high.

Medicinal uses. Asparagus is an excellent diuretic. Aspargine (that odor you smell when urinating) is antiseptic. Asparagusic acid is used to treat fluke infections, such as schistomiasis.

Dock *(Rumex orbiculatus, R. patientia, R. crispus)*

Description. The many varieties of dock are common weeds growing on disturbed ground, edges of fields, roadsides, and vacant lots. Leaves typically widest at base, narrow to tip, rounded at base; paper-like flower spikes; fruits 3-parted, brownish-to-red with 3 nutlets. Docks emerge in the spring, first as unfurling leaves, later the flower spike shoots up with smaller leaves attached. Flowers and,

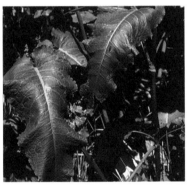

R. crispus

eventually, seeds cluster along the top several inches of the spikes. Swamp or water dock *(R. orbiculatus)* is found growing in water or along stream margins. It is stout and tall (to 6 feet) with a long root and flat, narrow, dark green leaves. Both curly dock *(R. crispus)* and yellow dock *(R. patientia)* have curly or wavy leaf margins.

Location. Entire United States, except extreme desert, southern California, and lower Florida.

Warning. *Contains oxalic acid and, like spinach, should not be eaten more than twice a week.*

Cooking tips. Leaves and seeds edible. Tender young leaves, as they emerge, are most edible. Older leaves are tough and bitter and should be cooked in two changes of water. Steam, sauté, or stir-fry young leaves. Season with ginger, soy, lemon juice, and sesame seed oil. Leaves are great with walnuts and raisins. Dock seeds are edible in late summer and autumn. Hulled seeds can be ground into flour and used as a soup thickener or as a flour extender in baked goods.

Medicinal uses. Curly dock and yellow dock are used by naturopaths and midwives as a tea to treat anemia and raise iron levels in pregnant women. Iron in this form does not cause constipation. Curly dock and yellow dock root are also used with vinegar to treat ringworm. All dock roots are laxative, bitter digestive stimulants.

Cinquefoil *(Potentilla canadensis)*
Silverweed *(P. anserina)*

Description. Leaves on long, jointed stolons (delicate stem-like appendages). Two types of leaves: oval or elliptical (which are much smaller and have sharply toothed leaflets up to 1¼-inch long). Small buttercup-like flower. Both of these species can be found on waste ground or in gravely or sandy habitats.

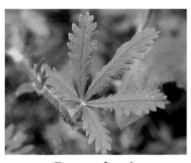

P. canadensis

Location. P. canadensis is found the eastern United States to the Mississippi. P. anserina is found on the West Coast.

Cooking tips. P. canadensis can be used to make a gold-colored tea that is high in calcium. For a quick roast, cook the leaves in a hot (covered) Dutch oven for two to three minutes. Pour boiling water over the leaves. P. anserina roots are edible. Gather the roots, wash them thoroughly, and steam in a wok. Native Americans steamed the roots in cedar boxes and served them with duck fat. To this day, the Ditidaht of British Columbia gather and prepare the roots in this traditional way.

Medicinal uses. Roots are rich in tannins and are used by some naturopathic physicians to treat diarrhea, Chrohn's disease, colitis, gastritis, and peptic ulcers. Use only under the supervision of a trained holistic health care practitioner.

Carrot,
Queen Anne's Lace
(Daucus carota)

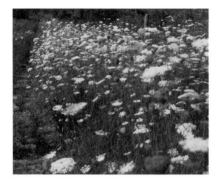

Description. Biennial. Fine, deeply dissected leaf. Second year's growth has white flower many call Queen Anne's Lace. Root smells and tastes like domestic carrot, but is tough and woody. High in vitamin A and fiber.

Location. Eastern United States, roughly to the Mississippi.

Warning. *Hemlock look-alike (see Appendix 1). Before using wild carrot, be certain that it has its characteristic carrot smell. Hemlock stems are purple-spotted or purple-blotched. When mature, hemlock is much taller than wild carrots. Remember Wild Plant Foraging Rule #1: When not certain of plant identification, follow the plant through a complete growth cycle or get expert advice before using.*

Cooking tips. Imparts a carrot-like flavor to vegetable stew. Eat soft tissue around root's pithy core. Florets can be stripped off head and sprinkled over salads. Also try them in meatloaf.

Medicinal uses. Root tea is antimicrobial, adiuretic, hypotensive, and a worm expellant. Animal studies show seed prevents ovum from implanting.

Burdock
(Arctium minus, A. lappa)

Description. Large leaf, looks like elephant ear; large taproot. *A. minus* has a smaller leaf, flower, and flower spike. Common garden nuisance. In June or July dig first-year roots of this biennial.

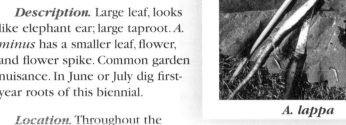
A. lappa

Location. Throughout the United States, except extreme mountain and desert regions.

Cooking tips. Peel roots and cut into thin strips. Boil strips in water, sesame seed oil, ginger, and soy sauce. If bitter, use two changes of water. Serve hot under a pat of butter and dollop of low-fat sour cream. Mock celery soup can be made with petioles of burdock. Add burdock, wild carrots, and wild onions to chicken stock. Cook, season, and serve. First-year young leaves can be scraped and eaten like celery.

Medicinal uses. Eighteenth-century treatment for gonorrhea and syphilis. Native Americans used for scurvy, sores, and rheumatism. Chinese use for tonsillitis, flu, and as poultice on boils and abscesses. Seed extracts lower blood-sugar levels. Traditionally, boiled root used to reduce inflammation, control bacteria infection, and treat skin conditions.

Bergamot, Bee Balm *(Monarda fistulosa)*

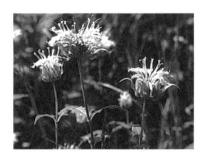

Description. Leaves paired, oval- to lance-shaped; lavender flowers, florets resemble war bonnets, with strong oregano odor and flavor. Typically found on well-drained soil, along roadsides and dry wood edges.

Location. Throughout the United States, except extreme mountain and desert regions.

Cooking tips. Eat young leaves raw, as they first emerge. Flowers have oregano-like taste. Use flowers in salads or as tea; excellent over sauces, especially Italian. Also try the flowers in your favorite meat marinade—

count on ½ cup of flowers to 2 cups of marinade. Infuse flowers and leaves in cold water with mint and lemon balm leaves. Refrigerate overnight.

Medicinal uses. Use the tea to treat colds, sore throats, fevers, and headaches. This expectorant prevents excess mucus, and soothes bronchial complaints, sinusitis, digestive problems, and flatulence. Rub tea over skin eruptions. Ancient Native Americans drank the tea to relieve arthritis pain.

Hawthorn *(Crataegus* spp.*)*

Description. Spiny shrubs to small, spiny trees; white flowers in terminal clusters, typically 5 petals; red berry fruit; leaves toothed, ovate, cut or lobed. Found in wetlands, gardens, along wood edges, lawns.

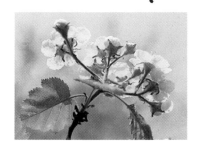

Location. Various species found throughout the United States.

Warning. *Uterine stimulate: May induce menstruation. Contra-indicated for pregnant women.*

Cooking tips. Sweet-sour flavor. Eat the fruit and flowers in salads, stews, soups, and tea. Try eating them right off the tree in season (August and early September). Dried hawthorn berries can be purchased at Oriental drugstores or markets.

Medicinal uses. Bioflavonoid-rich hawthorn has been used to improve peripheral circulation to the heart, extremities, and brain. In Europe and China hawthorn has long been used to treat heart disease. It is also used by naturopathic physicians and others to treat angina, cardiac arrhythmia, heart disease, high blood pressure, and intermittent claudication (leg pain caused by partially occluded coronary arteries). In China the dried fruits are decocted and used for treating irritable bowel and gall bladder problems. Only with your physician's knowledge and approval: Eat the fruits raw for circulatory stimulation, or simmer the new leaves and flower buds to make hawthorn tea to treat heart conditions. In China dried hawthorn berries are given to infants suffering from indigestion from improper nursing technique.

Jerusalem Artichoke
(Helianthus tuberosus)

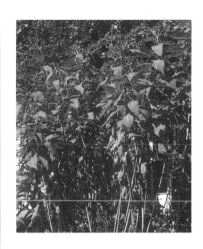

Description. Yellow sunflower; broad ovate, rough leaves, lower leaves opposite, upper leaves alternate; hairy stem; tuberous root. This plant can be found along roadsides. Add tubers to your garden, and they'll provide a substantial food source that continues to reproduce year after year. Harvest tubers in fall and spring.

Location. Throughout the United States.

Cooking tips. Tuber can be peeled, sliced, and eaten raw. Has taste similar to water chestnut. Also microwave, bake, or boil like a potato. This plant is worth looking for.

Medicinal uses. Tea made from flowers and leaves is a traditional treatment for arthritis. Inulin-rich tuber is slow to release sugars, making it a good food for diabetics.

Chicory *(Cichorium intybus)*

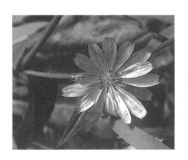

Description. Leaves lance-shaped, deeply cut, dissected margins, stiff midvein spine; blue flower. Common along the shoulders of rural roads.

Location. Throughout the United States, except extreme mountain and desert regions.

Cooking tips. Down in New Orleans the dried root of chicory is ground and blended with coffee. Young leaves are edible, although bitter. Try combining them with ½ cup of chicory blossoms and 1 pint of low-fat cottage cheese.

Medicinal uses. Occasionally used as a nerve tonic, liver tonic, bitters, laxative. May reduce inflammation.

Black Willow *(Salix nigra)*
Weeping Willow *(S. alba)*

Description. Tree or shrub; lance-like, fine-toothed leaves. Prefers wet ground.

Location. Throughout the United States.

Warning. Willow contains salicin. Too much salicin may be dangerous. Consult your physician before trying this tea.

Medicinal uses. Willow tea can be made from stems and leaves. Drop willow cuttings into hot water. Steep for 1 minute for a relaxing brew that may take the edge off an aching head. The salicin found in willow and in

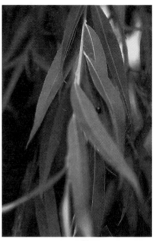

S. alba

many other plants is the natural chemical model for synthetic aspirin. Aspirin may help prevent acute infections, cancer, and heart attacks.

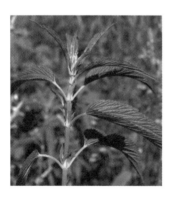

Stinging Nettle
(Urtica dioica)

Description. Hairy stem and leaves; hairs sting; leaves lance-like, sharply toothed. Common resident along roadsides, fields, and wooded areas. Fine, stinging hairs contain skin irritant that is destroyed when plant is cooked. Nettles are high in vitamins A and C, are fiber rich, and a great mineral source.

Location. Throughout the United States.

Warning. Don't confuse the hairy cells of stinging nettle with the thorny, poisonous horse nettle (see Appendix 1).

Cooking tips. Stinging nettle is one of my favorite foods. In the spring I sauté the young shoots with dandelions. In the summer and fall the new growth—the whorl of new leaves on the end of stems—can be picked, chopped, and stir-fried. Chopped leaves can be rolled up in a wonton with chopped celery, carrot, ginger root, and flax seeds. Steam wontons for 5 minutes, then dip in 4 tablespoons of low-sodium soy sauce and 2 tablespoons of sesame seed oil. Cook with wild carrot, wild leeks, dandelion greens, watercress, and soy sauce. Boil older plants, then throw away the plants and use nettle stock for soups or as a refreshing vitamin-rich drink. Plant can be harvested throughout the year. Simply cut off top new leaf generation for eating.

Medicinal uses. Tea may combat diarrhea. Diuretic in decoction. Herbalists rubbed whole plant over arthritic joints and muscles as counter-irritant. Freeze-dried nettles may relieve hay fever.

Woolly Mullein
(Verbascum thapsus)

Description. Large, hairy, Velcro-like leaf; yellow flower; biennial; prostrate first year, erect second year. Grows in vacant lots. Native Americans lined moccasins with the warm, woolly leaf.

Location. Throughout the United States.

Medicinal uses. Tea from leaves and flowers used as a folk or naturopathic remedy to treat coughs, colds, bronchitis, and other upper-respiratory problems. Hairy leaves used to rub out pain of stinging nettle. Mountain folkhealers use mullein flowers, Epsom salts, and vinegar to wash necrotic wounds of recluse spider bite.

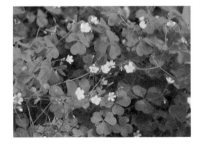

Yellow Sorrel, Wood Sorrel
(Oxalis stricta)

Description. Shamrock-like leaf, deeply dissected into 3 round lobes; yellow flower. Wood sorrel and garden sorrel leaves, flowers, and seeds have a sour taste. Common in many gardens.

Edible Wild Plants & Useful Herbs   **31**

Location. Eastern United States, roughly to the Mississippi.

Warning. *High in oxalic acid. Use this plant sparingly. Excessive consumption may inhibit the body's absorption of calcium.*

Cooking tips. Add yellow flowers, seeds, and leaves to salads—or brew them into a beverage.

Medicinal uses. The Chinese use the *Oxalis* species to clear fevers, resolve clots, and reduce swelling. Also used as snakebite treatment.

Sheep Sorrel *(Rumex acetoscella)*

Description. Thick, succulent, sour-tasting leaves; long, pointed, tapered tip, with short, pointed basal lobes. Found on waste ground, wood margins, gardens. Available spring and fall.

Location. Throughout the United States.

Warning. *High in oxalic acid (see yellow sorrel).*

Cooking tips. Prepare like wood sorrel. Eat sparingly.

Medicinal uses. This is one of the ingredients in the traditional Essiac anti-cancer formula that combines burdock root, sheep sorrel, red clover, rhubarb root, kelp, slippery elm bark, watercress and blessed thistle.

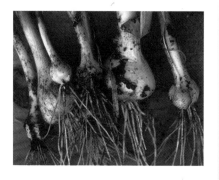

Wild Garlic
(Allium sativum)

Description. Long, narrow, pencil-like leaf stalk; flower head bears small green plantlets that drop off and propagate.

Location. Throughout the United States.

Cooking tips. Always cook wild garlic and wild onions to cleave inulin molecules to a more digestible sugar. Inulin is a polysaccharide, a stored-energy source typically found in roots and tubers.

Medicinal uses. Wild garlic, chives, and onions may reduce blood pressure, lower cholesterol, lower blood sugar, and protect you from acute infections such as a cold or the flu.

Day Lily
(Hemerocallis fulva)

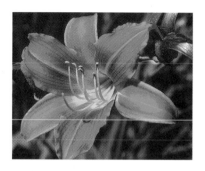

Description. Yellow, tuberous roots; long, narrow, lance-like leaves; orange lily flower. Found along roadsides. Transplant to clean soil away from auto pollution. Common in many gardens.

Location. Throughout the United States.

Warning. *Use plant only when in bloom. Early growth resembles poisonous Iris shoots (see Appendix 1); day lily's yellowish tubers are distinctive.*

Cooking tips. The strong-tasting flowers are flavonoid rich. Day lily petals can be teased apart from the whole flower and tossed in with salad greens. Flowers and unopened buds can be stir-fried or batter-dipped and cooked tempura style. Try the sautéed flowers wrapped in wontons, steamed. The Japanese Sauce (see page 19) makes a great wonton dip. Buds can be steamed, boiled, or deep-fried. Serve with butter or cheese sauce. Firm root tubers can be harvested all year. Add raw to salads or cook like a potato.

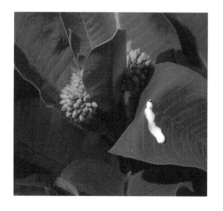

Milkweed
(Asclepias syriaca)

Description. Sticky white sap; large egg-like seed pods; large ovate leaves. Common milkweed is sometimes eaten as cooked vegetable—but the sap contains toxins.

Location. Eastern United States, roughly to the Mississippi.

Warning. *I have included milkweed as an edible plant because many people eat it. Like pokeweed, milkweed is potentially dangerous without special processing and cooking preparation. All parts of the plant may contain heart-stimulating cardiac glycosides. I recommend you not eat milkweed unless it is prepared by a knowledgeable and experienced forager. There are several species, some more edible than others. There is poor documentation on appropriate preparation. I would only eat this plant in a survival situation where no other food was available. See also Appendix 1.*

Cooking tips. All edible parts of this plant are best cooked. I eat the young shoots, unopened flower buds, and thrice-cooked seed pods. It is safest to steep plant parts in at least two changes (preferably three changes) of water to reduce cardiac glycoside, a potential toxin, content.

Medicinal uses. Sap used to treat warts, moles, and ringworm. Boiled roots used to treat sterility, asthma, and dysentery.

Ground Cherry, Lantern Plant
(Physalis pubescens, P. tomatilla)

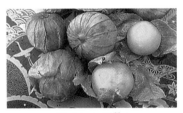

P. tomatilla

Description. Hairy stems and leaves; pale green plant. Sometimes called lantern plant because of the lantern-like husk. Ground cherries can be harvested when ripe, usually in August or September.

Location. Entire United States, except extreme desert, southern California, and lower Florida.

Warning. *Unripe berries may make a few sick. Avoid this fruit and other member of the nightshade family. The horse nettle is a toxic look-alike (see Appendix 1).*

Cooking tips. The Amish in my neighborhood pick wild ground cherries and bake them into wonderful pies. You can purchase this plant from Richter's (see Appendix 2). Plant the seeds in your garden, then harvest ground cherries in fall. By purchasing the plants from a reliable source and then planting them, you can be assured you are eating ground cherries and not a toxic look-alike, such as horse nettle. *P. tomatilla* are available in many Mexican markets.

Medicinal uses. Used by the Chinese as poultice over abscesses, and as a vermicide and cough sedative.

Goat's Beard
(Tragopogon pratensis)

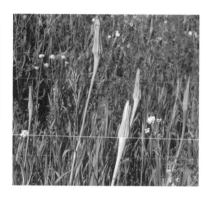

Description. Goat's beard looks like a large dandelion: yellow flowers; large, deeply and sharply serrated leaves.

Location. Entire United States, except extreme desert, southern California, and lower Florida.

Cooking tips. Root edible when boiled and then fried.

Medicinal uses. Apply cooled infusion of plant to boils. Use as a gargle for sore throat treatment.

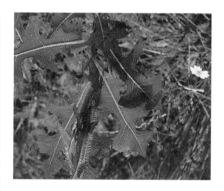

Prickly Lettuce
(Lactuca scariola)

Description. Lettuce-like; white, sticky juice in stems and leaves; leaves alternate, lance-like, toothed and spiny margin; small yellow flowers in clusters.

Location. Throughout the United States.

Cooking tips. Blanched leaves are bitter. Definitely won't impress dinner guests.

Medicinal uses. Was used as cough suppressant. About 200 years ago distilled scariola and wild opium *(Lactuca canadensis)* were used as a very weak, opium-like sedative.

Red Clover
(Trifolium pratense)

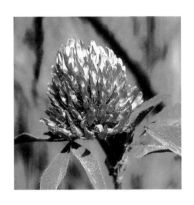

Description. Often three leaflets showing pale chevron; round flower head; rose-purple flower petals.

Location. Throughout the United States.

Cooking tips. Petals can be batter-fried or eaten raw in salads.

Medicinal uses. Tea from flowers is flavonoid rich, providing antioxidant, anti-cancer protection. Skilled herbalists used this plant to treat cuts, burns, and liver ailments. Integral part of the Essiac anti-cancer formula consisting of burdock root, slippery elm bark, rhubarb root, watercress, sheep sorrel, blessed thistle, red clover, and kelp.

Spiderwort *(Tradescantia virginiana)*

Description. Flower violet, three round petals, long golden stamens; long, lanced leaves. Common along roadsides.

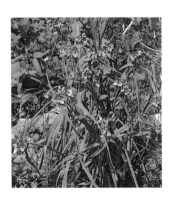

Location. Entire United States, except extreme desert, southern California, and lower Florida.

Cooking tips. The strong-tasting young shoots and leaves can be eaten, but are mucilaginous. The little flowers bloom every morning all summer long. I like them uncooked in an omelet or sprinkled in a floral salad.

Medicinal uses. Poulticed root rubbed on skin cancer. Tea for stomachache. Long leaves used to bind wounds. Antiseptic. The flowers may relieve congestion due to summer heat and humidity. The slimy texture should release and thin mucus, a reflex action due to the polysaccharides in the flower.

Comfrey
(Symphytum officinale)

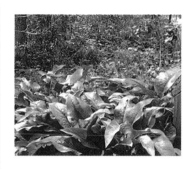

Description. Leaves large, elongated, hairy, prickly; stalks hollow, hairy; flower finger-like, pale white. Found on moist, low ground.

Location. This plant has escaped gardens and is found nationwide.

Warning. *This plant may be carcinogenic. May contain pyrrolizidine alkaloids that damage the liver. Avoid eating this plant, especially the roots. Dried leaves have lowest amount of the alkaloids. Although the alkaloids are concentrated in the root, they are found throughout the plant. I have included this plant as it was once a favorite of foragers and folk medicine practitioners. I do not recommend eating it.*

Medicinal uses. Plant parts demulcent, astringent. Native Americans used tea for dysentery, gonorrhea, and heartburn. Holistic practitioners use the herb internally to treat stomach ulcers and irritable bowel syndrome and externally to mend sprains and broken bones.

Peppermint *(Mentha piperita)*

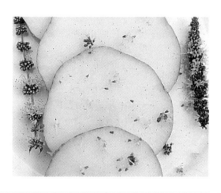

Description. Peppermint, like spearmint, found along wet lowlands, streams, and lakes. It has a square stem, like most members of the mint family, with opposite leaves, sharply serrated. Crushed plant has strong aromatic odor of mint.

Location. Eastern United States, roughly to the Mississippi.

Cooking tips. Use the flowers in salads and the leaves to flavor cold drinks such as cold infusion tea (sun tea). Used in many Middle Eastern foods. Try it in rice and tabouleh.

Medicinal uses. Oil used to treat colic. Tea used to treat colds, fever, and headache. Excellent digestive aid. Whole plant crushed and rubbed on skin to reduce pain and sensitivity.

Chamomile
(Matricaria chamomilla, Anthemis nobilis)

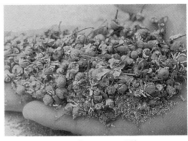

M. chamomilla

Description. Hairy stem; narrow leaflets divided into many segments; flower on long, erect stem, yellow/white florets. Aromatic. German chamomile *(M. chamomilla)* is the herb of choice, as it's more pleasant tasting than Roman chamomile *(A. nobilis).* Found in sandy soil in full sun.

Location. Eastern United States, roughly to the Mississippi.

Warning. *Over-dosage may cause vomiting. Similar to rag-weed pollen—may trigger allergies.*

Medicinal uses. Flower makes excellent tea—a soothing, relaxing brew sometimes taken for indigestion. Available over-the-counter. Tea used for treating children's colic (see physician first). Bioflavonoid rich; useful against hay fever and asthma. Use externally for eczema.

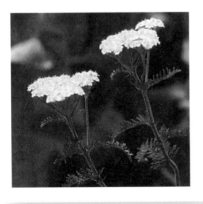

Yarrow, Milfoil
(Achillea millefolium)

Description. Creeping or erect herb. Leaves feather-like, slightly hairy, divided into fine leaflets; white or pinkish flower. Aromatic. Found in open sun or partial shade.

Location. Eastern United States, roughly to the Mississippi.

Warning. *Yarrow looks similar to poisonous hemlock (see Appendix 1). Get expert identification.*

Medicinal uses. Was used as poultice over wounds. Tea used to treat colds. Dried yarrow leaves cooked in lard makes an excellent wound dressing.

Asiatic Dayflower *(Commelina communis)*

Description. Common weed in many gardens. Erect stems collapse on themselves as they grow (up to three feet). Deep blue flowers, ½- to ¾-inch wide, two rounded petals (like Mickey Mouse ears) with a small white petal behind the pair. Flower's ovary sheathed in three green sepals; six yellow-tipped stamens. Fleshy, oblong leaves, 3- to 5-inches long, pointed tips. Leaves sheath stem.

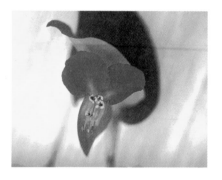

Location. Found nation-wide. Alien weed: originally from China.

Cooking tips. This free food comes up late every year. Young leaves and shoots can be added to salads. We get so many of these plants in our garden that I pull whole shoots, wash them, and add them to stir-fries. Entire flower is edible. As fruit matures, the seed capsule (tucked in the sepal sheath) is a crunchy treat. In late summer flowers keep coming. You can eat seed pods for a healthful dose of essential oils and phytosterols.

Medicinal uses. In China leaf tea is used as a sore throat gargle, for urinary infections, acute intestinal enteritis, and dysentery. Tea is also used to reduce fevers, as a detoxicant, and as a diuretic (to treat edema from join swelling and pain from arthritis). Flowers contain isoflavones and phytosterols. Seeds contain fatty acids and essential and non-essential amino acids.

Woodlands

Hepatica, American Liverwort
(Hepatica americana)

Description. Perennial plant; leaves on long hairy petiole, shaped like three lobes of liver; white, blue, or purplish flower appears early. One of the first flowers to bloom in March or April.

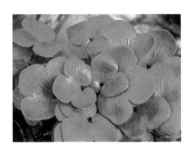

Location. Entire United States, except extreme desert, southern California, and lower Florida.

Warning. *Large amounts of hepatica are poisonous. Use is reserved for a skilled herbalist. See also Appendix I.*

Medicinal uses. Small amounts of roots and leaves used to treat indigestion and disorders of the kidneys, gall bladder, and liver. I have used a water extraction of the root to repel mosquitoes.

Skunk Cabbage
(Symplocarpus foetidus, Lysichitum americanum)

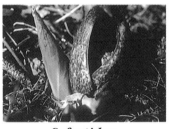

S. foetidus

Description. Plant smells like a skunk when damaged; leaves large, smooth margins; primitive spathe (flower) emerges before leaves. The plant is found in wet lowlands and woods. Not edible. Western skunk cabbage's *(L. americanum)* spathe is bright yellow.

Location. S. foetidus is found in the eastern United States, while Western skunk cabbage is found west of the Rockies.

Warning. *Skunk cabbage is poisonous and contains oxalate. Juice from the fresh plant may cause skin blistering and will severely burn digestive tract if eaten. Only experts* *should handle this plant. I have included this plant because it is a common woodland plant, is striking in appearance, and has a startling odor. Although its name suggests that it is edible, it requires exhaustive preparation in several changes of cooking water to yield mediocre results. Botanically, it is unique: It actually produces heat that often melts snow around its base. In Michigan it is the earliest flowering plant of spring. See also Appendix 1.*

Medicinal uses. Native Americans used *Symplocarpus* roots as a medicinal. First the roots were thoroughly dried to crystallize burning oxalate. Infusion or tea from the dried root was used as a mild sedative. The sap of *Lysichitum* was used to treat ringworm.

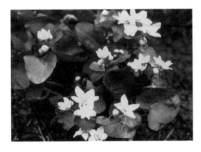

Marsh Marigolds, Cowslip
(Caltha palustris)

Description. Leaves ovate; distinctive fluorescent-yellow flowers. Thrives in sunlight to partial shade. Plants grow in low wetlands.

Location. Entire United States, except extreme desert, southern California, and lower Florida.

Warning. *In view of the caustic nature of this plant, best to avoid it. Use it as a survival food only.*

Cooking tips. Leaves eaten as a potherb in the spring before the flowers open. This is a risky practice, as it must be cooked in several changes of water. Leaves are extremely bitter and not worth the time and trouble.

Medicinal uses. Leaves used as laxative and cough syrup. Root used in decoction for colds.

Jack-in-the-Pulpit, Indian Turnip
(Arisaema triphyllum)

Description. Leaves compound, three leaflets, oval, smooth, lighter underside; distinctive primitive flower, spadix in pulpit-like spathe.

Edible Wild Plants & Useful Herbs   **41**

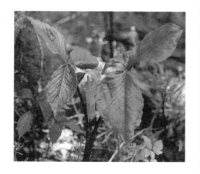

Indian turnip is found in rich soils, generally a woods or shady lowland.

Location. Entire United States, except extreme desert, southern California, and lower Florida.

Warning. *Do not eat fresh plant. Like skunk cabbage, it contains caustic oxalates when fresh and must be thoroughly dried before use. Not recommended. Handle with care: Calcium oxalate will cause painful burns in cracked skin or open sores. See also Appendix 1.*

Cooking tips. Native Americans sliced roots and dried them, deactivating calcium oxalate. Dried root was cooked and eaten like potato chips.

Medicinal uses. Plant parts used in treatment of cough, sore throat, and ringworm. Also as a poultice for boils and abscesses.

Mayapple
(Podophyllum peltatum)

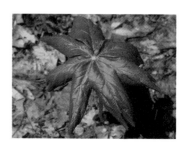

Description. Large pair of dissected, parasol-like leaves; white flower on petiole between leaves; yellow/green fruit. Mayapple is, for the most part, poisonous. The two large, parasol-like leaves shelter a white flower that bears an edible fruit when ripe in midsummer. Pick the fruit when soft and ripe.

Location. Entire United States, except extreme desert, southern California, and lower Florida.

Warning. *Except for the pulp of the ripe fruit, this plant is poisonous. See also Appendix 1.*

Cooking tips. Expert foragers carefully gather ripe fruit for use in pie fillings and jellies.

Medicinal uses. Etoposide, the active agent of mayapple, may be useful treating testicular and small lung cancer.

White Trillium
(*Trillium grandiflorum*)

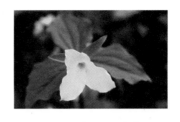

Description. Leaves, sepals, and flower petals in threes. There are several varieties of trillium. Leaves and red-to-purple flowers are edible but, for my taste, members of this genus are too pretty to eat. Trillium and toadshade (a red-flowered species) are excellent transplants. Locate in shade and rich soil.

Location. Entire United States, except extreme desert, southern California, and lower Florida.

Medicinal uses. Native Americans used *T. grandiflorum* root bark decoction for earsores, and splinters of wood soaked in root extraction were pricked through the skin over arthritic joints.

Ramps, Wild Leeks
(*Allium tricoccum*)

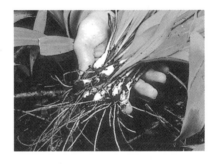

Description. Strong onion aroma; long, wide leaves grow directly from bulb. Found on banks and in wet woods.

Location. Eastern United States, roughly to the Mississippi.

Cooking tips. Leaves, stems, and bulbs are edible. Marvelous in stews and soup, or sautéed with soy sauce, extra virgin olive oil, and a little water to keep plants from sticking to pan.

Medicinal uses. Used as a tonic to combat colds. Disputed evidence that eating raw bulbs may reduce risk of heart disease. Chop leaves into chicken soup to potentiate this cold and flu fighter.

Fiddlehead Ferns
(*Matteucian* and *Ptereti* spp.)

Description. Fiddleheads are the unfurled, early-growth leaves of ferns (tightly wound like a fiddlehead).

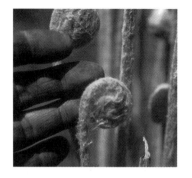

Location. Eastern United States, roughly to the Mississippi.

Warning. *Some ferns, such as bracken fern, may cause stomach cancer. Fiddleheads may also lead to thiamine problems. Best to avoid these plants.*

Cooking tips. Can be eaten raw or steamed. I prefer them sautéed or deep-fried. You can buy fiddleheads at Native American restaurants in Seattle and Vancouver. This is where you should begin your experience with eating ferns.

Wild Ginger
(Asarum canadense)

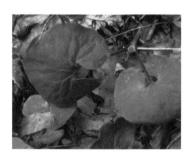

Description. Aromatic root, smells like ginger; two heart-shaped leaves; note the hairy stem and leaves; primitive flower emerges in May. Found on rich soil in moist woods.

Location. Entire United States, except extreme desert, southern California, and lower Florida.

Cooking tips. Crushed root can be added to salad dressings. When dried and grated it is an adequate substitute for oriental ginger. For the daring gourmet, try boiling the root until tender and then simmer in maple syrup. The result is an unusual candy treat.

Medicinal uses. Root traditionally used to treat colds and cough; antiseptic and tonic.

Sweet Cicely, Wild Anise
(Myrrhis odorata)

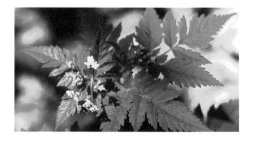

Description. Broken root smells like anise. Bright green, shiny leaves; small, white flowers in

44

umbels. Wild anise, commonly called sweet cicely, has a sweet anise odor and taste. Use as an anise substitute.

Location. Entire United States, except extreme desert, southern California, and lower Florida.

Warning. **Looks like hemlock (see Appendix 1).**

Cooking tips. Use root to spice cooked greens. Leaves can be added to salads.

Medicinal uses. Leaves occasionally eaten by diabetics as sugar substitute.

Partridgeberry, Squaw Vine *(Mitchella repens)*

Description. A tiny creeper with oval leaves, found at the base of trees in wet woods of the northern and central United States and Canada. Bland berry ripens to bright red by late summer.

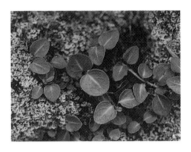

Location. Eastern, northern, and central United States.

Cooking tips. A tasteless trail food with little or no bulk—a hard-times survival berry, available all winter.

Medicinal uses. Pioneers used the dried leaf tea to treat menstrual pain and regulate menses. Aerial parts of plant were used as a cleansing, soothing wash for sore nipples and arthritis.

Wintergreen *(Gaultheria procumbens)*

Description. Evergreen; long oval leaves, finely serrated margins; drooping white flowers. The flower forms an edible berry that turns from white to red by late summer. Available all winter—if not gobbled up by late-season foragers.

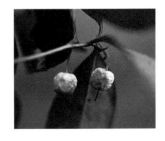

Location. Entire United States, except extreme desert, southern California, and lower Florida. There are several species of

Edible Wild Plants & Useful Herbs   **45**

this plant in North America. Creeping wintergreen, or checkerberry, is found in the eastern half of the United States.

Warning. *If taken internally, wintergreen oil is poisonous.*

Cooking tips. Add summer fruits to pancake and muffin mixes. Use the leaves to make a delicate tea or munch them (don't swallow) as a breath freshener.

Medicinal uses. Astringent and counterirritant. Never take oil internally. Tea from leaves has been used for flu and colds, and as a stomach alkalizer.

Spice Bush *(Lindera benzoin)*

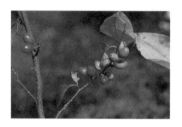

Description. Shrub found in rich woodlands and along streams. Grows to 15 feet, with numerous spreading branches. Smooth branches give off spicy odor when soft bark is scratched with thumbnail. Leaves smooth, bright green, pointed (widest near or above middle section), simple, alternate, deciduous, 2½ to 5½ inches long and 1½ to 2½ inches wide. Flowers small, yellow, in dense clusters along previous year's twigs. Fruits in clusters, widest in middle (somewhat football shaped, but with more rounded ends), start out green–bright red in autumn. Flowers appear in early spring, before leaves.

Location. Eastern United States, roughly to Mississippi River.

Cooking tips. In the spring I gather end twigs, tie them together with string, and throw them in a pot with leeks, nettles, mushrooms, and dandelions. Bundles of stems can be steeped in boiling water to make tea (sweeten with honey). Young leaves can be used in the same way. In the fall, try drying the fruits in a food dryer. Dry fruits are hard and can be ground in a coffee mill and used as a substitute for allspice.

Medicinal uses. Native Americans used the bark in infusion for treating colds, coughs, and dysentery. Tea made from the bark was used as a spring tonic. Bathing in this tea reportedly helps rheumatism. Tea made from the twigs was used to treat dysmenorrhea.

Cleavers, Bedstraw
(Gallium aparine)

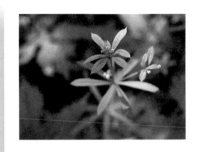

Description. Weak, slender stem; eight leaves in whorl; tiny white flowers. Found in woodlands, along streams, and in vacant lots.

Location. Eastern United States, roughly to the Mississippi.

Cooking tips. Also called bedstraw, cleaver leaves can be added to salads in early spring. Mature leaves are tough and must be cooked. Seeds of summer can be roasted and ground into coffee substitute. It's better than chicory but far short of coffee.

Medicinal uses. Diuretic. Tea used for skin diseases such as psoriasis, seborrhea, and eczema. Whole plant's juice is taken internally for kidney stones and cancer.

Grey Morel Mushroom *(Morchella esculenta)*
Black Morel *(Morchella elata)*

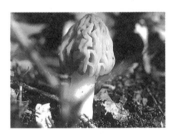

M. esculenta

Description. Convoluted grey or black brain-like flesh. Found from mid-April through May in many wooded areas. Convoluted brain look is distinctive, but there are some dangerous look-alikes.

Location. Eastern United States, roughly to the Mississippi.

Warning. *Many mushrooms are deadly. Seek positive identification from an expert before eating.*

Puffball Mushroom
(Calvatea gigantea)

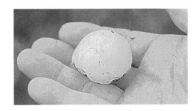

Immature mushroom

Description. Softball-to-basketball-size mushroom; fleshy white throughout. Puffball is found on rich soil in shady areas.

Location. Eastern United States, roughly to the Mississippi.

Warning. *Before eating, cut open and be certain flesh is white and not yellow. Also avoid this plant if gills or a rudimentary stem are inside.*

Cooking tips. Can be cooked and eaten like an edible mushroom. Prepare sliced puffball in satay sauce, then stir-fry with vegetables and tofu. Slices can also be sautéed in butter.

Avalanche Lily, Yellow Avalanche Lily
(Erythronium grandiflorum)

Description. Leaves lance- and ellipse-shaped, narrowing at base; deeply buried, edible corm; single yellow flower (sometimes two) on 7- or 8-inch stem (July). Found in alpine meadows and high slopes in western mountains. Similar to, and from the same genus as, the trout lily and the white dogtooth violet of the eastern United States.

Location. Mountain west, primarily the Sierras and Rockies.

Warning. *The corm contains polysaccharide inulin, and thus must be cooked to be edible.*

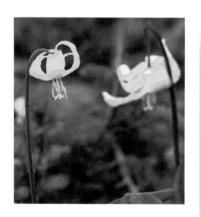

Cooking tips. Reaching the corm is a difficult dig, and much effort is needed. Native Americans wrapped the bulbs in cattails and reeds, then cooked them in an earth-filled pit over which a fire was burned. Ten to twelve hours in the pit would render the corms both edible and delicious.

Medicinal uses. I believe the inulin-rich bulb would be helpful to diabetics. (In Japan the inulin in burdock root is used to treat diabetics.)

Spring Beauty *(Claytonia caroliniana)*
Indian Potato *(C. lanceolata)*
Mountain Potato *(C. tuberosa)*

Description. Approximately 7 inches tall; narrow, lance-shaped leaves die off after bloom; flowers 1-centimeter across, light pink to white or white with pink veins, in loose terminal clusters, numbering from 3 to 18. Plant grows from ground where they are attached to an acorn-size, fleshy corm. Emerge and bloom in early spring. Found

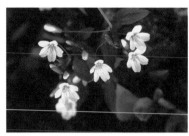

C. caroliniana

in rich, moist woods throughout the east and across the northern tier of states and the mountainous west.

Location. Entire United States, except extreme desert, southern California, lower Florida, and the Prairie states.

Cooking tips. The brown-skinned corm is edible. Peel the skin, wash, and eat raw or cooked. Try it on the grill with roasted vegetables. Roll the corm in olive oil, then roast for about 8 minutes until browned. Flowers are edible but bland.

Trout Lily *(Erythronium americanum)*

Description. Trout lily or white dog-toothed violet (*E. albidum*) has mottled leaves and small, yellow lily-like flower. Avalanche lilies (of the mountain west) are close relatives with edible bulbs.

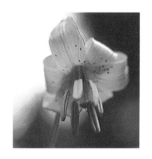

Location. Eastern United States, roughly to the Mississippi.

Cooking tips. Young leaves may be boiled for 10 minutes and eaten, but they are poor tasting. The tuberous root is also edible after lengthy boiling. The real beauty of this plant is in the eyes of the beholder—as a foodstuff it's best left alone.

Medicinal uses. Tea from root used to reduce fever. Crushed leaves used as poultice over ulcers.

Clintonia, Corn Lily
(*Clintonia borealis, C. uniflora*)

Description. Waxy leaves. Near look-alike of trout lily.

Location. Entire northern United States. *C. borealis* is found in east, while *C. uniflora* is found in west.

Warning. *Know your foraging ground. Unfurled corn lily leaves look like other inedible leaves.*

Cooking tips. Corn lily is edible but, like the trout lily, it's best to leave this inferior foodstuff alone. Pick young leaves before they unfurl. Chop into salads, or boil and serve with butter, salsa, and a splash of soy sauce.

Medicinal uses. Native Americans used leaves as poultice over wounds, sores, and burns. Tea from root used as mosquito repellent.

American Ginseng *(Panax quinquefolium)*

Description. Straight, erect stem, with 2 or 3 leaf stems; 5 to 11 leaves per stem. American ginseng root, a prized medicinal in China, sells for about $300 per pound. Commercially cultivated.

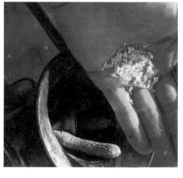

Location. Eastern United States, roughly to the Mississippi.

Cooking tips. The Chinese cook the root in chicken soup. They also eat the berries. Dried root can be ground in an old-fashioned sausage grinder.

Medicinal uses. Ginseng root's active ingredients are called saponins (glycosides). Some saponins raise blood pressure, others lower it; Some raise blood sugar, some lower it. Obviously, more research is needed. Today saponins from ginseng are being tested in preliminary studies as an anti-cancer chemotherapy.

Evening Primrose
(Oenothera biennis)

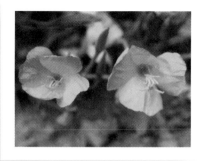

Description. Biennial, second year erect plant; yellow flower; leaves lance-shaped, pointed tip, fine-toothed margin. Evening primrose is found in fields bordering wooded areas.

Location. Eastern United States, roughly to the Mississippi.

Cooking tips. The flowers, roots, and seeds are edible. Dip flowers in egg whites, roll them in sugar, then deep-fry. Also try cooking them in a stir-fry or spreading them in salads.

Medicinal uses. Plant parts contain Gamma Linolenic Acid (GLA). GLA may prevent acne, alcoholism, obesity, and schizophrenia (as yet unproven). My wife has had success relieving PMS with the oil of this plant's seeds.

Candied Evening Primrose

....

2 tablespoons high-proof alcohol (such as Everclear)
1 egg white
sugar

Whip together alcohol and egg white. Dip flowers. Sprinkle a thin layer of sugar on a cookie sheet. Fill a salt shaker with sugar, then sprinkle the sugar over the egg white–laden flowers. If you're handy with chopsticks, you can rotate the flower as you coat it with sugar. Lay the flowers on the cookie sheet and let them dry. Try candied flowers in tea or cordials, or use to garnish a dessert plate. All flowers can be candied. Also try this recipe with rose petals and violets. Yields two dozen flowers.

Ground Nut *(Apios americana)*

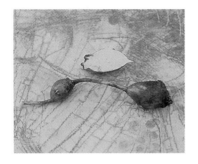

Description. Climbing, pea-like plant vine; numerous tubers along length of root; leaves alternate, compound, feather-like; seeds in long pods. Ground nut grows on wet ground, along the fringes of streams, bogs, and thickets. Easily transferable to your garden, where they can be harvested in the autumn or spring.

Location. Entire United States, except extreme desert, southern California, and lower Florida.

Cooking tips. Seeds are edible. Cook them like lentils. Tubers of *Apios* are 15 percent protein—a great potato substitute. Native Americans established settlements near this staple—a high-protein foraging food.

Sassafras
(Sassafras albidum)

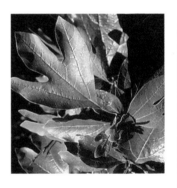

Description. Small tree with aromatic limbs, leaves, and roots. The leaves usually have two or three lobes and are alternate. There are many sucker plants growing adventitiously from the parent plant.

Location. Southeastern and southern United States.

Warning. *Sassafras oils may be carcinogenic (contains traces of carcinogen safrole). Use judiciously.*

Cooking tips. Boil root, sweeten, and drink.

Medicinal uses. Sassafras tea used as a diuretic and stimulant. Leaves and bark made into a tea and rubbed on the body may work as a mosquito repellent. Decoction from root was used as a tea substitute during Colonial times.

Pawpaw *(Asimina triloba)*

Description. Small tree (10 to 25 feet) growing on river banks, along streams; often a secondary growth under taller trees. Leaves are alternate, simple, large (up to 12 inches), narrow at base and broad near tip.

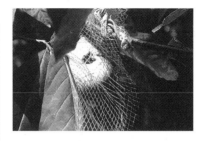

Location. Southeastern and southern United States.

Cooking tips. Large fruit can be eaten raw. Or remove seeds, cook like pudding, and blend with yogurt.

Medicinal uses. An anti-cancer substance has been isolated from pawpaw that is more than 1,000 times as potent as the synthetic drug adriamycin.

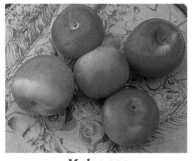

Malus **spp.**

Apple, Crab Apple *(Malus* and *Pyrus* spp.)

Description. Small trees to 30 feet; flowers white, rosy white; fruit smaller than domestic apples. Some species have thorns.

Location. Throughout the United States.

Cooking tips. Sour, acid taste. Cook with sugar or honey. Make preserve with raspberries, blueberries, or blackberries.

Medicinal uses. Fruit can be cooked and eaten for colds.

Oaks and Acorns *(Quercus* spp.)

Description. This is a large genera with species worldwide. Note: The best way to get acquainted with and learn how to identify oaks is to visit an arboretum, where the oaks are labeled for easy identification.

Location. Throughout the United States and southern Canada.

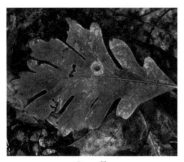
Q. alba

In the United States, I prefer acorns from the oaks that have rounded instead of pointed leaf lobes. White oak, bur oak, swamp chestnut oak, and chestnut oak are good examples from the eastern United States. The chinquapin oak, or yellow chestnut oak, also has sweet acorns. Out West look for live oak, blue oak, and Oregon white oak. Oaks with pointed leaves have more tannins and are too bitter to consume, even after special preparation.

Cooking tips. All oak nuts can be improved by an overnight soaking in fresh water (to leach out bitter-tasting tannins). Native Americans would shell, crack, or smash the acorns, then place them in a skin bag and soak them in a stream for a day or two to remove the tannins. A quick solution in the kitchen is to puree the acorn meat in water. Using a blender, combine one cup of water with every cup of nut meat. Blend thoroughly. Then press the water out of the nut meat through cheese cloth (or a clean pair of nylons or a white sock). I like the acorn puree on baked potatoes, over tomato sauce, in all baking recipes, or out of hand as a snack.

Medicinal uses. White oak has tannin-rich bark. While bitter tasting, tannins are also antiseptic and astringent. Native Americans and pioneers made tea from the bark and used it to treat mouth sores, burns, cuts, and scrapes. Many considered the bark a panacea. The Iroquois scraped powered bark from healed-over broken oak branches and sprinkled it over the navel of infants to heal the area after removal of the umbilical cord.

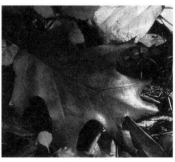
Q. rubra

They also used red oak bark decoction for diarrhea. Once again, the tannins account for the reported effectiveness of this remedy.

Sugar Maple *(Acer saccharum)*
Red Maple *(A. rubrum)*
Big Leaf Maple *(A. marcrophyllum)*

Description. Tree leaves resemble basic form of Canada's national emblem, typically 3 lobes (red maple leaves have distinctive red petioles); tree crowns are broad and rounded in the open; bark is smooth when young and furrows with age; seeds have characteristic helicopter-blade appearance and fly accordingly.

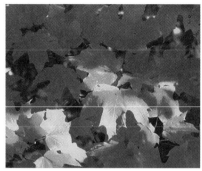

A. saccharum

Location. Various species found throughout the United States and southern Canada.

Cooking tips. Seeds may be eaten, but are poor tasting. Pluck the seeds from the helicopter blade husk and cook or stir-fry like peas.

Medicinal uses. Maple syrup is a glucose-rich sugar substitute with the added benefit of numerous minerals. Use it as a sweetener in place of sugar (which has no minerals). Traditionally, maple syrup has been used to flavor and sweeten cough syrups. The unfinished fresh sap is considered a mineral-rich tonic. I store a couple gallons in the freezer and keep one in the refrigerator as a water source that—for flavor and nutrition—beats bottled spring water.

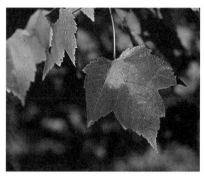

A. rubrum

Maple Sap Tap

Maple sugar and maple syrup from the winter and spring sap is what these trees are all about. For taps or information on where they can be purchased, contact a maple sugar mill near you.

Using a brace and a ⅜-inch bit, drill through the bark until you hit hardwood. Clean the hole thoroughly, then use a hammer to drive in the tap. For trees under 10 inches wide, use only one tap. For larger trees you may use two or three taps in a circle around the tree. Use a covered pail to collect the sap. If you're going to boil down the sap on an open fire, make sure that your wood is dry as smoke will give the syrup an undesirable flavor. I use three pans over a long, narrow fire pit, pouring the sugar water from pan to pan as it cooks. Pan number one receives the fresh water from the trees, pan two receives the reduced water from pan one, and pan three receives the further reduced water from pan two. Pan three, of course, will have the thickest, richest water. Boil the syrup in pan three until it is thick enough to coat a spoon.

Sap flows best on warm sunny days after a freezing night. In southern Michigan tapping begins in late January and continues until mid-April when the sap runs dark, thick, and stingy.

A few other trees that can be tapped for sap include: black walnut, and white, black, and yellow birch. Grape vines climbing high in the forest canopy can also be cut in the spring to provide copious amounts of mineral-laden water.

Mountains, Plains, Deserts & Seacoasts

This section identifies a few of the more common edible wild plants found in unique environments. Each geographic location in the United States and Canada has endemic plant life that may not be found elsewhere. When traveling in mountains, deserts, plains, and coastal areas, it's a good idea to pack along an edible plants book for that specific locale.

MOUNTAINS, PLAINS & DESERTS

Jojoba *(Simmondsia californica)*

Description. Shrub. Seed capsules burst in early fall, disgorging oily, chocolate-colored edible seeds.

Location. Mountain west, primarily the Sierras, and mountain borders into desert southern California.

Cooking tips. Seeds eaten raw or cooked. Roasted and ground seeds are whipped in cooked egg yolks until paste forms. Boil in milk, sugar, and a little water. Add a drop or two of vanilla extract to flavor. Drink hot.

Medicinal uses. Native Americans used oil for growing hair and treating cancer and kidney problems. Oil has been applied to body and head sores and is reported to be emetic.

Miner's Lettuce *(Montia perfoliata)*

Description. Leaves form cup or saucer around stems; delicate, small white flowers. Found in moist, shady places. High in vitamin A.

Location. Pacific coastal range, east to plains.

Cooking tips. Cook like dandelion greens or eat leaves and stems raw. Best with vinegar-laced salad dressing.

Indian Bread Root, Prairie Turnip
(Psoralea esculenta)

Description. Low-lying, hairy herbs of the prairie. Long-stemmed leaves, compound, divided into five fingers; flowers in dense, blue spike (each floret looks like small pea blossom). Edible part is 1- to 2-inch tuberous root.

Location. Prairie.

Cooking tips. Eat raw, sliced in salad with vinegar and oil dressing. Roots can be dried and preserved. Add dried root to soups and stews.

Medicinal uses. High in starch (may be 70 percent starch). Psoralea genus used to treat psoriasis (PUVA) and some forms of cancer (Psoralen/photophoresis).

Prickly Pear, Indian Fig *(Opuntia* spp.*)*

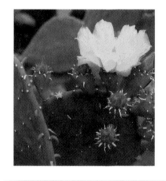

Description. Desert and prairie cactus. Spreads along ground on dry land in sandy soil. Broad but thin, spined, fleshy, pear-shaped but flattened segments; fruit pear-shaped, rounded; yellow flower blooms in March and April.

Location. Desert.

Warning. *Although I have eaten the flowers of several species of prickly pear and I have seen Mexicans eat the flowers in Del Rio, Texas, I cannot find any documentation on their safety. Until I discover whether or not prickly pear flowers can be eaten as food, I do not recommend them as food.*

Cooking tips. Harvest carefully, wear gloves. Peel or flame away spines. Slice "leaf" into segments and stir-fry, deep-fry, or roast over an open fire. Pulp of ripe fruit can be removed and made into jelly. I have eaten the flowers.

Medicinal uses. Leaf pad, split in half, makes an excellent compress over wounds. Native Americans in the Southwestern desert areas use a prickly pear compress over snake, scorpion, and spider bites.

Mesquite *(Prosopis juliflora, P. pubescens)*

Description. Woody tree or shrub of arid regions. Compound, feather-like leaves; seed pods resemble green bean pods.

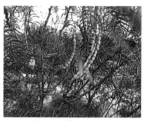

P. pubescens

Location. Desert.

Warning. *May cause dermatitis.*

Cooking tips. Wood used to cook and flavor meats. Seed pods edible, juicy, sweet when ripe, very seedy.

Medicinal uses. Native Americans of the Southwest treat adult-onset diabetes by including mesquite pods, beans, and prickly pear in their traditional diet.

Agave, Century Plant, Mescal *(Agave* spp.*)*

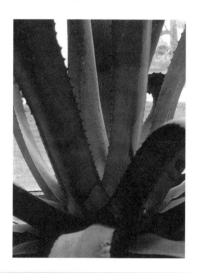

Description. Long sword-like, stiff, fibrous leaves shooting skyward in circular cluster; 10- to 15-foot flower stalk grows from leaf cradle; clusters of yellow flowers.

Location. Desert.

Cooking tips. Young bud of plant can be cut out. Cut entire bud from leaves as it emerges. Trim away leaves and flower tips. Prepare fire in large pit lined with stones. Let large fire burn down to coals, then put bud in ashes. Cover bud with hot stones and ashes, and bury in dirt. Open the pit and recover the cooked bud ten to twelve hours later. Cut away charred covering to expose sticky, sweet, pineapple-tasting interior. Note: You may need help from the local native population to prepare the plant correctly.

Medicinal uses. Plant fruit is made into native drink, mescal. Agave sap was used to seal and heal an axe wound in conquistador Cortez's thigh.

Almost all marine seaweeds are safe to consume, and the two questionable varieties are easy to avoid: foul-tasting lyngbya, a thin, hair-like species that clings to mangrove roots in warm waters; and desmarestia, which is found in deep, open waters and contains sulphuric acid and imparts an unpleasant lemon-like taste. Therefore, avoid mangrove-clinging seaweeds and deep open-water varieties.

Because of limited space only three popular edible seaweeds are covered—by no means the limit of your foraging choices.

Kelp
(Laminaria spp.*)*

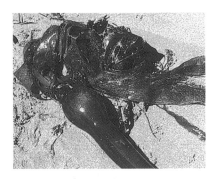

Description. A brown seaweed that can grow to more than 100 feet in length. Large frond-like leaves; stem can be thick as a human's wrist; air-filled bulbs or bladders hold plant erect in water. Plant is often torn loose and washed ashore after storms. Note: Gardeners are encouraged to spread seaweeds of all types on their organic gardens. Containing over 90 minerals, marine algae are a wonderful addition to the garden. Excellent for fiber. Contains most minerals humans need.

Location. Found along West Coast, from California to Alaska.

Cooking tips. Wash the plant in clean water. Soak in weak wine vinegar or lemon juice until pliable. Air-dry in sun. After drying, scrape off blue-green surface layer. Thick white core can be chopped, shredded, or ground. Best cooked in soups and stews. Dry the shredded parts for later use. I have dried various seaweeds by spreading them on my car windshield in full sunlight.

Medicinal uses. Improves yolk color when fed to chickens. Good source of iodine (important clotting agent). Kelp salt prevents muscle cramps.

Nori, Laver, Porphyra *(Porphyra* spp.*)*

Description. Rose-pink to red-brown with aging; flat, blade-like, irregular shape to 20 inches; satin sheen, thin, elastic. Nearly 36 percent protein. High in iodine and vitamins A and C.

Location. Mid-tidal zone.

Cooking tips. Forage in late spring. Sun-dry, then store in airtight canning jars or plastic bags. Use it fresh, seasoned and tenderized in soy sauce. Dry and flake into baked goods, or use in soups and stews.

Medicinal uses. May lower blood cholesterol levels (as yet unproven).

Alaria, Wakame *(Alaria marginata)*

Description. Grows to 6 feet tall; olive-brown to green; attached by short stem (stipe) and holdfast cell; short paddle-like sporophylls just below edible frond blades. Do not cut away sporophylls when harvesting—this procedure guarantees the life and future of your alaria supply. High in essential trace elements. Good source of pantothenic acid, and vitamin C and B vitamins.

Location. Found on rocks in lower tidal zones.

Cooking tips. Dry plant. Can be restored with water to near-fresh condition. Wrap reconstituted alaria leaves around rice and meats, cook in casseroles, or simmer in pot roast. Great in mushroom soup. Especially good when used in chicken soups and stews.

Narrow-Leafed Seaside Plantain, Goose Tongue
(Plantago maritima)

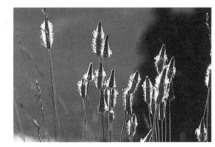

Description. Long, narrow, lance-shaped leaves growing from basal whorl; no basal sheath; leaves with thick longitudinal ribs. Appearance similar to narrow-leafed garden plantain *(P. lanceolata)*.

Location. West Coast of North America.

Warning. *Goose tongue can be confused with arrow grass. Arrow grass leaves are flat on one side and round on the other, with sheaves at the base of the leaves. Goose tongue leaves have prominent ribs and are more flattened. If you cut the goose tongue leaf in cross section, it would appear flat or slightly V-shaped. The characteristic plantain spike of goose tongue is distinctive. Remember Wild Plant Foraging Rule #1: Follow these two plants through an entire season before eating goose tongue.*

Cooking tips. Succulently salty and mineral rich. Eat it fresh and raw. Can also be used as a stuffing for salmon. Mix it with finely sliced kelp and sauté it with olive oil and water. Then stuff the mixture in the cavity of a cleaned and washed salmon and steam the fish in a reed basket or in a Chinese basket steamer over a pot of boiling water until done.

Medicinal uses. Fresh leaves and fresh juice considered anti-inflammatory and antimicrobial. Native American healer Patsy Clark chews the leaves and applies them over wounds. In Germany the leaves are simmered in honey for 20 minutes to treat gastric ulcers.

Beach Pea *(Lathyrus japonicus)*

Description. A marine coastal dweller. Leaves compound, even-numbered, six to twelve leaflets typical, tipped with curling tendril typical of pea family; opposite leaflets 2.5-inches long; fruit pea pod-like, hairy, approximately 2.5-inches long.

Location. Found among driftwood and dunes in sandy upper areas of beach.

Warning. *Many members of the pea family are potentially toxic. Make positive identification, eat only small amounts, and follow all foraging rules.*

Cooking tips. Native Americans cooked the seeds in seal oil. Cook them with salmon. The new growth (stalks of spring) can be stir-fried, boiled, or steamed. After beach peas flower, tender young pods can be cooked and eaten like snow peas.

Medicinal uses. The Chinese used this Pacific Rim wild food as a tonic for the urinary organs and intestinal tract.

Appendix 1

Poisonous Plants & Poisonous Look-alikes

What follows is only a partial listing of poisonous plants in the United States. For a more comprehensive discussion refer to the books listed in Appendix 2: Recommended Books and Videos & Other Resources. Always keep the phone number of your poison control center in your wallet and your car.

American Liverwort
(Hepatica americana)

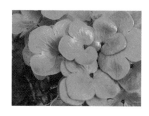

Kidney- or liver-shaped leaves with hairy petioles; first flower of spring. Burning alkaloid, requires special preparation for consumption. Use reserved for skilled pharmacist or herbalist. See also page 40.

Arrow Arum
(Peltandra virginica)

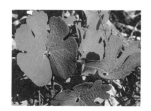

Arrow-shaped leaf, pinnate veins; green primitive flower; grows in water. Some argue the burning alkaloids may be dried out of the seeds and roots. Even so, the bitter taste of the prepared plant is unfit to eat. All parts of this plant, including the flower and mature fruits, are poisonous.

Bloodroot
(Sanguinaria canadensis)

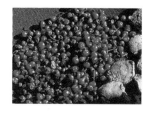

Plant's underground rhizome exudes a red "sap" when broken. Plant has a single, deeply dissected leaf; single white flower. Juice of plant is skin and eye irritant. Eating moderate quantities may be fatal.

Blue Flag Iris
(Iris spp.)

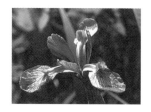

Sword-like leaves; purple, blue, or yellow flower; rhizome. Causes diarrhea, vomiting, and dermatitis.

Datura, Jimson Weed
(Datura stramonium)

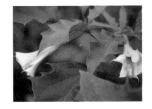

A large plant with spiny stems, spiny fruit pod, spined leaves, and spiny flowers. Hallucinations, delirium, and violent actions result from eating plant parts. Rarely fatal.

Death Camas, Poison Sego
(Zigadenus spp.)

A sego lily look-alike. 1.5 feet high; grass-like; yellow or white flowers growing along central flower stalk. Has onion-like bulb but no onion-like odor. All parts toxic. May cause vomiting, headache, dizziness, and convulsions.

Dutchman's-Breeches
(Dicentra cucullaria)

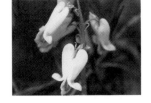

Deeply dissected, carrot-like leaves; white flower looks like "bloomers" or man's breeches. Tuber is most poisonous. Causes convulsions and breathing difficulties, but is rarely fatal.

Hellebore, False
(Veratrum viride)

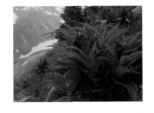

Large, ovate, stalkless leaves, clinging and spiraling up sturdy stem; flowers yellow-green, in branched clusters. Grows in wet, swampy areas. Western variety of hellebore grows on open mountain slopes. May cause asphyxia, convulsions, and death.

Horse Nettle
(Solanum carolinense)

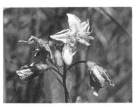

Spiny stems and leaves. Leaves coarse, irregular, large-toothed; white flower; fleshy, yellow berry fruit. Alkaloid, solanum. Causes nausea, vomiting, and stomach and bowel pain.

Jack-in-the-Pulpit,
Indian Turnip *(Arisaema triphyllum)*

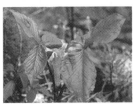

Flower has characteristic spathe and spadix like preacher in a pulpit. Calcium oxalate crystals burn when eaten fresh. See aslo page 41.

Mayapple
(Podophyllum peltatum)

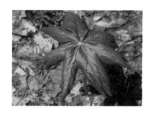

A plant of the woods. Parasol-like leaf, deeply dissected; single white flower; yellow/ green fruit. Serious cases of plant ingestion may lead to coma and death. See also page 42.

Milkweed
(Asclepias syriaca)

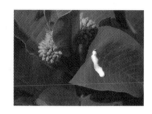

Large ovate leaves; stomach-shaped fruit pod. Plants exude milk-like sap when damaged. Overdose of galitoxin (milkweed toxin) has caused death in livestock. Eat shoots, flowers, and seed pods only with the guidance of an expert. Various species are more toxic than others. Proper cooking technique can destroy the potentially toxic cardiac glycosides. See also page 33.

Nightshade, Bittersweet
(Solanum dulcamara)

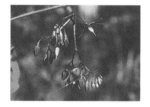

A climbing vine with purple rocket-shaped flowers, bearing a reddish-orange fruit. Leaves lobed, alternate. Rarely fatal.

Poison Hemlock
(Conium maculatum)

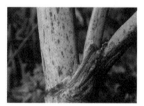

Purple-spotted stems. Large plant, white flowers in many branched flower heads (umbels). Be careful, many edible look-alikes such as parsley, carrot, wild anise, parsnips and other members of the carrot family. Toxin, conine. Causes respiratory failure and death.

Poison Ivy
(Toxicodendren radicans)

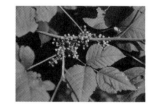

A climbing vine or shrub. Hairy stem; leaflets in threes; white or pale yellow berries. Contact may cause dermatitis. Jewelweed *(Impatiens capensis)* is a good treatment for poison ivy rash.

Poison Oak
(Toxicodendren diversiloba)

A small shrub. Resembles poison ivy (leaves more lobed). Contact causes dermatitis.

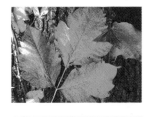

Poison Sumac
(Rhus vernix)

Shrub with compound leaves; 7 to 15 leaflets; white fruits instead of red fruit of sumac. Causes dermatitis.

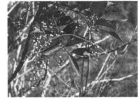

Pokeweed
(Phytolacca americana)

Ovate leaves, pointed at tip; reddish-purple stems; clusters of purple-colored fruit. Grows on waste land. Rarely fatal, but can cause cramps and vomiting. See also page 23.

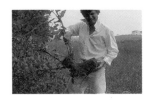

Skunk Cabbage
(Symplocarpus foetidus)

Wetlands dweller. Primitive fleshy plant; large ovate leaves; smells like skunk when torn or damaged; primitive flower (spadix and spathe). Terrible burning, bitter taste. Rarely fatal. See also page 40.

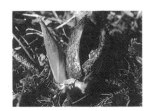

Water Hemlock
(Cicuta maculata)

Inhabits wetlands. Has sharply toothed leaves, similar to poison hemlock in appearance. Looks like many edible members of carrot family. Beware: Convulsions and death will occur a few hours after consumption.

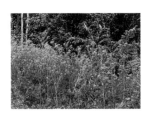

Appendix 1

Appendix 2

Recommended Books, Videos & Other Resources

•••

Videos

Jim Meuninck has a free catalog of several one-hour videos that identify and demonstrate the use of edible and medicinal wild plants. Call Jim Meuninck at (616) 699–7061 or e-mail jmeuninck@aol.com.

Cooking with Edible Flowers and Culinary Herbs, Jim Meuninck and Sinclair Philip (60 minutes/VHS, 1990).

Diet for Natural Health, Jim Meuninck, Candace Corson MD, and Nancy Behnke Strasser RD. (60 minutes/Video with computer database, 1999). One diet for disease prevention and weight control.

Edible Wild Plants, Jim Meuninck and Dr. Jim Duke (60 minutes/VHS 1988). One hundred useful wild herbs.

Herbal Preparations and Nutritional Therapies, Jim Meuninck (60 minutes/VHS, 1999).

Little Medicine: The Wisdom to Avoid Big Medicine, Jim Meuninck and Theresa Barnes (60 minutes/VHS 1997).

Meuninck's Medicinal Plant Index, Jim Meuninck (CD ROM, 1999). Interactive media with world wide web linkages covering over 500 herbs, edible plants, edible flowers, and medicinal plants.

Native American Medicine, Jim Meuninck, Patsy Clark, and Theresa Barnes (60 minutes/VHS, 1997).

Natural Health with Medicine Herbs and Healing Foods, Jim Meuninck and Ed Smith, James Balch (60 minutes/VHS, 1992).

Trees, Shrubs, Nuts & Berries, Jim Meuninck and Dr. Jim Duke (60 minutes/VHS, 1990). Video field guide.

Books

Field Guide to Edible Wild Plants, by B. Angier (Stackpole Books, 1974).

It's the Berries, by Liz Anton and Beth Dooley (Garden Way Publishing Book, 1988).

Michigan Trees, by Burton Barnes and Warren Wagner (University of Michigan Press, 1986).

Shellfish & Seaweed Harvests of Puget Sound, by Daniel Cheney and Thomas Mumford (Puget Sound Books, 1986).

Handbook of Edible Weeds, by James A. Duke (CRC Press, 1992).

Handbook of Medicinal Herbs, by James A. Duke (CC Press Inc., 1988).

Handbook of Northeastern Indian Medicinal Plants, by James A. Duke (Cardamon Publications, 1986).

CRC Press Handbook of Nuts, by James A. Duke (CRC Press, 1989).

Field Guide to North American Edible Wild Plants, by Thomas Elias and Peter Dykeman (Van Nostrand Reinhold Company, 1982).

Medicinal and Other Uses of North American Plants, by Charlotte Erichsen-Brown (Dover Publications, 1989).

An Instant Guide to Edible Plants, by Pamela Forey and Cecilia Fitzsimons (Bonanza Books, NY 1986).

Eastern/Central Medicinal Plants, by Steven Foster and James Duke (Houghton Mifflin, 1990).

Edible Native Plants of the Rocky Mountains, by H.D. Harrington (University of New Mexico Press, 1967).

Sturtevant's Edible Plants of the World, by U.P. Hedrick (Dover Books, 1972).

An Ethnobotanical Guide to Medicinal Wild Plants of the Prairie, by Kelly Kindscher (University Press of Kansas, 1992).

Traditional Plant Foods of Canadian Indigenous People, by Harriet Kuhnlein and Nancy Turner (Gordon and Breach, 1991).

Edible Wild Plants, by Oliver Medsger (Collier Books, 1966).

Medicinal Plants of the Pacific West, by Michael Moore (Red Crane Books, 1993).

Sea Vegetables, by Evelyn McConnaughey (Natureagraph Publishers Inc., 1985).

Plants of Coastal British Columbia, by Jim Pojar (Lone Pine, 1994).

Edible Wild Fruits and Nuts of Canada, by Nancy Turner (National Museums of Canada, 1979).

American Indian Medicine, by Virgil Vogel (University of Oklahoma Press, 1970).

Western Forests, by Stephen Whitney (Alfred A. Knopf, 1988).

Seed and Plant Resources

For catalogues and information on seeds and plants, contact the following:

Richter's Herb Catalogue (905-640-6677; Web site: www.richters.com). A free catalog of edible and medicinal plant seeds and live plants.

American Botanical Council (512-331-8868). Ask for their Herbal Education Catalog.

J.L. Hudson, Seedsman Catalog (Star Route 2, Box 337, La Handa, CA 94020). Rare and unusual seeds.

Seeds of Change (505-438-8080). Free catalog.

Horizon Seeds (541-846-6704). Rare wild plants, both edible and medicinal.

Index

BASIC ✳ ESSENTIALS™

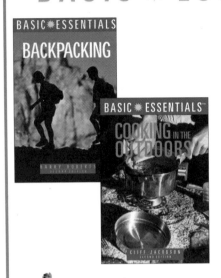

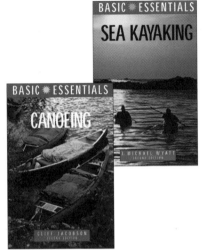